HANS BERGER

ON THE ELECTROENCEPHALOGRAM OF MAN

HANS BERGER
ON THE
ELECTROENCEPHALOGRAM OF MAN

The Fourteen Original Reports on the Human Electroencephalogram

TRANSLATED FROM THE ORIGINAL GERMAN
AND EDITED BY

PIERRE GLOOR

Professor of Clinical Neurophysiology, McGill University, Montreal (Canada)

ELECTROENCEPHALOGRAPHY AND CLINICAL
NEUROPHYSIOLOGY

SUPPLEMENT NO. 28

ELSEVIER PUBLISHING COMPANY

AMSTERDAM/LONDON/NEW YORK

Electroenceph. clin. Neurophysiol., **1969,** *Suppl. 28*

ELSEVIER PUBLISHING COMPANY
335 JAN VAN GALENSTRAAT
P.O. BOX 211, AMSTERDAM, THE NETHERLANDS

ELSEVIER PUBLISHING CO. LTD.
BARKING, ESSEX, ENGLAND

AMERICAN ELSEVIER PUBLISHING COMPANY, INC.
52 VANDERBILT AVENUE
NEW YORK, NEW YORK 10017

LIBRARY OF CONGRESS CARD NUMBER: 75-80081

STANDARD BOOK NUMBER 444-40739-1

WITH 175 ILLUSTRATIONS

PRINTED IN THE NETHERLANDS

Preface

It was while holding a National Research Council, Rockefeller Foundation fellowship at the Sorbonne in 1932 that my attention was drawn to a remarkable series of publications by an obscure German psychiatrist in Jena entitled "Über das Elektrenkephalogramm des Menschen". Working with Ali Monnier on the electrical properties of nerve fibres with the newly developed cathode ray oscilloscope he had just imported from the laboratories of George Bishop, Herbert Gasser, and Joseph Erlanger in St. Louis where he had held a Rockefeller Foundation fellowship a few years before, we were highly skeptical of the possibility of recording anything of significance from the surface of the brain, in view of the enormous complexity of action potentials which must be coursing in all directions in the multitude of nerve cells and fibres of the brain. Alfred Fessard was working next door, in the laboratories of the Collège de France, also struggling with a primitive cathode ray oscilloscope, studying the rhythmic properties of decalcified nerve fibres.

It seemed highly unlikely at that time that the simple rhythmic waves, the "Alpha- und Beta-Wellen" of Hans Berger, could possibly represent the true electrical activity of such complex nerve tissue as the cerebral cortex, especially in man, recorded not by an experienced electrophysiologist but by a psychiatrist with rather crude and simple apparatus, as compared to the vacuum tube amplifiers we had so carefully put together to operate the cathode ray oscilloscope. Upon returning to the United States in 1933 to work with Leonard Carmichael of Brown University, and to establish neurophysiology laboratories at the Bradley Hospital, still with the support of the Rockefeller Foundation, my attention was again drawn to Berger's work by a review which appeared in the *Archives of Neurology and Psychiatry* brought to my attention by Arthur Ruggles. We then heard that Adrian was beginning to take Berger's work seriously. Since Howard Andrews had already built a good high sensitivity amplifier oscillograph apparatus, Carmichael and I decided that we might waste a little time during the summer of 1934 checking some of Berger's findings. It was fortunate that our first two subjects, Carl Pfaffmann, a graduate student, and myself happen to have a good regular alpha rhythm, for we failed to get much alpha from Leonard Carmichael or from Howard Andrews.

We were immediately able to confirm many of Berger's findings, to begin a whole new field of research in these hospital laboratories. At the same time, Alex Forbes, Pauline and Hal Davis, and Fred Gibbs and William Lennox were beginning their work in Boston. Consequently, the second part of my doctorate thesis defended in Paris in 1935 was on the subject of the electroencephalogram. It was on this occasion that I first visited the laboratories of Professor Hans Berger in Jena. This was an unforgettable experience, to be always cherished in the years to come, for I was profoundly impressed by this inspired and inspiring, humble, honest, friendly, distinguished and courageous man, and his most charming and elegant wife, Mrs. Hans Berger. Hitler was just appearing over the horizon in these days, and the

v

fearful dangers of the Nazis was among the many subjects discussed in the intimacy of their beautiful home, in addition to the exciting long story of Berger's careful painstaking work, beginning before the first world war, how he persisted in spite of technical difficulties and the criticism of skeptical colleagues, making use of the many patients with skull defects resulting from this war, to prove that the electrical waves recorded from the intact skull were truly representative of the electrical activity of the brain beneath. This had to be done while engaged in his Professorial duties as Chief of Psychiatry at the University of Jena, Head of the psychiatric clinic and hospital, as well as engaging in clinical practice. We exchanged samples of E.E.G. tracings we had taken in our respective laboratories. We kept in touch by correspondence, and met again in Paris only once two years later, to renew what had become a close personal friendship. Hitler's war then came between us, and what we had feared together in Jena came to pass. But Hans Berger and his good and faithful wife remained true to the high ideals they had stood for all their life, being heartbroken by what was happening to their country. His resistance to the Nazis cost him his life, but won him the deep admiration and respect of all, as a great human being who cared more for his ideals than for his life. How fortunate to have such a man as the founder of electroencephalography.

For those who have come to work in the field of electroencephalography in later years, the name of Berger may mean only a vague point in history. He even refused to allow Adrian to commemorate his work by calling alpha waves the "Berger rhythm". His publications were hard to read in German. This translation, so carefully done by Dr. Gloor, is not only a splendid tribute to the man and his work, but for the first time, makes this historical beginning of electroencephalography available to all. It is well worth careful reading, for in it is reflected the character of a great man, beloved by all those who were privileged to know him.

The translation of Berger's work into English has not been an easy task. His writings reflected not only the classic formal elaborate style of prewar German scientific writing, but he added his own personal variations which reflected his own psychiatric and philosophical thinking, the deep lying motivation for his interest in the development of electroencephalography. He was convinced that careful investigation of the workings of the brain by objective scientific methods would lead eventually to an understanding of the mind itself, its normal functions in sleep and waking, and its derangements in mental disease.

We are extremely fortunate in having the English translation done by Dr. Gloor whose native tongue was German, but who is equally fluent and educated in English, and whose own interests and scientific competence are so similar, in many respects, to those of Hans Berger. In his own words Dr. Gloor "was faced with the difficult task of retaining as far as possible the very personal style of Hans Berger, which reveals so much of his personality, without doing undue violence to the proprieties of style of English writing ... I hope the end result is a happy compromise between the all too ponderous German ... and the somewhat cold crispness of scientific English". I feel sure that the readers of this book will agree that Dr. Gloor's conscientious efforts have succeeded brilliantly, and have also made Berger's work, as well as Hans Berger, familiar to many who would never have been able, otherwise, to have this opportunity.

It is particularly fitting, it seems to me, that this translation of Berger's work was undertaken on the initiative of The American E.E.G. Society and the International Federation of Societies for Electroencephalography and Clinical Neurophysiology in order to provide a commemorative volume on the occasion of the Seventh International Congress held in San Diego, September 1969, just 40 years after the first publication of Hans Berger's "Über das Elektrenkephalogramm des Menschen". At this Congress Lord Adrian, who was largely responsible for the initial introduction of Berger's work to the English speaking world, delivered the opening address on "The Discovery of Berger" in which the beginnings of electroencephalography were beautifully portrayed from a distinctly personal point of view in the elegant but simple manner so characteristic of Lord Adrian. This volume provides a splendid memorial of this occasion.

HERBERT H. JASPER

Translator's Foreword

The plan to translate Hans Berger's papers on the human electroencephalogram into English took shape gradually over the past few years. This project was first suggested to me by Dr. Charles Henry of Cleveland, who never tired of emphasizing how little most electroencephalographers and neurophysiologists know about the work of the man who discovered and first studied the human electroencephalogram. Subsequently the American EEG Society and the International Federation of Societies for Electroencephalography and Clinical Neurophysiology became interested in this plan. Thanks to their enthusiastic support, I decided to proceed with this difficult task. It was a labor of love, and as the work progressed it grew more so, since I became increasingly fascinated with the original thinking and the arresting personality of one of the great neurological scientists.

The first question which arose was that of the choice of material that should be translated. Berger published 102 papers and monographs during his scientific career. (They are listed in an appendix to his obituary, written by H. Boening in the *Archiv für Psychiatrie und Nervenkrankheiten* in 1941). Twenty-eight of these 102 publications deal with the EEG; all are written in German, except for two small papers, one in Spanish and the other in English. It seemed logical to choose for translation Berger's 14 reports on the EEG which carry the common title "Über das Elektrenkephalogramm des Menschen". These 14 reports form a natural unit. They contain Berger's first descriptions of his original observations and experiments on the electroencephalogram. In them he develops his ideas and theoretical concepts on the electrical activity of the human brain. His other publications on the EEG contain no new observations or conclusions and their material is wholly derived from that first presented in the 14 papers. This is also true for the monograph published in the *Acta Nova Leopoldina*, in which Berger sums up his work on the human electroencephalogram.

The translation of Berger's work into English presented many problems. The difficulty did not only arise from the very different syntactic structure and stylistic requirements of the English and German languages, but even more so from Berger's personal style of writing. Berger's writing is complex and the sentence structure, from the translator's point of view, often forbiddingly tortuous. The danger was therefore very real that by staying too close to the intricate and slightly old fashioned style of the German text, one would produce unreadable English; on the other hand, there was the danger that the solicitude of rendering Berger's writing in contemporary scientific English would destroy the peculiar flavor of the original text which is so revealing of the personality of its author and of the temper of his time. The solution obviously lay in a compromise which, I hope, has preserved enough of Berger's original style without jarring the sensitivities of the contemporary English reader. Often it would have been easy to paraphrase the original text and to weed out many of the qualifying statements which Berger felt compelled to include in his writing.

Some of the readers might perhaps wish I had done so in order to produce a more easily flowing text. I believe, however, that Berger should be allowed to speak to the English reader as much as possible in his own style, for to do otherwise would destroy an ingredient of his writing which from the point of view of the medical historian is essential. Some of the problems which arose from the translation are briefly discussed in a set of Translator's Notes appended to this volume. They are referred to in the text by the letter "T" followed by the appropriate number. In the proofreading of the semi-final draft and in the preparation of the final text I had the good fortune to be generously assisted by Dr. Frederick Andermann, by Dr. Charles Henry and by Dr. Francis McNaughton to whom I owe a great debt of gratitude for their patient work and for their many excellent suggestions.

In preparing the introductory chapter on "Hans Berger and the Discovery of the Electroencephalogram", I drew on many of Berger's own writings, but the chapter owes much to other published sources which are listed in the bibliographical references appended to it. I also received valuable personal information on Berger's life and work from Mrs. Ursula Berger, Prof. Richard Jung, Dr. M. Schrenk, Mr. W. Keuscher and Prof. Herbert Jasper, all of whom I wish to thank for their many enlightening comments and contributions. Particularly valuable source material were the excerpts from Berger's diary and experimental protocols which were published for the first time in Prof. R. Jung's contribution to the *Jenenser EEG Symposion* entitled "Hans Berger und die Entdeckung des EEG nach seinen Tagebüchern und Protokollen". It is our good fortune that Berger's detailed diary, which he started in his 18th year of life and which contains entries until 10 days before his death, has been preserved, with the exception of the volumes for the years 1897–1910 which unfortunately have been lost. Dr. M. Schrenk of Freiburg im Breisgau is now in the process of analyzing this unusually rich source of information and I hope that means will be found to enable him to publish this material together with a definitive biography of Hans Berger.

Mrs. Ursula Berger, Prof. R. Jung and Dr. R. Werner have also generously supplied me with some historical photographs which are pertinent to the early period of electroencephalography and of which some are included as plates in this volume. I am also indebted to Mr. W. Keuscher, Hans Berger's former technician, who was able to provide me with valuable information concerning some of this historical material.

I wish to thank Mrs. Eugenie Reens, Miss Marianne Steiner, Mrs. Elizabeth Campbell and Miss Ann-Marie Crosby who have typed the various drafts and the final text of the manuscript. I also gratefully acknowledge the financial support for clerical work which I received from the Canadian Society of Electroencephalographers. Last but not least, I want to thank my wife and my children for the patience with which they accepted the fact that in order to carry out this project I had to spend increasing amounts of my free time immersing myself in the fascinating world of Hans Berger.

Montreal, December 1968   P. Gloor

Contents

Hans Berger and the Discovery of the Electroencephalogram

"ἐν τῷ ἐγκεφάλῳ εἶναι τὸ ἡγεμονικόν,
in the brain is the guiding principle" (Hans
Berger, quoting Alcmaeon of Crotona in
his Rectorial Address given on July 18, 1927).

The publication in 1929 of the first paper on the human electroencephalogram
by Hans Berger was an event for which the scientific world was not prepared. One
can readily appreciate this, if one recalls that physiology was then only beginning to
understand more clearly the principles of excitation and conduction in peripheral
nerves, thanks to the work of Gasser, Erlanger, Biedermann, Adrian and others.
Central nervous system physiology in the 1920s was little more than functional
neuroanatomy. Only Sherrington in his work on the spinal cord had begun to come
to grips with true physiological principles of central nervous system function. These
principles, however, were still derived from observations of events taking place outside
the central nervous system, such as the carefully measured pull or relaxation of muscles
in response to well defined stimuli. It was therefore not surprising that in 1929
hardly anyone took notice of the rather peculiar scientific contribution of a not very
well known German professor of psychiatry at Jena who, leapfrogging across all the
intermediate stages which a careful Sherringtonian approach to the study of the
physiology of the central nervous system would have called for, addressed himself
directly to the electrophysiological investigation of the most complex functions of the
human brain. No one realized that Berger had written the opening chapter of a
totally new and exciting era of neurophysiology. By resolutely turning away from the
then fashionable preoccupation with morphology, the minutiae of cerebral localization and an exclusive concern with basic electrophysiological mechanisms, he led the
way to the investigation of the dynamics of brain function. As a clinician he was ill
prepared to undertake such an ambitious task and one might well ask why he chose
to leave the beaten paths followed by his contemporaries and what induced him to
search for ways of studying the electrical activity of the human brain. To answer
these questions we need to know Berger's personal aspirations, the goals he had set
himself and how his scientific concepts and aims grew out of the intellectual climate
of late 19th century Germany in which he received his education.

THE LIFE AND WORLD OF HANS BERGER

Hans Berger was born on May 21, 1873 in the small town of Neuses near
Coburg in Northern Bavaria. His father was a physician who stimulated his early
interest in the natural sciences. His mother was the daughter of the German poet

[1]

Friedrich Rückert, who is also known for his studies on oriental philosophy. Undoubtedly Berger's interest in philosophy and poetry owed much to the influence of his mother. Hans Berger received his pre-university education at the "Gymnasium Ernestinum" in Coburg, at a time when Germany, politically, culturally and scientifically had risen to the pinnacle of her power. The intellectual climate of the period shaped Berger's intellectual outlook. German thinking at that time was based on the belief in the ultimate unity of human learning, or "Wissenschaft", a term for which there is no exact English equivalent. "Wissenschaft" is more than science, it includes the humanities, philosophy, even theology and thus encompasses all forms of higher learning. To this day Germany never experienced to the same degree, as other European nations did, the dichotomy between science and the humanities, the "two cultures" syndrome. A striving for universal, undivided truth inspired much of German scientific thinking in the 19th Century and was at the root of the phenomenal blossoming of philosophy in that country. The intellectual credo of this era was probably best expressed by Goethe in his *Faust*:

> "That I may detect the inmost force
> which binds the world, and guides its course"

Hans Berger was a natural heir to this tradition. He could not be satisfied with being only a scientist; he had to be a scientist-philosopher.

This broad intellectual outlook developed early in his youth. In his late teens, while still attending the Coburg "Gymnasium", he set down the aims of his life in his diary. He writes of his plans to study mathematics and the natural sciences in order to become an astronomer. However, he adds that he does not want to neglect "die schönen Wissenschaften", *i.e.* the humanities and philosophy, and thus become "an ossified philistine". During these adolescent years he also became interested in the relationship between the body and the mind through his reading of Schroeder van der Kolk's book *Leib und Seele* ("Body and Soul") which he had found in his mother's library.

When Berger graduated from the Coburg "Gymnasium" in 1892 he followed his first inclination, and enrolled as a student of astronomy at the University of Berlin. A year later, in 1893, he volunteered for service in the German army. During his military training, he had an experience which gave his life its decisive orientation and launched him on his search for the answer to the age-old question of the interrelationship between psychical events and physical processes. In 1940, in his last publication *Psyche* he described this experience as follows: "As a 19 year old student, I had a serious accident during a military exercise near Würzburg and barely escaped certain death. Riding on the narrow edge of a steep ravine through which a road led, I fell with my rearing and tumbling horse down into the path of a mounted battery and came to lie almost beneath the wheel of one of the guns. The latter, pulled by six horses, came to a stop just in time and I escaped, having suffered no more than fright. This accident happened in the morning hours of a beautiful spring day. In the evening of the same day, I received a telegram from my father who enquired about my well being. It was the first and only time in my life that I received such a query. My oldest sister, to whom I had always been particularly close, had occasioned this telegraphic enquiry, because she had suddenly told my parents that she knew with certainty that I had suffered an accident. My family lived in Coburg at the time. This is a case of spontaneous telepathy in which at a time of mortal danger, and as I contemplated certain death, I transmitted my thoughts, while my sister, who was particularly close to me, acted as the receiver". Thus, Berger's decision to abandon the study of astronomy and to devote himself to the elucidation of the relationships between the psychical and the physical world was prompted by this curious event which convinced him of the reality of telepathy.

It is a testimony to his objectivity as a scientific investigator that in his writings on the electroencephalogram he never succumbed to the temptation to suggest that the electrical oscillations of the brain which he had discovered could represent the physical basis of telepathy. When this suggestion was made by others, he rejected it without hesitation, as the final paragraph of the last of his 14 reports on the human electroencephalogram shows.

After his release from military duty in 1893, Berger took up the study of medicine, first in Würzburg and later in Berlin, Munich, Kiel and Jena. He received his doctorate in medicine at Jena in 1897. After his graduation he became a junior staff member at the Psychiatric Clinic of the University of Jena, which was directed by Otto Binswanger. Except for military service during the first world war, Berger worked without interruption at the Jena Psychiatric University Clinic from 1897 to his retirement in 1938.

He had the good fortune to find at the clinic an able mentor in the person of Ziehen, who shared his interest in psychophysiology. At that time there were few investigators who had any interest in this field. After a promising start with the pioneering work of Weber, Fechner, Helmholtz, Hering and Wundt, earlier in the 19th Century, psychophysiology had fallen into disrepute among neurologists and psychiatrists. Two new approaches had become fashionable, the neuroanatomical approach of Gudden, Meynert, Flechsig, Forel and von Monakow, and the functional approach as exemplified by the work of Kraepelin, Bleuler, Janet, Freud, Adler and Jung. Berger felt no attraction for either of these two avenues of research. The former was not functional enough to satisfy his psychophysiological interests and the latter, in his eyes, lacked a firm foundation in the natural sciences which he always believed to be indispensable for the understanding of brain function and its relation to mental processes. Thus, from the start, he chose the difficult role of being an outsider, a position in which he was to remain for the rest of his scientific career.

In spite of his psychophysiological interests, however, Berger's first scientific research work still followed the beaten path of neuroanatomy. His first publication which appeared in 1898 in *Ziehens Monatsschrift* was entitled "Degeneration der Vorderhornzellen des Rückenmarks bei Dementia paralytica" ("Degeneration of the anterior horn cells of the spinal cord in dementia paralytica"). His interest in psychophysiology, however, soon surfaced. In the opening paragraph of his fourth paper "Experimentell-anatomische Studien über die durch den Mangel optischer Reize veranlassten Entwicklungshemmungen im Occipitallappen des Hundes und der Katze" ("Experimental anatomical studies on the retardation of development of the occipital lobe of the dog and cat, resulting from a lack of visual stimuli"), he mentions the heuristic doctrine of psychophysical parallelism which inspired this piece of research. It was published in the *Archiv für Psychiatrie und Nervenkrankheiten* in 1900. Although morphological in its technique, it aimed at the elucidation of relationships between sensation and its material substrate in the brain.

In July 1901, Berger received his first academic appointment with the rank of "Privatdozent". In the same year he published the results of his first physiological research entitled *Zur Lehre von der Blutzirkulation in der Schädelhöhle des Menschen* ("On the circulation of the blood in the cranial cavity of man"). Adopting Mosso's technique of plethysmographic recording from a pulsating skull defect in a patient who had undergone a trepanation, he studied the action of a variety of drugs known to affect mental function and cerebral circulation, such as chloroform, cocaine, morphine and amyl nitrite. Berger hoped that he would be able to use changes in brain circulation as indicators of material cerebral processes associated with mental events. His hope that this method would provide useful information concerning psychophysical relationships, however, remained unfulfilled as he readily admits in the preface to this publication. However, in spite of his disappointment, he continued to use the technique of cerebral plethysmography and published a second monograph on his findings entitled *Über die körperlichen Äusserungen psychischer Zustände* ("On bodily manifestations of mental states"). It carried the subtitle of "Further experimental contributions to the knowledge of the circulation of the blood in the cranial cavity of man" and appeared in two parts, the first in 1904 and the second in 1907. These two volumes contained observations on the cerebral plethysmogram and on its responses to a variety of psychological states such as attention, various affects and sensory stimuli. Much later he returned briefly to plethysmographic recordings of the brain when he proved that the oscillations of the electroencephalogram are independent of the cerebral pulse wave. Figures 1, 2 and 3 of his 3rd report on the electroencephalogram of man show excellent curves of the cerebral plethysmogram recorded simultaneously with the electroencephalogram and the electrocardiogram (see p. 97 and 98).

It was at the time when he was pursuing these studies on the cerebral plethysmogram that he first became interested in recording the electrical activity of the brain. He was familiar with the pioneering work in experimental animals which had been carried out by Caton, Fleischl von Marxow, Beck and Cybulski. We do not know what aroused his interest in cerebral electrophysiology, for unfortunately the volumes of his diary covering the period from 1897 to 1910 have been lost. Perhaps it was caused by his realization that the plethysmographic technique was an inadequate tool for psychophysiological research. In any event, in 1902 he attempted for the first time to record the electrical activity of the cerebral cortex in the dog. Several other experiments were carried out between 1902 and 1910, but none were too successful. In 1910 he received some assistance from Dr. Stübel, who worked at the Physiological Institute of the University under Biedermann, one of the leading electrophysiologists of the time. The first records were taken with a Lipmann capillary electrometer. Later the small Edelmann string galvanometer was used. In his first paper on the electroencephalogram published in 1929 Berger briefly described these experiments.

In 1910 he decided to abandon this line of research, because of the paucity of positive results. The entry in his diary of November 30, 1910 vividly expresses his disappointment with these studies: "Of nine experiments, one success and even this one rather doubtful, because in this case skin currents could not be excluded in the experiment. One can therefore not say that I gave this thing up lightly. Eight years! Trying always, time and again." A few days later he noted: "I definitely plan to finish up the experiments on the cerebral cortex of dogs", and adds: "Observations on man".

During the years in which Berger made his first attempts at electrical recording from the cortex of animals, he pursued still another line of research. He studied the changes in temperature of the cerebral cortex which occurred in response to a variety of sensory and emotional stimuli. He also measured the temperature changes occurring during mental work and under the influence of drugs known to affect mental processes, such as anesthetics and morphine. The opportunity to carry out this research presented itself since Neisser and Pollack had introduced the method of cerebral puncture as a diagnostic procedure in neurology and neurosurgery. This method had been designed to aid in the diagnosis and localization of brain tumors. Before the era of contrast neuroradiology, it served as a useful guide for the surgeon who contemplated the extirpation of a cerebral tumor and who wished to have some information as to its extent and histological structure. Berger used this opportunity to introduce very fine precision thermometers into the brains of a number of patients in whom this diagnostic procedure was being carried out. He complemented his human observations by a series of experiments carried out on a chimpanzee which he had purchased specifically for this purpose. The results of these studies were published in 1910 in a monograph entitled *Untersuchungen über die Temperatur des Gehirns* ("Investigations on the temperature of the brain"). The section of the monograph in which Berger discusses the significance of his findings is extremely enlightening. Nowhere else does he state as positively his conviction that psychophysical relationships will ultimately become explainable in terms of the basic laws of physics.

In 1910 a young technical assistant, Baroness Ursula von Bülow, joined the staff of the clinic. She helped Berger in experiments on the psychogalvanic reflex, which he was then carrying out. One year later, Hans Berger and Ursula von Bülow were married. In 1912, their only son, Klaus, was born and between 1914 and 1921, they had three daughters, Ruth, Ilse and Rosemarie. The outbreak of the first world war in 1914 interrupted both Hans Berger's scientific studies and his harmonious family life. He served on the western front in the military hospital at Rethel. His duties as an army neuropsychiatrist left him enough time to read his beloved philosophers, among them Spinoza and Kant and many works of literary and historical interest. He also reflected much on his plans for his future research in the light of what he read, as is attested by numerous entries in his diary.

After the end of the war, Berger returned to Jena. Germany was at that time in the throes of revolutionary change. The old patterns of life had been shattered and the future looked grim and uncertain. Binswanger resigned as director of the Psychiatric University Clinic and returned to his native Switzerland. The university authorities selected Berger as his successor and appointed him to the chair of psychiatry at the University of Jena. Administrative and clinical duties prevented Berger, during the next few years, from resuming his research activities. It was during these years that his interest in the study of the electrical activity of the brain re-awakened. In 1920 he made his first unsuccessful attempt at recording the electrical activity of the brain from the scalp of a bald medical student. Only in 1924 did he find sufficient time to resume his investigative work in earnest. Once again Berger changed his methods of research. He attempted to stimulate the cortex of patients with skull defects by applying an electrical current to the skin covering the defect. His friend and colleague Guleke, who was Professor of Surgery at the University of Jena and who had a particular interest in neurosurgery, willingly put at his disposal a number of patients who had undergone palliative trepanations. It is not immediately apparent how these cortical stimulation experiments related to Berger's fundamental interest in psychophysiology. A passage he had written 14 years earlier in the concluding pages of his monograph on temperature studies of the brain, explains the rationale of these new experiments: "From a general physiological point of view and according to the two phases of the metabolism, one can divide the processes in the living sub-stance, including those in the cerebral cortex, into processes of dissimilation [breakdown] and assimilation. Hering was the first to make this distinction. It can be shown that the psychical processes are associated with the phase of dissimilation, as I already emphasized elsewhere. For we know that when the electrical current acts upon elec-trolytes, including the tissues of the human body, it produces a breakdown. In the course of brain operations, one frequently subjects the exposed cortex of the awake patient to the action of the electrical current. A report has just appeared which describes stimulation experiments carried out on the postcentral gyrus of man by an English investigator[1]. The stimulation elicited very definite touch sensations in the fingers of the contralateral hand; thus the stimulating effect, that is the breakdown or the dissimilation phase, corresponds to the sensation of touch." The main purpose of these stimulation experiments therefore was to elicit subjective sensations. Berger's hope was that this might give him some clue as to the nature of the relationship between the physicochemical events produced by the electrical stimulus and the mental processes as revealed by the patient's subjective experience. Undoubtedly, the availability of many patients with skull defects, in whom the pulsating surface of the brain was separated from the stimulating electrodes only by a few millimeters of tissue, reactivated Berger's interest in recording the electrical activity of the brain. This idea which flashed through his mind, and was to lead to the most momentous decision of his life, is recorded in very brief and partially stenographic form, in one of the protocols of his stimulation experiments. The entry is dated June 2, 1924 and reads: "The idea to search for cortical currents in humans with palliative trepanations ..." Berger had finally embarked upon the road that would lead him along a tortuous path strewn with many obstacles to ultimate success and fame. He was 51 years old at the time, an age when few scientists start a new successful research career leading to truly original discoveries (Plate 1).

---

[1] The "English" investigator was none other than Harvey Cushing.

From many points of view, Berger was ill-prepared for his new task. He had only little electrophysiological experience. It was derived from a series of mostly unsuccessful experiments which he had carried out more than 14 years earlier. His knowledge of physics and instrumentation was limited, as he honestly admits in his first paper on the human electroencephalogram. Berger seems to have received no help from his colleague Professor Biedermann who was an excellent electrophysiologist and was Chairman of the Department of Physiology at Jena. Two factors may have contributed to this lack of cooperation. It is probable that Biedermann, like all the electrophysiologists of his time, saw no particular merit in Berger's research. Berger may have sensed this critical attitude and therefore was probably unwilling to approach Biedermann with any request for advice and assistance. It is of interest that Biedermann's name never appears among the many electrophysiologists whose work he quotes in his papers. Berger's shyness and his difficulty in sharing with others what interested him most passionately may also have prevented him from seeking Biedermann's advice. Fortunately, the same lack of communication did not exist between Berger and Professor Esau, who headed the Institute of Physics. Esau and two of his associates, Wien and Dietsch, advised Berger on many occasions and helped him with problems that arose from his instrumentation.

The instruments available to Berger were not well suited for the research he was contemplating (Plates 2 and 5). He carried out his first electrical recordings from skull defects in 1924 by using the large Edelmann string galvanometer, an instrument which had been designed to record electrocardiograms. In 1926 he acquired the new Siemens coil galvanometer, an apparatus which was also used in electrocardiography (Plate 5). Later, in 1932, the Siemens Company constructed an oscillograph with amplifier for him. This instrument had adequate gain and in contrast to the earlier galvanometers was a voltage measuring, rather than a current measuring device. All these instruments were used with an optical recording system. The electrical oscillations deflected a mirror upon which a light beam was projected. The deflections of the light beam were proportional to the magnitude of the electrical signals. The movement of the spot of the light beam was recorded on photographic paper moving at a speed of 3 cm/sec. Sometimes slower speeds of 1.5 cm/sec or 2.3 cm/sec were used. The paper width was 12 cm. The lengths of the records varied between about 2.5 and 7.5 meters.

Berger remained faithful to his old recording instruments, even when newer and better equipment, such as the cathode ray oscillograph or Tönnies' ink-writing oscillograph became available. Whether he persisted in the use of his old instruments because he was used to them, or because he lacked the funds necessary to purchase more modern equipment remains an open question. In the 1930s, Berger entertained the hope that Siemens could provide him with a multiple oscillograph system, but this hope remained unfulfilled. Thus to the end of his career, whenever he wished to record with more than one channel at a time, he was forced to use simultaneously the Siemens oscillograph and the coil galvanometer. Because the gains of the two instruments were very different and because it was difficult to put the light spots of the two systems in precise vertical alignment, many of his double recordings look rather odd and were not fully satisfactory from a technical point of view, a fact of which he was well aware.

Berger experimented with a variety of recording electrodes (Plate 4). At the beginning he used mainly the DuBois-Reymond type of non-polarizable clay electrodes. These electrodes were placed on the skin over skull defects in patients who had undergone palliative trepanations or who had sustained a cranial injury during the first world war (Plate 3). Later he used needle electrodes inserted epidurally in the region of the skull defect or a variety of metal surface electrodes made of malleable leadplates, lead foil or silver foil. In subjects with intact skulls he usually placed one electrode in the frontal, the other in the occipital region.

With these relatively primitive methods Berger relentlessly pursued his aim of recording the electrical activity of the human brain. He persisted in his attempt in spite of many difficulties and repeated disappointments. Fortunately, the records taken during this early period have been preserved for posterity in the "Hans Berger Archives" at the University of Freiburg im Breisgau. Leafing through these early records, one can only marvel at the determination and singlemindedness with which Berger pursued his goal, for most of the early tracings show little more than a straight line with only the very occasional slight deflection, which could hardly be interpreted as convincing evidence of cerebral activity. It is therefore not surprising that Berger often nearly despaired and frequently thought of abandoning his studies on the electrical activity of the human brain. However, his faith was finally rewarded and he obtained results which he could trust. The slow struggle which led him to his final conviction of the reality of the human electroencephalogram, his hopes and fears, the moments of discouragement and despair are vividly described in his diary and in his experimental protocols. Many excerpts of these have recently been published by Jung in the *Jenenser EEG Symposion*.

The first indication that he might succeed in recording the electrical activity of the human brain came early, when on the 6th of July 1924 he observed small, tremulous movements of the galvanometer string while recording from the skin overlying a bone defect in a 17 year old patient, named Zedel, who previously had been one of his subjects for his cortical stimulation experiments (Plate 3). Zedel had been operated earlier by Guleke because he was suspected of having a brain tumor. In his first paper on the human electroencephalogram Berger briefly described this case as his first successful recording of an EEG. However, from his experimental protocol we know that he did not fully trust this observation, but it encouraged him greatly. On the same day he recorded in his diary his joy at the prospect of continuing with this type of research: "Cortical currents (circulation, temperature, electrical processes!) and the hope so beautifully expressed by Mosso[1], which I experience time and again when I apply precise measuring instruments to the brain. A type of work which agrees well with me and my whole — psychophysiological — attitude". At

---

[1] In his diary Berger does not specify what he and Mosso hoped to learn from such experiments. Towards the end of his 3rd report on the human EEG, however, he makes it clear that Mosso's hope, which he shared, was that by applying exact measuring instruments to the brain, "we may learn to recognize the physical bases of consciousness" (See page 129).

the time of these early studies Berger already used the term "electroencephalogram" in his diary. But for several years he still had doubts about the cerebral origin of the electrical oscillations he recorded. As late as 1928, one year before publication of his first paper on the electroencephalogram, he was almost ready to abandon his electrical recording studies. On the 11th of July 1928, he wrote in his diary: "Plans! I feel the need for creative scientific work. For many years I have worked in vain on the presumed EEG. What now? Abandon EEG!"

The first recordings on human subjects were carried out in a small annex of the clinic, the Hufeldhaus. A few years later the recording instruments were transferred to the main building and housed in a room adjacent to the antechamber of the director's office (Plates 5 and 6). Berger's interest in the human electroencephalogram was very much his private affair and was not allowed to interfere with the efficiently organized daily work of the clinic. Only a few of his collaborators had any knowledge of his work, either because they were used as subjects for his recording or because they assisted him in the experiments as was the case for Hilpert, and later Lemke and Lembcke. None of these men, however, later continued to work in the field of electroencephalography, although two of them, Hilpert and Lemke, became chairmen of university departments, Hilpert in Greifswald and Lemke in Jena after Berger's retirement, and would have had ample opportunity to do so. Mr. Keuscher, Hans Berger's technician, was the only other person in the clinic who was deeply involved in the work on the human electroencephalogram. The recordings were always carried out between 5 and 8 p.m., after the daily work of the clinic had come to an end. All electrical machinery and equipment in the main and adjacent buildings were turned off in order to avoid electrical interference by stray currents. Fortunately the main supply line to the clinic was fed by DC-power and this certainly contributed to Berger's success in preventing electrical interference in most of his recordings.

The publication of Berger's first paper on the electroencephalogram of man in 1929 had little impact on the scientific world. It was either ignored or regarded with open incredulity. Even Berger himself, after the publication of his first report, was not completely free of doubts about the validity of his findings, but in spite of this he forged ahead with his work and published further contributions to the study of the electroencephalogram in a series of papers which followed upon each other at relatively short intervals. Except for his second paper, published in the *Journal für Psychologie und Neurologie*, all his reports entitled "Über das Elektrenkephalogramm des Menschen" appeared in the *Archiv für Psychiatrie und Nervenkrankheiten*. As he advanced in his research, he became increasingly more sure of himself and convinced of the significance of his discovery.

The tragedy of this period of his life was that although he had finally succeeded in making a significant scientific contribution, the scientific world around him consistently denied him his well-deserved recognition. He remained lonely and isolated in his interests and even later, when others like Kornmüller and Tönnies, at the Kaiser Wilhelm Institute in Berlin-Buch, confirmed his findings, he was often criticized and not taken seriously. There were many reasons for this lack of recognition and this widespread skepticism. One source of the resistance against the acceptance of

Berger's findings was to be found among the expert neurophysiologists. Those who were at home among the axons and who studied their action potentials just could not believe that regular oscillations of quasi sinusoidal form could represent the electrical activity of an organ as complex as the human brain and that such activity could be recorded from the scalp. Adrian and Matthews in their 1934 paper on the "Berger rhythm" admit that initially they had been very skeptical about the validity of Berger's work. In the introduction to their paper they wrote: "During the same period a number of workers have recorded the potential changes which take place in the exposed cortex of animals. Their findings have been difficult to reconcile with Berger's as the potential changes have been much less regular and have rarely shown any sign of a persistent rhythm at 10 a second. Our own work on animals (Adrian and Matthews 1934) led in the same direction. We found it difficult to accept the view that such uniform activity could occur throughout the brain in a conscious subject and as this seemed to be Berger's conclusion, we decided to repeat his experiments." This skepticism was reinforced by the common assumption that Berger, a psychiatrist, was an unlikely person to make such a striking discovery.

Berger's personality was another factor which made it difficult for his contemporaries to accept his discovery at face value. Kolle and Ginzberg, both pupils of Berger, describe him as shy and reticent. He had difficulties to communicate with others at a warm personal level. His sensitive and humane private personality, which appears so vividly from his diary, was not easily perceptible to the people with whom he worked. His warm and refined inner self was hidden behind a façade of sternness and iron self-discipline. He impressed his collaborators as an authoritarian whose foremost interest was to run his clinic according to a strict, meticulous and almost military routine and who demanded the same devotion to detail from his subordinates. To his assistants and residents he appeared unimaginative; Ginzberg calls him "static". Berger's daily work followed a time-table of clocklike regularity. He arrived at the clinic every day punctually at 8:00 A.M. At 9 o'clock on the dot he began his daily conference with his assistants and residents, who had to report all the minutiae of what had gone on during the preceding 24 hours. The conference was followed by ward rounds until noon. After lunch he joined his wife and children for a walk over the hills surrounding the city. At 4:00 P.M. he was back at the clinic and saw his private patients in his office until 5:00 P.M. The hours from 5:00 P.M. to 8:00 P.M. were devoted to his research. After supper Mr. Schlöhmilch, an intelligent long term patient who worked as his secretary, came over to the director's residence for two hours of dictation.

During his daily conferences with his staff Berger dealt almost exclusively with routine clinical and administrative problems. Scientific matters were relegated to another conference held every Saturday afternoon between 5 and 7:00 P.M. During these two hours of what the staff jestingly referred to as "Klughusten" (which literally translated means "wise coughing") patients with problems of special scientific interest were presented and their cases discussed. To his staff Berger seemed to be mostly interested in neurological localization problems and it is somewhat misleading if he is only described as a psychiatrist. He was more of a neurologist and his residents and colleagues admired his skill in making correct localizing neurological diagnoses. Berger made a point of attending all neurosurgical operations performed by his colleague Guleke on patients in whom he had identified the location of a brain tumor on the basis of clinical signs alone. Berger was the first to introduce diagnostic neuro-radiology in Germany and it is therefore surprising that he never attempted to use the electroencephalogram as a localizing diagnostic tool.

Though recognized as an excellent neurologist by his staff and colleagues, he never struck them as an innovator. In their eyes his obsessive devotion to routine overshadowed all other qualities. This made it nearly impossible for those who knew him to suspect that in the privacy of his research laboratory, Berger was on the verge of making a revolutionary scientific discovery. Berger was particularly reticent about what interested him most intensely. Thus he did not share with his associates his intellectual excitement about the discovery of the electroencephalogram. Ginzberg, who worked for three years as a resident on Berger's service, relates that even in his own clinic after the first paper on the electroencephalogram had already been published "no one with the exception of Hilpert had the remotest idea of electro-encephalography". Thus even to his closest collaborators he seemed to be an unlikely man to make as momentous a discovery as that of the human electroencephalogram. It is truly amazing how his most absorbing scientific interests and his personal dreams and aspirations which are so clearly revealed in his diary and which can even be sensed in his publication, could remain so thoroughly hidden from his closest associates. What a contrast between the public and the private man!

An additional factor which contributed to Berger's difficulties and to the lack of recognition for his work was the political situation of the time. Berger's early publications on the EEG appeared when Hitler rose to power and when the Nazi party gradually took over control of all aspects of German life. The University of Jena was badly affected by the blight of Nazism, both in its faculty and student body. Berger disliked the Nazis and they retaliated by disparaging his work. Those who acted in this manner were not only party functionaries, but also scientists who had espoused the new political credo. Berger was distrusted by those in power and was even forced to submit to censorship the few papers which he presented abroad, as for instance the one he gave at the International Congress of Psychology in Paris in 1937. It is therefore not too surprising that his contribution to science was underrated in his native Germany, even more than elsewhere.

The year 1934 marked the end of Berger's tragic isolation, thanks to Adrian's and Matthews' publication on the "Berger rhythm". Adrian, whose competence as a neurophysiologist could not be questioned, fully confirmed Berger's observations and thus put the seal of scientific respectability upon his work. Soon interest in the electroencephalogram discovered by Berger quickened in all countries of the Western World, except in Germany. Berger's name became famous among neurophysiologists the world over. Beaudoin, Durup and Fessard in France, Brémer in Belgium, Grey Walter in Great Britain, Gibbs, Lennox, Jasper, Davis, Travis and Loomis in the United States followed in his footsteps, confirmed his results and carried them further by introducing newer and better recording methods. In 1937, Berger attended the

International Congress of Psychology in Paris where to his surprise he found himself to be an international celebrity. "In Germany I am not so famous", he is reported to have remarked on this occasion. The Paris Congress marked the high point of his career. He was now 64 years old (Plate 8).

Although the international scientific community had finally accepted him into their ranks, tragedy awaited him in his own homeland. A year after the meeting in Paris he was subjected to the most humiliating experience of his life. While making rounds in his clinic, on the 30th of September 1938, he was called to the telephone. He was informed abruptly that on the next day, the 1st of October, he was to retire from his post as chairman of the department and turn the clinic over to his successor. Strictly speaking the decision of the University authorities was legal, since Berger had attained retirement age. However, the manner in which this decision was communicated to him was a deliberate insult and represented the final outrage to which he was subjected by the Nazis who by then had assumed full control of university affairs. Shortly after Berger's retirement, his laboratory was dismantled. He retired to the small town of Bad Blankenburg in Thuringia. His last years were sad and tragic. He was deprived of any opportunity to pursue his scientific research. He saw his country led into a murderous war by a government for which he had no respect. Understandably, he became increasingly despondent. He developed a severe depression which, even though he was a psychiatrist, he mistook for a cardiac condition. On the 20th of May 1941, he wrote his last entry in his diary: "Tuesday, on my desk at 10 o'clock. I try again and again to get out of bed having been laid up for more than eight weeks. I have behind me days of despair in which I yearningly wished for my early end. I have sleepless nights during which I keep brooding and struggling with self-accusations. I am unable to read or work in any organized way, but I want to force myself, for like this it is unbearable ... All the loved ones write to me so kindly and send me good wishes and flowers. B.B.v.E. and also Mrs. v.L., Ursula and Ruth look after me so touchingly. I am often so full of despair and impatience. I have read all papers on the EEG and made abstracts. Kornmüller is reprimanded often and from many sides. I have read Napoleon's memoirs (10 volumes), which interested me very much. I have wonderful flowers near my bed which make my heart heavy, — but be patient, little brother." Here Berger's diary ends. Ten days later in the depth of his depression he took his own life. He was laid to rest behind the Friedenskirche in Jena, near the place where he had worked for over 40 years.

HANS BERGER'S PSYCHOPHYSIOLOGICAL CONCEPTS

Berger's work on the human electroencephalogram can be understood only if one realizes that for him the study of the electrical activity of the human brain was a means to an end. Berger was not particularly interested in the electroencephalogram as an electrophysiological phenomenon, nor was he interested in its applications as a diagnostic tool in neurology or psychiatry. The electroencephalogram absorbed his interest for one single reason only: he believed that in it he had found the key which would unlock the secret of man's nature as a psychophysical being. He believed that in the EEG he was able to discern some well defined and measurable physical properties which represented true expressions of mental processes.

Berger's approach to psychophysiology had its roots in some fundamental scientific concepts discovered in the course of the 19th Century. Three of these were particularly important to him: (i) the law of conservation of energy, (ii) the total dependence of biological processes upon physicochemical mechanisms which fully obeyed the law of conservation of energy and thermodynamics, and (iii) the knowledge gained from clinical observations that mental processes were completely dependent upon brain function. It was however obvious that the brain–mind problem would not yield as readily to interpretation in terms of physicochemical laws as other problems of physiology had done. There was no easy way to account for mental processes in a scientifically satisfactory manner in terms of the known principles of physics and chemistry. Was it possible that psychophysiology transcended the limits of our physicochemical world? Was it perhaps conceivable that the brain could be the only organ in which the two sides of the equation of energy turnover would not balance and where some functions, apparently those that were most highly developed, escaped the laws of conservation of energy? Or, on the contrary, could physical processes be found which were directly correlated with mental activity, not only in a qualitative, but also in a quantitative way? These were the questions which preoccupied 24 year old Hans Berger when he entered Binswanger's clinic in 1897, and which he pursued with dogged singlemindedness throughout his entire scientific career. The persistent search for this elusive connection between the material and the psychical world, which he firmly believed could ultimately be described in terms of observable and measurable physical or physicochemical phenomena, was the underlying motive for all his scientific studies, including those on the human electroencephalogram.

Nowhere did Berger express more clearly where he stood on these fundamental scientific and philosophical issues of the mind–brain problem than in his short monograph *Psychophysiologie in 12 Vorlesungen* ("Psychophysiology in 12 lectures") published in 1921. In this slim volume Berger first critically reviews the various ideas which have been proposed to explain psychophysical relationships. The oldest and most pervasive of all has been the dualistic view. It postulates the separate existence of a material body and an immaterial soul. The concept of mutual interaction between the physical and the mental, which is inherent in the dualistic proposition, is, of course, derived from our immediate, subjective every day experience. We all know that what goes on in our mind can result in physical action directed towards our environment; conversely, physical changes taking place in our environment enter our consciousness and modify our thinking and feeling. Psychophysical dualism is therefore a natural, one may even say a logical outgrowth of the way we experience the world in which we live. Berger then goes on to show that in spite of these attractive features, psychophysical dualism can hardly be accepted within the framework of modern natural sciences, for it is incompatible with the law of conservation of energy. Psychophysical dualism presupposes that the immaterial mind, which is not subject to physical laws, can intervene in physicochemical processes which are energy-dependent and take place in the brain, for instance when we perform volitional movements.

The incompatibility of psychophysical dualism with fundamental physical laws led to the attempt to explain psychical events exclusively in physicochemical terms. Berger, in agreement with Wundt however, finds it difficult to accept this simple materialistic theory, since it conflicts with the empirical fact that the mind and the body are linked in a relationship of mutual interaction. Berger refuses to accept the notion that mental processes are merely byproducts of physicochemical processes in the brain. Such a concept would make it impossible to explain how the mind in its turn can cause physicochemical changes, as for instance when it induces the cortical processes that lead to a volitional movement.

Berger finds it equally difficult to accept the theory of psychophysical parallelism which was very fashionable in his day and which to many seemed to offer a satisfactory solution to the dilemmas raised by both the dualistic and the classical materialistic theories. Briefly, psychophysical parallelism postulates that physical processes in the brain and psychological processes in the mind are always proceeding in parallel, but just as two parallel lines never intersect, it was believed that the physical and the mental processes never interact directly, although they always retain a well defined relationship to each other as two parallel lines do. This solution of the dilemma did not appear very satisfactory to Berger. To him it was only the old dualism in a new disguise, shorn of its most attractive feature, namely mutual interaction of the mental and the physical world. In spite of all his reservations, he was however prepared to test the usefulness of psychophysical parallelism as a heuristic principle. He defined the principle by the following axiom: "Material processes in the cerebral cortex proceed in parallel with mental processes". However, he made it clear that he did not regard all cortical processes as being endowed with mental qualities. In his work on the electroencephalogram he attempted to identify those processes which correspond to mental activity and to distinguish them from those which do not. He also attempted to define the conditions which these material cortical processes have to fulfil in order to assume mental qualities. However, for him, psychophysical parallelism was only a temporary conceptual crutch. He did not believe in its fundamental premise which implied an absence of interaction between mental and physical processes. He accepted as an empirical fact that interactions between psychical and physical processes do occur, together with the implication that psychical factors had to be included within the chains of causality of physical events. On the other hand, he also subscribed without reservations to the principle of conservation of energy and to its full applicability to biological phenomena, including those of the brain. He believed that the conflict between these two propositions could be resolved by adopting the notion of "psychical energy" which had been developed around the turn of the century by some philosophers such as Külpe and Lasswitz, by the Danish psychophysiologist Alfred Lehmann, and which had also been accepted by the famous physical chemist Ostwald. In developing his ideas on psychical energy, Berger borrowed heavily from the work of Alfred Lehmann. In his 12th lecture on "Psychophysiology" he wrote: "Alfred Lehmann also supported the assumption that a specific psychical energy exists. He designates as psychical energy that energy developed in the central nervous system with which a psychical phenomenon is immediately associated. This form of energy, in addition to several other energy forms, originates during brain activity; it is a special form of energy. According to Lehmann, this energy must first of all possess physical characteristics and must also be measurable as physical energy. Secondly, it must obey the law of conservation of energy. When psychical energy originates, an equivalent amount of other forms of energy must disappear. Psychical energy is generated through the transformation of physical energy and can be reconverted into the latter. However, not every transformation of energy within the brain leads to the formation of psychical energy." Ostwald believed that psychical energy was the most highly developed and rarest form of energy, which could only originate in very complex organs such as the cerebral cortex. Berger hoped that by means of sufficiently accurate measurements of the energy turnover in the brain, the amount of psychical energy could be calculated by extrapolation. Since the only source of energy in the brain is chemical, the problem from a conceptual point of view appeared simple: in the brain chemical energy is transformed into heat, electrical energy and psychical energy. Initially he assumed that electrical energy would ultimately be transformed into heat and therefore, precise measurements of heat production in the brain while it was engaged in mental activity could be used to measure psychical energy indirectly. This reasoning formed the basis for his study on brain temperature published in 1910.

The final chapter of this monograph in which Berger discusses the significance of his experimental measurements is extremely revealing of the manner in which he hoped to approach the solution of the riddle of psychophysical relationships. It is therefore worthwhile to summarize briefly how he attempted to calculate the energy equivalent of psychical energy. He started his calculations by establishing the amount of energy that would be necessary to raise the temperature of the cortex by 1°C. He arrived at this figure by taking into account the total volume of human cerebral grey matter, its specific weight and its specific heat. The value he found was 348,435 cal (which is equivalent to 1,459,963,600 ergs or 14.89 kgm). He then introduced into his calculations some experimental values obtained in man. Thus during the excitatory stage of chloroform narcosis, he had observed a temperature increase in the cortex of 0.08°C per minute which corresponds to an energy value of 7.6 kgm per minute. He found a similar value during awakening from anesthesia and considered it to be an acceptable value for the resting energy production of the brain. During the continuous performance of arithmetic, he found in the cerebral cortex of one subject during the first 3 minutes a temperature increase of 0.07°C, which amounts to an energy production of 3.474 kgm per minute. In the following 7 minutes, the increase was less, only 0.01°C or 0.213 kgm per minute. He extrapolated these figures to an 8 hour period of concentrated mental work and arrived at a value of 122 kgm. In analogy to what is known from other organs, especially muscle, he assumed that heat production represents only 40% of the total energy produced by living tissue. Thus an additional 60% must be transformed into other forms of energy. The value for 8 hours of mental work therefore had to be corrected to 305 kgm. This represents only 0.03% of the total metabolic energy requirement of a 16 hour waking day in which no physical work is performed. Berger commented that it is not surprising that many investigators who measured the total energy turnover of the human organism during mental work were unable to demonstrate any significant increase over the resting metabolic rate since the value he had calculated was well within the margin of error inherent in such experimental procedures.

He then proceeded to the final step, the quantitative definition of the maximum value of psychical energy. Mental work over a period of 8 hours requires 305 kgm. This amounts to 0.51 kgm per minute or 50,031,000 ergs per minute; 40% of this amount is dissipated in the form of heat, and 60% is available for other forms of energy, including psychical energy. This corresponds to 0.306 kgm per minute or 30,018,600 ergs per minute. This amount of energy contains, among others, the portion which is equivalent to psychical energy. In what proportion this energy amount is divided between psychical energy and other non-thermal energy forms cannot be established and thus it was only possible to say that the amount of psychical energy produced in the brain during mental work cannot exceed the value of 0.306 kgm per minute.

In spite of the ingeniousness of the calculations their end result led into a blind alley. Indeed the quantitative determinations provided little insight into the true complexities of psychophysical interactions, and must have appeared singularly unsuited for elucidating the more detailed aspects of such interactions, as exemplified by attention, conscious perception, ideational activity and the disturbances of mental function encountered in diseases of the brain, psychoses and various forms of intoxication. For these purposes, a more flexible and differentiated research method was required. Berger found it in the electroencephalogram.

BERGER'S WORK ON THE HUMAN ELECTROENCEPHALOGRAM

As scientific documents Berger's fourteen papers on the electroencephalogram of man are unusual in more ways than one. Their style is complex, the sentence structure is elaborate and studded with often unnecessary details. Even in German they are not easy to read. The style betrays the fact that the papers were dictated by Berger to his secretary Mr. Schlöhmilch in the late evening hours. They frequently read more like an oral presentation of the stream of consciousness type rather than carefully edited written essays. In this respect the fourteen papers on the electroencephalogram are quite different from Berger's earlier publications, such as his lectures on Psychophysiology, which were written in a lucid, crisp and easily flowing style. More so than in his earlier publications he injected into these papers his personal feelings. Indeed one always senses his intense personal involvement in his work and through his writing one readily perceives his conscientious, meticulous and obsessive personality.

Thus in his early papers on the electroencephalogram, he shares with us the many doubts about the significance of his findings and the worries these caused him, but he also lets us participate in his joy of discovery and in his pride in having established a scientific truth. Scientific objectivity does not prevent him from expressing his deep human concern for people, as appears so vividly for instance in the 9th report when he describes his experiment on hypoxia in which the subject, Dr. W., unexpectedly lost consciousness. His moral rectitude is clearly evident from his refusal to follow the suggestion made to him that he should study the gradual extinction of the electrical activity of the brain in a dying person. His honesty and his fairness to other workers with whom he disagreed, as well as his modesty concerning the limitations of his own knowledge and skill are clearly revealed in his writings. He also makes it clear that he never regarded his own hypotheses as sacred cows. There was, however, a passionate desire not to be misunderstood, which explains many of the repetitions and the numerous qualifying statements which lace his writings. From our present vantage point, we may regret that he thus broke up what otherwise might have been a smooth flow of ideas. We must, however, realize that Berger felt on the defensive not only because he was often openly or secretly criticized, but also because he was acutely aware of his technical limitations as an electrophysiologist. He therefore felt obliged to deal with these criticisms in his papers. He also used them to vent his feeling of annoyance towards some of his critics who, he felt, had treated him unfairly. His tone is particularly testy in his last report published in 1938, for even at this late date, some critics persisted in dismissing his findings as artefacts. Berger rarely attended scientific meetings where he would be forced to take part in personal debates. He took cover behind the printed page when he wanted to engage in a scientific argument. When not in the physical presence of his opponents, he felt free to criticize them, to show the weakness of their arguments and to forcefully restate his own case.

Berger's first paper on the electroencephalogram published in 1929 is in many ways the most fascinating one of the series. Step by step he retraces the long and often arduous path that led him to the conviction that he had indeed discovered the electroencephalogram of man. Having demonstrated that regular electrical current oscillations can be recorded from the dura of skull defects and from the scalp of a subject with an intact skull, he proceeds in a number of carefully designed experiments to show that these current oscillations cannot be attributed to cerebral pulsations, to the cerebral blood flow, to the electrocardiogram, to blood flow through scalp vessels, to skeletal or smooth muscle artefact, to eye movements or to the electrical properties of the skin. Particularly elegant is the observation on his son Klaus made by means of the pulse telephone which demonstrated that the pulse wave of the scalp vessels bears no relationship at all to the electroencephalogram. Equally convincing are the records shown in the third report in which the cerebral plethysmogram was recorded simultaneously with the electroencephalogram from the same skull defect. The independence of the two curves is particularly well shown in these records. These were very important observations, for many of Berger's critics, and initially even Berger himself, suspected that the electrical oscillations recorded from skull defects or from the scalp could be of vascular rather than cerebral origin. In the third report, Berger finally succeeded in providing formal proof of the cerebral origin of the electrical current oscillations he had discovered. In a patient subjected to a diagnostic procedure, he recorded directly from the cerebral cortex and the underlying white matter and was able to show that the characteristic oscillations of the electro-encephalogram originated in the cortex and not in the white matter.

The series of experimental observations in which, step by step, Berger proved the cerebral origin of the EEG can serve as a model of well conceived, logically designed and carefully executed scientific experiments. To this day and age his critical and questioning attitude towards his own findings and the care with which he assembled all the necessary evidence to buttress his hypothesis, can still serve as an inspiring example of how scientific research ought to be conducted.

Having proved to his own satisfaction that the electroencephalogram did indeed originate in the cerebral cortex, Berger felt free to pursue his real interest, namely to use this new recording method for the investigation of psychophysical relationships. The second report describes his first observations dealing with this question which he continued to pursue in all his subsequent publications on the human electro-encephalogram.

Berger started from the observation, which he made very early, that the alpha waves disappear upon eye opening. He soon realized that other sensory stimuli, such as touch, pain and noise, elicited the same responses. This finding came as a complete surprise to him, for on the basis of the experimental work in animals reported by Caton, Fleischl von Marxow, Beck and Cybulski, he expected to find the opposite, namely an increase in the amplitude of the cerebral oscillations. He therefore had a great deal of difficulty in accepting this observation as evidence of a true cerebral response. His further studies disclosed that this response in the electro-encephalogram occurred not only with sensory stimuli, but that identical changes were elicited by voluntary movements or merely by the intention to perform such movements, and were encountered also during intellectual work, as *e.g.* when performing mental arithmetic. He also established that the responses habituate when identical sensory stimuli are repeated. He concluded from these observations that the response is a correlate of attention and represents a generalized reaction of the brain.

From a physiological point of view, he interpreted his observations as follows: He assumed that a sensory stimulus produces a localized increase in the potential oscillations in the corresponding sensory center. Since the human sensory cortical areas are inaccessible to scalp or even to dural recordings, this local increase could not be detected in such recordings. Drawing upon ideas developed by Pavlov and by Wundt, he then postulated that this localized center of activity exerts a generalized inhibitory effect upon the remainder of the cerebral cortex. This inhibition manifests itself by a disappearance of the alpha waves and by a flattening of the electroenceph-alogram.

Berger realized that this concept was highly theoretical, especially since he had been unable to demonstrate a crucial element of the hypothesis, namely the localized increase in the cerebral electrical oscillations in the active sensory center. He was therefore very pleased when, in 1932, Kornmüller and Fischer reported that they had indeed observed high voltage potential oscillations in sensory areas in response to the appropriate sensory stimuli.

Berger concluded from these observations that the alpha waves represented the concomitants of psychophysical processes taking place in the brain and that under certain circumstances these can be associated with conscious mental processes. He was reinforced in this belief by his observation that the alpha waves disappeared during chloroform narcosis, that they were absent in post-ictal coma, that they were not yet developed in the immature brain of the newborn infant, and that the duration of the alpha waves was greatly increased in patients with organic brain lesions which were associated with mental changes. However, he also soon realized that during manic-depressive psychosis and schizophrenia, as well as in many mental defectives, the electroencephalogram was normal. These observations disturbed him and the explanations he gave as to why normal records were obtained in some of these conditions are somewhat contrived.

Berger now attempted to define more clearly the psychophysiological significance of the mechanism of attention which he had proposed on the basis of his observations on the human electroencephalogram. He assumed that the psychophysical activity which manifests itself in the alpha oscillations of the electroencephalogram originates in the three superficial cortical layers (Plate 7). On the basis of some neurohistological characteristics, von Monakow, Berze and others had postulated that these superficial cortical layers represented the material substrate in which mental processes take place. Berze called this superficial part of the cortex the "intentional sphere" and, following von Monakow's suggestion, he assumed that it functioned as a whole and did not show any evidence for localization of specific functions. This was in contrast to the organization of the three deeper cortical layers, which Berze called the "impressional sphere" and which was thought to be organized according to the principle of topographical representation of functions. In it sensory and motor fields are represented as well as the central depositories of engrams. Berger assumed that the principal oscillations of the electroencephalogram, the alpha waves, represented the physiological activity of Berze's "intentional sphere" and that this explained the ubiquity of the alpha rhythm, its near perfect synchrony between the two hemispheres and its global response to stimuli arousing attention. He believed that in the inattentive, but conscious state, this activity proceeds automatically and is characterized by the presence of generalized alpha activity involving all areas of the cerebral cortex. This represents what Berger, in his last report, aptly described as the "passive EEG". It corresponds to a passive mental state in which the mind is driven by spontaneously arising thoughts and images. As soon as a sensory stimulus attracts our attention, or as soon as we concentrate upon a particular mental task, the psychophysical activity of the cortex ceases to be diffuse and is concentrated upon the area involved in the performance of the momentary mental task. In the case of a sensory stimulus, this activity involves the appropriate sensory receiving area. In this active region the psychophysical activity is enhanced and exceeds the critical magnitude for conscious experience which Berger equated with Fechner's "internal threshold". The concentration of psychophysical activity in a local area which results from its circumscribed enhancement, coupled with its generalized inhibition in areas around the center of activity, represents the physiological basis of focussing of attention. The diffuse inhibitory process manifests itself in the electroencephalogram by the arrest of alpha activity. Consciousness is narrowed, mental activity is no longer passively driven and, to use the terminology which Berger introduced in his last paper, we are now dealing with an "active EEG".

Berger believed that psychophysical activity always involved the entire extent of the three superficial layers of the cortex. He repeatedly emphasized that in psychophysical activity the cerebrum acts as an undivided whole ("ein einheitliches Ganzes") and that this activity represents a unitary process. By this he did not imply, however, that this generalized activity is necessarily undiversified. In the "passive EEG" it is relatively undifferentiated and unstructured. In the case of attention to a sensory stimulus, however, a topographic patterning develops. A local increase in psychophysical activity is associated with generalized inhibition of the cortical psychophysical mechanism outside the active center. Thus this represents a global response of the cerebral cortex. In mental work the centers of activity shift and wander over the cortical surface as mental activity progresses through successive stages. The momentary centers of activity are, however, always surrounded by widespread inhibition. In this sense the concept of the brain acting as a whole is, as Berger put it, complementary to the principle of functional localization. In his Rectorial Address entitled "Über die Lokalisation im Grosshirn" ("On localization in the cerebrum") which he delivered on the 18th of July 1927 he summed up his views on the subject: "It is probable that in general during wakefulness the entire cortex is in a certain state of readiness, or if I may use a metaphor, it behaves as if it were energized by [electrical] power. However, only in very specific areas, now in one place and then in another, power is drawn for the performance of functions."

Although he initially believed that conscious experience is impossible unless psychophysical activity exceeds a certain fixed threshold, he later modified this view and assumed that there is no absolute threshold for the emergence of consciousness. He postulated that a psychophysical process can only become conscious if the corresponding physiological process in an area of cortex is clearly differentiated from the activity taking place in the surrounding regions. A potential gradient must exist between the active center and the areas which surround it. The absolute magnitude of the ongoing cortical activity, however, is unimportant for the development of conscious experience. Only the ratio between the magnitude of the cortical activity in the active center and that going on in its surroundings determines whether the process enters consciousness or not. Thus, for the genesis of conscious phenomena, it is not at all necessary that the psychophysical activity anywhere should be markedly elevated, the only prerequisite is that the local process should emerge clearly from the continuously and automatically ongoing activity in the cortex surrounding it. He was led to this concept from his observations in barbiturate anesthesia, where to his surprise he found that cortical activity everywhere was enhanced in amplitude. Since he interpreted the high voltage activity as a result of exaggerated alpha activity in which individual alpha waves fused into slow waves, he was first at a loss to understand why such an increase in what he believed to be psychophysical activity should be associated with the unconsciousness of the anesthetic state. He concluded that under the conditions of barbiturate anesthesia, gradients in the cortical psycho-physical activity no longer exist and therefore consciousness is impossible. The concepts which Berger introduced into cortical neurophysiology here are none other than the principle of lateral or surround inhibition and that of signal-to-noise ratio. These concepts have assumed outstanding importance in our current thinking on perceptual physiology and information theory, although in neurophysiology we now apply them at a microphysiological rather than at the macroscopic scale in which Berger envisaged them.

Berger believed that the potential differences which develop in the psycho-physical activity of the cortex during conscious states are short-lived. They soon become equalized. He assumed that the equalization process corresponds to the psychical event. Here he returned to his old speculations on psychical energy and its relationship to physical energy forms and put forward the tentative hypothesis that during such an equalization process, electrical energy may be tranformed into psychophysical energy. He assumed that the latter is soon reconverted into some form of physical energy which induces structural alterations in the fabric of the central nervous system. Thus through conscious experience and the temporary conversion of physical into psychical energy which is associated with it, the central nervous system is continuously being restructured and psychophysical processes are laid down in material form. In this way, each organism undergoes its own individual and irrevers-ible historical evolution. This notion that electrical activity in the brain could lead to structural changes in the nervous system and thus form a basis for learning, would even at the present time put Berger among the most avant-garde neurobiologists. It matters little that his ideas in this regard were based on almost pure speculation, for we are hardly that much further advanced in this field today.

In his 12th report, published in 1937, Berger modified his conceptual model of psychophysical activity. He felt compelled to alter his views in the light of the findings published by Dusser de Barenne and McCulloch who had shown that after thermo-coagulation of the three superficial cortical layers, rhythmic cerebral potentials still originated from the deeper cortical layers. Berger therefore no longer felt justified in localizing the alpha generating mechanism to the upper cortical layers. He still believed however that psychophysical function involved the three superficial cortical layers. He therefore concluded that the beta waves, which till then he had considered to be related to brain metabolism, were the concomitants of psychophysical activity. He was reinforced in this belief when he observed excessive amounts of rapid activity in the EEG of manic patients and in other states of mental excitation. Unfortunately the presumed increase in beta activity turned out to be 50 cycle artefact. Berger freely admitted his error and published a note to this effect, but he was convinced that new observations, which he made after he had detected his earlier mistake, were free of artefact and thus supported his new concept. However, in these later years, the extreme caution which he had exercised during his earlier studies had given way to some degree of overconfidence and many of the observations of this period are not fully valid. His new revised conceptual model of psychophysical cortical activity also lacks the freshness and originality of the earlier one.

In his studies on the human electroencephalogram, Berger repeatedly touched on basic neurophysiological and neuropharmacological problems. He also commented on the characteristics and on the importance of EEG changes in a variety of pathological states. However, he approached these questions exclusively from the point of view of his own personal interest in psychophysiology and it is evident that he was not primarily interested in the basic neurophysiology, neuropharmacology or in the clinical pathology of the electroencephalogram. Nevertheless he was the first to make many pertinent observations in these areas and to develop some theoretical concepts about the origin and the regulation of the EEG in normal and pathological states.

He regarded the alpha waves as the result of membrane potential oscillations of cortical nerve cells located beneath and between his two recording electrodes. Initially he was inclined to attribute the beta waves to structural elements other than nerve cells, such as the glia, the cerebral blood vessels or perhaps the neuropil. He believed that the alpha waves reflected the specific neural functions of the brain, whereas the beta waves only reflected fundamental metabolic and nutritional processes common to all tissues (Plate 7). Later, however, he modified this view and suggested that the alpha waves were generated by the large pyramidal cells of the deeper layers of the cortex and that most of the beta waves, especially the shorter ones, originated in the small superficial cortical neurons.

Berger was impressed by the synchronization of the electrical oscillations generated by the two cerebral hemispheres and conceived of the EEG as reflecting a uniform wave of activity sweeping in a sagittal direction over both hemispheres. He assumed that this cortical activity was regulated by a thalamic center, which also kept the activity of cortical neurons within certain bounds. When thalamic control lessened or was abolished, as for instance during sleep, barbiturate anesthesia, anoxia, insulin coma or generalized cerebral seizures, cortical activity became disinhibited, excessive and disorganized. The fine structuring of potential gradients necessary for conscious experience was no longer possible, hence the loss of consciousness common to these states.

Over the years, Berger recorded the EEG in a great variety of pathological states. He was the first to describe the presence of slow waves in the EEG associated with many kinds of cerebral lesions. He interpreted them as slow alpha waves and was unwilling to accept the term delta waves. He recognized that in vascular lesions, when the disease process had run its course and had become inactive, the electroencephalogram could revert to normal. He interpreted this as evidence that the electroencephalogram only reflected "generalized disturbances of function of the brain" ("allgemeine Betriebsstörungen").

Berger made many interesting observations on epilepsy. He demonstrated the profound depression of the electrical activity in post-ictal coma. To his great chagrin he never obtained a satisfactory recording of a generalized tonic-clonic convulsion. He did record, however, a number of minor seizures associated with loss of consciousness. Some of these probably were psychomotor attacks. They were associated with flattening of the electroencephalogram. He also made the observation that absence attacks were associated with high voltage 3/sec discharges in the EEG. His record, however, showed only large amplitude, regular 3/sec slow waves with no spike components. Berger waited several years before he published this observation, because he initially suspected that the high voltage oscillations were artefacts. Berger was also the first to describe high voltage, abrupt, potential oscillations in the inter-ictal EEGs of epileptic patients, the paroxysmal sharp waves of today's EEG terminology, and he interpreted them correctly as an indication of a predisposition to seizures.

His speculations about the mechanism of generalized seizures are interesting, since they reveal him as an early "centrencephalist". He postulated that generalized attacks originate from an area in the diencephalon which produces a sudden disconnection of the cortex from its thalamic control center. The consequence of this was intense generalized cortical disinhibition, which may lead to an epileptic attack. His concepts on this matter are however based only on very few empirical facts and his conclusions are far fetched and not very convincing.

His most valuable contribution to the electroencephalogram in epilepsy is his detailed description of an observation in a patient with general paresis and focal motor seizures which he published in his 7th report. This patient showed high voltage sharp waves which occurred in relation to localized jerks of the right hand and which Berger correctly localized to the left central region. He clearly demonstrated in beautiful records that the discharges in the electroencephalogram preceded the movements of the hand. The simultaneous recording of the EEG and of the hand movements by means of the pulse telephone which had been placed in the patient's palm is a particularly elegant proof of this relationship. Berger concluded that the electrical discharges in the left central region were responsible for the clonic jerks of the right hand. He was thus the first to prove the correctness of the Jacksonian hypothesis that clinical epileptic manifestations result from excessive discharge of grey matter in an area of the brain related to the function involved in the clinical seizure. It is of interest that Berger neither on this nor on any other occasion ever mentioned Hughlings Jackson's work. One wonders why he remained unfamiliar with Jackson's writings. In Jackson he would have found a kindred spirit with whom he could have shared his intense interest in the philosophical aspects of neurology and a common devotion to Herbert Spencer's philosophical ideas.

When Berger published his last paper on the human electroencephalogram, in 1938, the new approach to the study of brain function which he had inaugurated in 1929 had gathered momentum in many centers both in Europe and in the United States. Thanks to his pioneering work a new diagnostic method had been introduced into medicine. Physiology had acquired a new investigative tool. Clinical neurophysiology had been liberated from its exclusive dependence upon the functional anatomical approach and electrophysiological exploration of complex functions of the central nervous system in the neurophysiological laboratories had received a major impetus. The work of the lonely pioneer in Jena had finally received its well deserved recognition. Many of those who undertook the study of the electroencephalogram were able to bring a far greater technical knowledge of neurophysiology to bear upon the problems of the electrical activity of the brain than Berger had ever been able to do. Nevertheless to this day the community of neurological scientists has not ceased to look with respect and affection to the father of electroencephalography who, through his lonely struggle, often in tragic isolation and against overwhelming odds, initiated this new era of neurophysiology.

P. GLOOR

BIBLIOGRAPHY

ADRIAN, E. D. and MATTHEWS, B. H. C.: The Berger rhythm. Potential changes from the occipital lobes in man. *Brain*, **1934**, *57*: 355–385.

BERGER, H.: Degeneration der Vorderhornzellen des Rückenmarks bei Dementia paralytica. *Ziehens Mschr. Psychiat. Neurol.*, **1898**, *3*: 1–30.

BERGER, H.: Experimentell-anatomische Studien über die durch den Mangel optischer Reize veranlassten Entwicklungshemmungen im Occipitallappen des Hundes und der Katze. *Arch. Psychiat. Nervenkr.*, **1900**, *33*: 521–567.

BERGER, H.: *Zur Lehre von der Blutzirkulation in der Schädelhöhle des Menschen.* Gustav Fischer (Publ.), Jena, **1901**.

BERGER, H.: *Über die körperlichen Äusserungen psychischer Zustände. Weitere experimentelle Beiträge zur Lehre von der Blutzirkulation in der Schädelhöhle des Menschen.* Gustav Fischer (Publ.), Jena; *I. Teil* **1904**, *II. Teil* **1907**.

BERGER, H.: *Untersuchungen über die Temperatur des Gehirns.* Gustav Fischer (Publ.), Jena, **1910**.

BERGER, H.: *Psychophysiologie in 12 Vorlesungen.* Gustav Fischer (Publ.), Jena, **1921**.

BERGER, H.: *Über die Lokalisation im Grosshirn.* Jenaer akademische Reden. Heft 4. Gustav Fischer (Publ.), Jena, **1927**.

BERGER, H.: Über das Elektrenkephalogramm des Menschen. *Arch. Psychiat. Nervenkr.*, **1929**, *87*: 527–570.

BERGER, H.: Über das Elektrenkephalogramm des Menschen. Zweite Mitteilung. *J. Psychol. Neurol.*, **1930**, *40*: 160–179.

BERGER, H.: Über das Elektrenkephalogramm des Menschen. Dritte Mitteilung. *Arch. Psychiat. Nervenkr.*, **1931**, *94*: 16–60.

BERGER, H.: Über das Elektrenkephalogramm des Menschen. Vierte Mitteilung. *Arch. Psychiat. Nervenkr.*, **1932**, *97*: 6–26.

BERGER, H.: Über das Elektrenkephalogramm des Menschen. Fünfte Mitteilung. *Arch. Psychiat. Nervenkr.*, **1932**, *98*: 231–254.

BERGER, H.: Über das Elektrenkephalogramm des Menschen. Sechste Mitteilung. *Arch. Psychiat. Nervenkr.*, **1933**, *99*: 555–574.

BERGER, H.: Über das Elektrenkephalogramm des Menschen. Siebente Mitteilung. *Arch. Psychiat. Nervenkr.*, **1933**, *100*: 301–320.

BERGER, H.: Über das Elektrenkephalogramm des Menschen. Achte Mitteilung. *Arch. Psychiat. Nervenkr.*, **1934**, *101*: 452–469.

BERGER, H.: Über das Elektrenkephalogramm des Menschen. Neunte Mitteilung. *Arch. Psychiat. Nervenkr.*, **1934**, *102*: 538–557.

BERGER, H.: Über das Elektrenkephalogramm des Menschen. Zehnte Mitteilung. *Arch. Psychiat. Nervenkr.*, **1935**, *103*: 444–454.

BERGER, H.: Über das Elektrenkephalogramm des Menschen. Elfte Mitteilung. *Arch. Psychiat. Nervenkr.*, **1936**, *104*: 678–689.

BERGER, H.: Über das Elektrenkephalogramm des Menschen. Zwölfte Mitteilung. *Arch. Psychiat. Nervenkr.*, **1937**, *106*: 165–187.

BERGER, H.: Berichtigung. *Arch. Psychiat. Nervenkr.*, **1937**, *106*: 508.

BERGER, H.: Über das Elektrenkephalogramm des Menschen. Dreizehnte Mitteilung. *Arch. Psychiat. Nervenkr.*, **1937**, *106*: 577–584.

BERGER, H.: Das Elektrenkephalogramm des Menschen und seine psychophysiologische Deutung. *XIème Congr. Int. Psychol. Paris*, **1937**, *1*: 220–226.

BERGER, H.: Über das Elektrenkephalogramm des Menschen. Vierzehnte Mitteilung. *Arch. Psychiat. Nervenkr.*, **1938**, *108*: 407–431.

BERGER, H.: Das Elektrenkephalogramm des Menschen. *Acta Nova Leopoldina*, **1938**, *6*: 173–309.

BERGER, H.: *Psyche*. Gustav Fischer (Publ.), Jena, **1940**.

BOENING, H.: Professor Hans Berger — Jena. *Arch. Psychiat. Nervenkr.*, **1941**, *114*: 17–24.

FISCHGOLD, H.: *Hans Berger et son temps. Actualités Neurophysiologiques* (A. M. MONNIER, Ed.), 4th series. Masson et Cie., Paris, **1962**: 197–221.

FISCHGOLD, H.: Sources de l'électroencéphalographie. Chapter in "*Von Boerhaave bis Berger*" (K. E. ROTHSCHUH, Ed.). Gustav Fischer (Publ.), Stuttgart, **1964**: 225–242.

GINZBERG, R.: Three years with Hans Berger. A contribution to his biography. *J. Hist. Med. allied Sci.*, **1949**: 361–371.

JUNG, R.: Hans Berger und die Entdeckung des EEG nach seinen Tagebüchern und Protokollen. *Jenenser EEG Symposion* (R. WERNER, Ed.). VEB Verlag Volk und Gesundheit, Berlin, **1963**: 20–53.

KOLLE, K.: Hans Berger. 1873–1941. Chapter in "*Grosse Nervenärzte*". *21 Lebensbilder* (K. KOLLE, Ed.). Georg Thieme (Publ.), Stuttgart, **1956**, *1*: 1–6.

WERNER, R.: Hans Berger zum Gedächtnis. *Jenenser EEG Symposion* (R. WERNER, Ed.). VEB Verlag Volk und Gesundheit, Berlin, **1963**: 13–19.

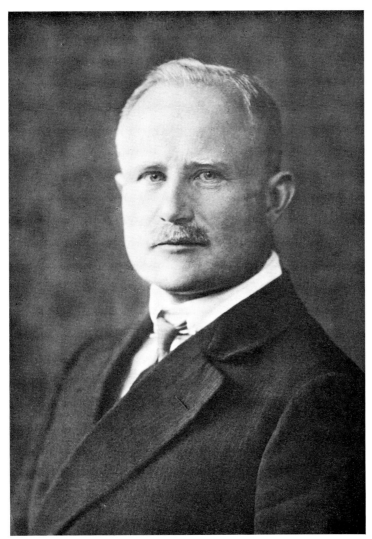

Plate 1

Hans Berger at the age of 52 (1925), one year after he began his work on the human electroencephalogram. (Courtesy of Mrs. Ursula Berger).

Plate 2

The first EEG recording apparatus used by Berger to record the string movements of the Edelmann string galvanometer. (Courtesy of Mrs. Ursula Berger). The numbers were added to the original photograph by Mr. W. Keuscher, who was Hans Berger's technician. In a letter Mr. Keuscher gave the following informations on this instrument: "This is a recording apparatus which stood in the 'Hufeldhaus'. The string galvanometer made by 'Edelmann', Munich stood in front of the recording apparatus. At the beginning we recorded muscle currents in patients with trepanations until, in the presence of Prof. Hilpert, small oscillations occurred in the resting string of the galvanometer, the hour of birth of the EEG ..."

"In the recording apparatus shown in the picture, *no film* was used, but a roll of silver bromide paper, 5 to 6 cm in width. These exposed curves ran into a metal box and were unrolled and developed in the dark room. Original records of this kind exist in the Archives of Prof. Jung ... The curve appeared on a dark background [see Figure 1 of first report, p. 42], in contrast to later records in which, because of the mirror, the curve appeared black on a light background..."

"*Number 1* is the crank driving the motor. *Number 2* indicates the markers made of fibers, I believe they were blades of straw cut to the desired size. *Number 3* was a switch. If I turned it to the right, the recording paper moved and ran into the metal box. *Number 4* was a graduated lens. Through it when it was opened the string of the galvanometer was projected upon the photographic paper. *Number 5* was the diaphragm and the marker for the individual curves from 1 to ?. *Number 6* was the famous box into which the exposed paper glided. There was a sliding bar fixed to the box which after the end of the experiment simultaneously cut off the record and closed the slit. *Number 7* was the time marker, a tuning fork with a period of 1/10 of a second which, however, was provided with a clock work and which when necessary had to be wound up."

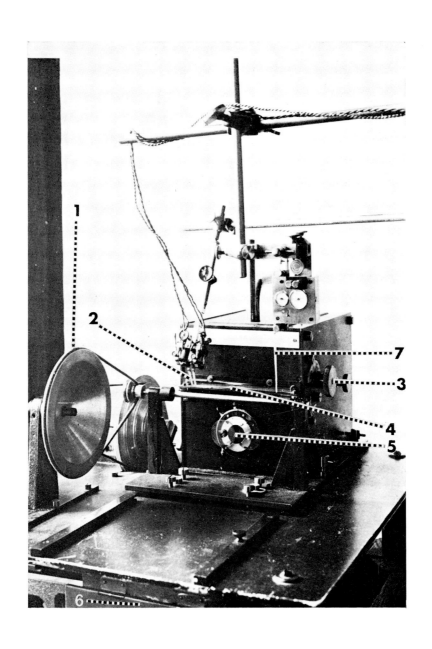

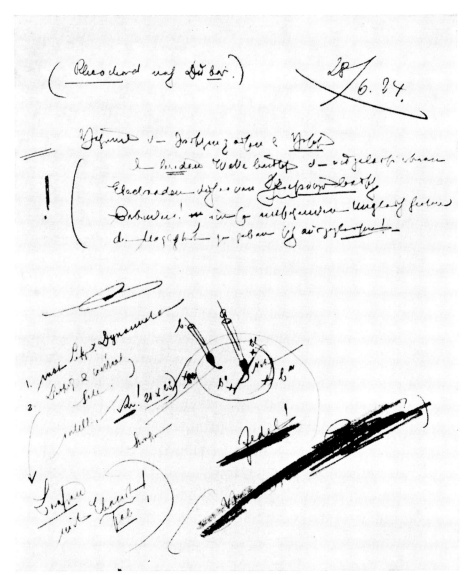

Plate 3

Berger's protocol of his experiment carried out on the 28th of June 1924 on his patient Zedel, in which current oscillations originating from the human brain were observed for the first time. The drawing outlines the area of the skull defect and the position of the non-polarizable clay electrodes. (From R. Jung, *Jenenser EEG Symposion*. V.E.B. Verlag Volk und Gesundheit, Berlin, 1963).

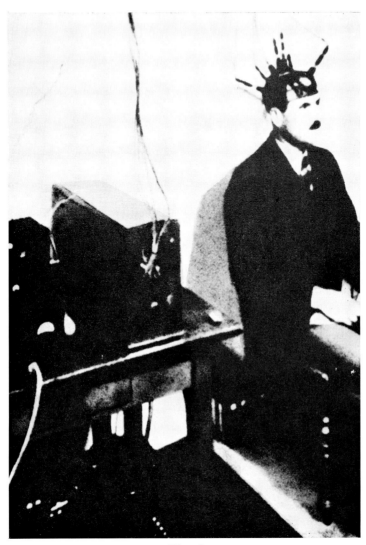

Plate 4

Photograph of one of the first attempts at recording the electroencephalogram in man. According to Mr. Keuscher this patient was investigated at the very beginning of Hans Berger's studies on the human EEG. The patient had a left-sided trepanation and the record was taken with silver electrodes (1 cm in diameter) which had been glued to the scalp with adhesive tape. This was apparently the only time that the record was taken while the patient was in a sitting position. No current oscillations could be demonstrated in this man. Later patients were always examined while they were lying on a couch. Unfortunately no photograph of such an EEG recording seems to exist. (Courtesy of Mrs. Ursula Berger).

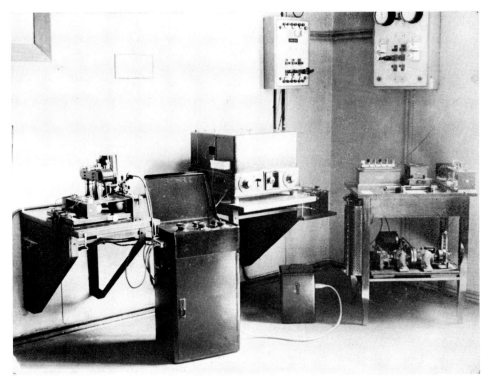

Plate 5

Hans Berger's EEG laboratory in the main building of the University Clinic of Jena with the equipment used between 1926 and 1931. The double coil galvanometer stands on the left side. On its right is the recording apparatus with the camera. On the extreme right is the equipment for the resistance measurements. The subject lay on a couch on the left side of the coil galvano-meter. (From R. Werner, *Jenenser EEG Symposion*. V.E.B. Verlag Volk und Gesundheit, Berlin, 1963).

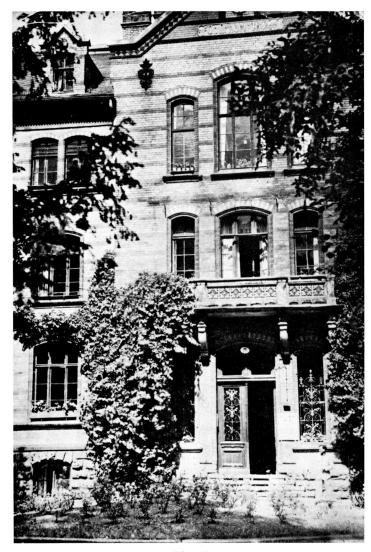

Plate 6
Main entrance of the Psychiatric University Clinic in Jena as it appeared in Hans Berger's days. The window on the first floor on the left side is that of the antechamber of the Director's office in which Hans Berger carried out his EEG recordings and which housed the instruments shown in plate 5. (Courtesy of Mrs. Ursula Berger).

Plate 7

Sketch made by Hans Berger in his protocol book in which he outlined his conception of the processes giving rise to alpha and beta waves and to their disturbances in various pathological states. The text, partially stenographic, in Hans Berger's own handwriting reads as follows:

"Thoughts, 21.9.31. In the cortex always two processes present!

1. $\psi\varphi$ [psychophysical]. α process. Nutrition! β process. These are the organic conflagrations of Mosso. Normal!

2. Unconsciousness. Processes α. β.

3. Preparation for epileptic seizure. State of impending attack! α. β.

4. Epileptic seizure. α. β. Intracerebral temperature rise, 0.6° Mosso, i.p. [personal observation?] 0.36° in man. According to Mosso not always the case however".

(From R. Jung, *Jenenser EEG Symposion*. V.E.B. Verlag Volk und Gesundheit, Berlin, 1963).

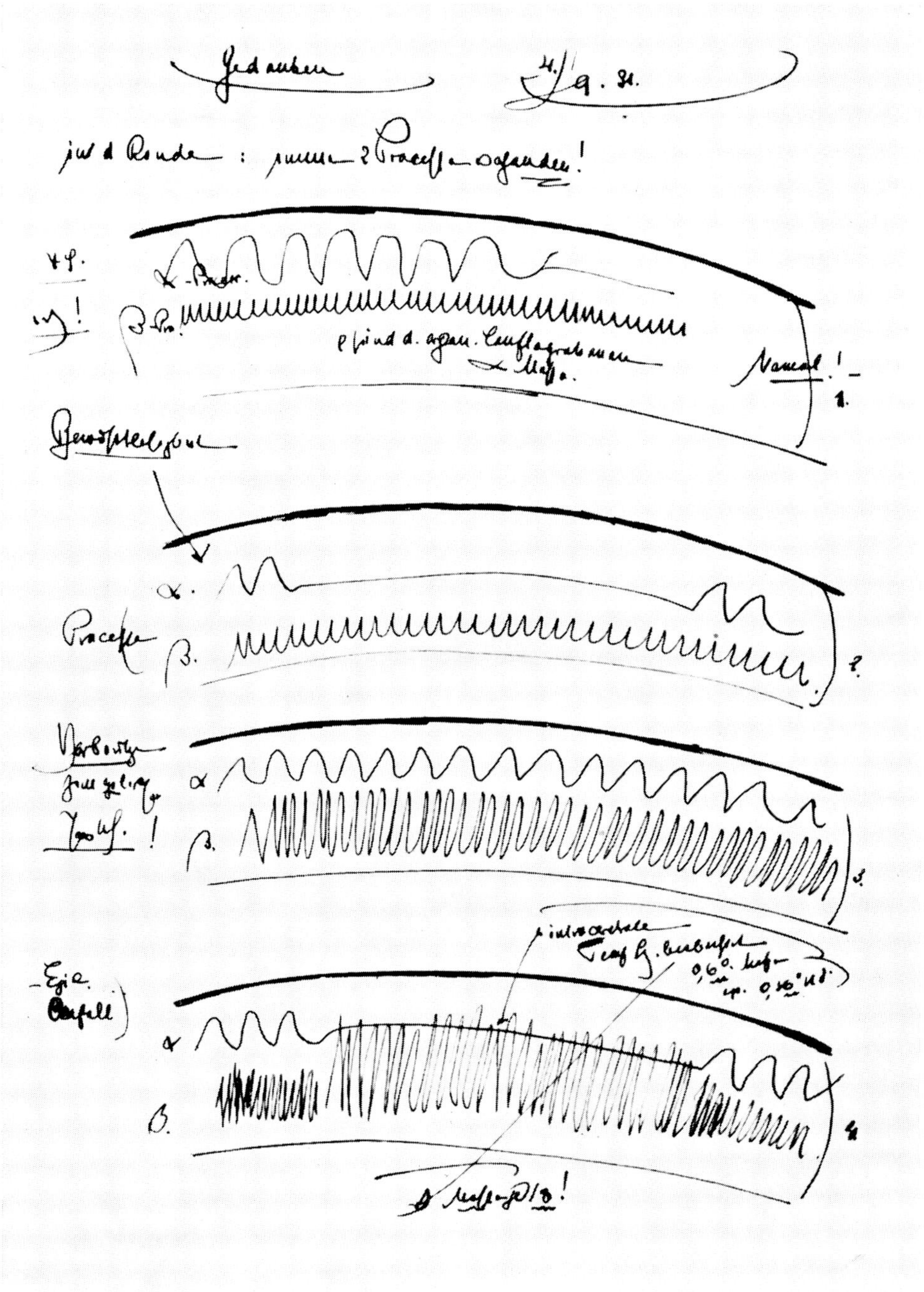

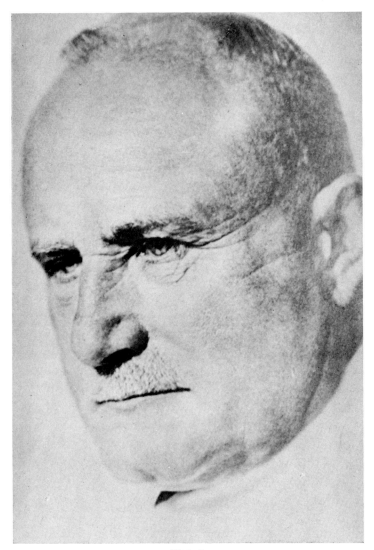

Plate 8
Hans Berger at the age of 63 (1936), two years before his retirement. (Courtesy of Mrs. Ursula Berger).

I

On the Electroencephalogram of Man

by Professor Hans Berger, Jena

(With 17 figures)

(Received April 22, 1929)

[Published in *Archiv für Psychiatrie und Nervenkrankheiten*, **1929**, *87*: 527–570]

As *Garten*[1], who in all likelihood can be regarded as one of the greatest experts in electrophysiology, has rightly emphasized, one cannot be far from the truth if one ascribes to each living plant or animal cell the ability to produce electrical currents. Such currents are called bioelectric currents, because they accompany the normal manifestations of life of the cell. They are, I presume, to be distinguished from currents artificially produced by injuries which were designated under the terms of demarcation currents, alteration currents or injury currents[T2]. It was to be expected as a matter of course that bioelectrical phenomena should be demonstrable also within the central nervous system, since it represents such an enormous cell aggregate and in fact this demonstration was made relatively early.

Caton[2] as early as 1874 published experiments on rabbit and monkey brains, in which non-polarizable electrodes were either applied to the surface of both hemispheres, or in which one electrode was placed on the cerebral cortex and the other on the surface of the skull. The currents were recorded with a sensitive galvanometer. Distinct current oscillations were found which became accentuated especially upon arousal from sleep and when death was imminent, but after death decreased and later completely disappeared. *Caton* already was able to demonstrate that strong current oscillations occurred in the cerebral cortex when the eye was exposed to light and he surmised that perhaps these cortical currents could be used for the purpose of localization within the cerebral cortex.

In 1883 *Fleischl von Marxow*[3], using non-polarizable electrodes and a sensitive galvanometer, first observed that in various animals, when records were taken from two symmetrically placed points on the surface of the cerebral hemispheres, only slight or no deflections at all occurred at first, but that with peripheral stimuli, *e.g.*

---

[1] *Garten*: Die Produktion von Elektrizität. *Wintersteins* Handbuch der vergleichenden Physiologie, Volume 3, 2nd half, p. 105[T1].

[2] *Caton*: Brit. med. J., **2**, 278 (1875); abstract in Zbl. Physiol., **4**, No. 25 (1890). According to *Bechterew*: Die Energie des lebenden Organimus, p. 102. Wiesbaden, 1902.

[3] *Fleischl von Marxow*: Gesammelte Abhandlungen, p. 410. Leipzig: J. A. Barth, 1893; and Zbl. Physiol., **4** (1890).

by exposing the eyes to light, one could obtain clear-cut deflections when the electrodes were located in the region of *Munk's* visual centers. Chloroform administration abolishes the occurrence of deflections on the galvanometer in response to peripheral stimulation. If one allows the animal to wake up from the narcosis, current oscillations in response to peripheral stimulation reappear in the cerebral cortex. He succeeded in recording these currents not only from the exposed cerebral cortex, but also from the dura mater and even from the calvarium divested of its periosteal covering. He stressed that one has to exercise great care to prevent cooling of the cerebral cortex and adds: "It may even become possible, by taking records from the scalp, to perceive the currents generated in our own brain by various mental acts".

A. *Beck*[1] also worked on the cerebral cortex of the dog, using non-polarizable clay electrodes and *Hermann's* galvanometer. He made the important observation that a current of variable strength is present *at all times*, when any two points on the cortical surface are interconnected. The oscillations of this current do not coincide in time with respiration or the movements of the pulse and are also independent of movements of the animal. This current disappears during narcosis. Upon stimulation of peripheral sense organs, *e.g.* of the eye by magnesium light, a strong current oscillation occurs in the contralateral occipital lobe, thus making it possible to define the dog's visual area by means of these potential oscillations.

In 1892 *Beck* and *Cybulski*[2] published additional studies carried out in monkeys and dogs. Using a sensitive galvanometer, they again found that when two points of the cerebral cortex were connected, a current of varying strength was present all the time. A relationship of its oscillations with pulse and respiration could not be demonstrated. They took great pains to show in particular that the currents originate in the cortex itself and are not conducted from elsewhere. Thus, *e.g.*, passing strong currents through the scalp, while the cerebral electrodes remained applied, did not elicit any movement of the galvanometer needle. Upon local stimulation of the cerebral cortex a local alteration of the cortical currents took place. Upon stimulation of the forelimb a current oscillation was induced in the area of the cruciate sulcus; upon illumination of the eye a similar change occurred in the occipital lobe. These electrical changes in the cerebral cortex were easiest to elicit in monkeys and were all the more pronounced, the closer the stimulus resembled those stimuli that usually affect the animal under normal conditions. Thus, *e.g.* a slight touch of the hand influences the galvanometer more strongly than pinching of the skin. The authors believe that these electrical phenomena in the cerebral cortex correspond to the simple mental states[T3].

Gotch and *Horsley*[3] performed experiments on cats, rabbits and monkeys. They used non-polarizable clay electrodes and *Lippmann's* capillary electrometer. They interconnected various parts of the cerebral cortex. At rest currents were almost

---

[1] *Beck, A.*: Die Bestimmung der Lokalisation der Hirn- und Rückenmarksfunktionen vermittels der elektrischen Erscheinungen. Zbl. Physiol., **1890**, No. 16.

[2] *Beck* and *Cybulski*: Weitere Untersuchungen über die elektrischen Erscheinungen der Hirnrinde der Affen und der Hunde. Zbl. Physiol., **6**, 1 (1892).

[3] *Gotch* and *Horsley*: Zbl. Physiol., **1889**; J. Physiol., **1890**.

totally absent, but upon each peripheral stimulation a current oscillation took place.

Danilevsky[1,T4] in 1891 observed current oscillations in the cerebral cortex of dogs in response to peripheral stimulation.

Upon *Bechterev*'s suggestion *Larionov*[2] in 1899 and *Trivus*[3] in 1900 used the current oscillations originating in the cerebral cortex to localize the auditory and visual areas of the dog, without being able to make any significantly new observations in the course of these studies.

Tcheriev[4] carried out similar studies in 1904. He became convinced that these currents were in all probability dependent upon the movement of the blood in the cerebral vessels and that they were therefore not caused by the state of activity of the central nervous system.

In 1912 *Kaufmann*[5] experimented on 24 dogs and took records with non-polarizable electrodes and a *Wiedemann* galvanometer. He was able to demonstrate unequivocally the physiological origin of the electrical phenomena and to refute *Tcheriev's* view. He succeeded in recording these currents also from the surface of the skull bone. He likewise saw *at all times* spontaneous oscillations of the cortical current and succeeded in demonstrating changes occurring upon peripheral, *e.g.* visual stimulation.

Pravdich-Neminsky[6] in 1913 recorded the cortical currents in the dog for the first time with the string galvanometer and observed the influence of peripheral stimuli which, however, were at first limited to electrical stimulation of the sciatic nerve.

In 1919 *Cybulski*[7] in collaboration with a coworker also studied the action currents of the cerebrum in dogs and monkeys by means of the string galvanometer. They could only confirm *Beck's* and *Cybulski's* earlier observations.

Finally, in 1925 *Pravdich-Neminsky*[8] published a larger study in Pflügers Archiv. He points out that such continuous phenomena as the spontaneous oscillations of the cerebral cortical currents had not been observed by all investigators, but only by *Beck*, *Danilevsky* and *Kaufmann*. His own investigations were carried out in dogs. Records were taken with non-polarizable clay electrodes and the large *Edelmann* string galvanometer. In addition to the "electrocerebrogram", the cerebral pulsations and the blood pressure were also recorded. *Neminsky* also became convinced that *Tcheriev* was incorrect in asserting that a simple physical relationship exists between the electrical phenomena in the brain and the friction of the blood

[1] *Danilewski*: Zbl. Physiol., **5**, No. 1 (1891).

[2] *Larionow*: Über die corticalen Hörzentren. Schriften der Klinik für Nerven- und Geisteskrankheiten, St. Petersburg, 1899.

[3] *Triwus*: Die negativen Stromschwankungen in der Hemisphärenrinde des Gehirns. Thesis, St. Petersburg, 1900.

[4] *Tschirjew*: J. Physiol. et Path. gen., **4**, 671 (1904); Arch. Anat. u. Physiol., **1913**, Physiol. Abt., p. 414, especially p. 442 and 447.

[5] *Kaufmann*: Elektrische Erscheinungen in der Grosshirnrinde. Rev. Psych. Neur. u. exper. Psychol. (Russian), **17**, 403 (513) (1912). Abstract Z. Neur., **6**, 1130 (1913).

[6] *Prawdicz-Neminski*: Elektrische Gehirnerscheinungen. Zbl. Physiol., **1913**, No. 18, 915.

[7] *Cybulski*: Zbl. Physiol., **1919**, 406.

[8] *Prawdicz-Neminski*: Zur Kenntnis der elektrischen und der Innervationsvorgänge in den funktionellen Elementen und Geweben des tierischen Organismus. Elektrocerebrogramm der Säugetiere. Pflügers Arch., **209**, 362 (1925).

on the walls of the cerebral vessels, etc. In the electrocerebrogram recorded with the *Edelmann* string galvanometer, he was able to distinguish waves of first and second order. Of those of the first order there were 10–15 in one second, of those of the second order, there were 20–32 in one second. *Neminsky* was also successful in recording such oscillations from the dura, as well as from the bone of the skull, just as from the cortex itself.

Most of the authors cited here considered these "cortical currents" as the expression of the activity of the cerebral cortex of the animal, because they increase with functional involvement of the cortical centers and disappear during narcosis or at death. It is useful to distinguish between the *current present at all times*, which can be recorded from the cerebral cortex, and its *alterations under the influence of peripheral stimuli*. The latter current oscillations are particularly sensitive and disappear easily upon cooling of the cortex and for otherwise not wholly explainable reasons. Whether the interpretations given by the authors are in fact correct, is still by no means established. *Garten*[1] expressed the opinion that the electrical phenomena in the central nervous system, in accordance with the complicated structure of the latter, may be explained in a variety of ways. According to him, if an action current is observed, the first question that arises is whether this action current originates from the myelinated nerve fibers, or whether it is caused by excitation of many unmyelinated fibers of the grey matter, or by excitatory processes of the ganglion cells in the cortex or in deep-lying nuclei. *Garten* adds: "The conditions will become especially complicated in studies on the *cerebral cortex*, because there we have to expect simultaneously action currents of very different systems which at times may be active and at other times may be at rest".

I myself worked in 1902 with *Lippmann's* capillary electrometer. Using boot-shaped clay electrodes[T5] and *Fleischl von Marxow's* procedure, I attempted to record currents from symmetrical locations in the two cerebral hemispheres of the dog. In five experiments, in one cat and four dogs, it was possible to carry out the experiment as designed without technical flaws, but several other experiments failed. In these five experiments oscillations of the electrometer, which did not depend upon external stimuli, were found when the electrodes rested on the brain surface of the unanesthetized animal. Once they were also recorded from two points on the dura which still covered the two cerebral hemispheres. On the other hand, in contrast to *Fleischl von Marxow's* observations, it was possible in only one of these five experiments to demonstrate the occurrence of current oscillations upon stimulation of peripheral sense organs; upon stroking the dog's forepaw a very pronounced current oscillation occurred each time on repeated occasions. Because at that time I was particularly interested in the effect exerted by peripheral stimuli upon these currents recorded from the cerebral cortex, I abandoned the experiments.

Subsequently, in 1907 I performed once again an experiment on a dog, with the capillary electrometer, without, however, being able to observe the hoped for current oscillations upon stimulation of peripheral sense organs.

---

[1] See footnote 1 on p. 37.

Then, in 1910 I tried with the small *Edelmann* string galvanometer to obtain currents from symmetrical points of the cortex, using non-polarizable boot-shaped clay electrodes. Even though at rest, *i.e.*, without the influence of external stimuli, one saw at all times exceedingly small oscillations of the string, larger deflections again failed to occur in any of the dogs investigated, either upon touching the paw, or upon illuminating the eye, or even under the influence of strong auditory stimuli, although the animals were not anesthetized.

Then last year, at a time when my observations on man, which I shall report below, were already available, I again performed three experiments on dogs[1]. In these I used the large *Edelmann* string galvanometer and the double-coil galvano-meter of Siemens and Halske, the latter with particularly sensitive inserts[T6]. The dogs used in these experiments had received 1.5 grams[T7] of Veronal by mouth about five hours before the experiment; then in addition, one hour before the beginning of the preparatory operation, they received 0.03–0.05 grams of morphine subcutane-ously. In accordance with *Einthoven's* suggestion for the recording of the electro-cardiogram in the animal, and in order to avoid cooling of the cerebral cortex, I sub-stituted freshly amalgamated tiny zinc plates for the non-polarizable clay electrodes which I had used before. The zinc plates were introduced into the subdural space through a slit in the dura. They measured 12 mm in length and 4 mm in width; their four corners were rounded off to avoid injuries; to them was soldered the well in-sulated connecting wire; they had a surface area of 25 sq.mm. After they had been inserted through the slit in the dura, through which they were just able to pass, they were advanced into the subdural space far enough to come to rest in the laterally sloping region of the skull. Thus their surfaces were firmly applied to the pia-arachnoid covered cortex and they were pressed against the dura and the bone by the pulsating brain. The trephine opening, which was kept as small as possible, was enlarged with a *Lüer's* rongeur only to the extent necessary to permit easy introduction of the tiny zinc plates, and was then completely filled with the wax customarily used in brain operations in man. The well insulated wire was led through this mass of wax. The wire itself was surrounded by wax, and the skin was then closed with a few sutures over the trephine opening. Thus, the brain was in no way exposed to drying or cooling.

In accord with the above findings quoted from the literature it was found that when these electrodes were applied over two areas of the same hemisphere, or also when they rest upon the right and left hemisphere, a current exhibiting considerable oscillations is present at all times.

Figure 1[2] shows a record of the continuous cerebral current oscillations[T9], which were recorded from the right and the left hemisphere of an approximately four year old female dog by means of the tiny amalgamated zinc plates and the large *Edelmann* string galvanometer. The legend of the figure gives additional details con-

---

[1] In all investigations carried out since 1924 to be reported here, Privatdozent Dr. med. *Hilpert* always helped me by word and deed, for which here too I express to him my most sincere thanks.

[2] All figures are reproductions of original records at a *reduced* size.

cerning the type of recording, the resistance and other similar items. One recognizes in Figure 1 larger oscillations of longer duration and smaller ones of shorter duration.

Using exactly the same arrangement, the current oscillations that can be picked up from the cortex of the two hemispheres were recorded with the coil galvanometer of Siemens and Halske which for my purposes is much more sensitive. Figure 2 shows

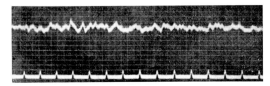

Fig. 1. Four year old female dog; amalgamated tiny zinc plate electrodes in the subdural space, right and left. Large *Edelmann* string galvanometer. Platinum string of 10,800 Ohm. Condenser inserted in the circuit[T8]. Resistance in the electrode circuit = 360 Ohm, 10 mm = 0.001 Volt. At the top: curve recorded from the brain; at the bottom: time in 1/5ths sec.

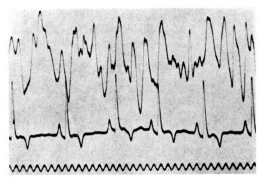

Fig. 2. The same female dog as in Figure 1 and the same cerebral recording. Siemens and Halske double-coil galvanometer. At the top: the curve recorded from the cerebrum; below: the electrocardiogram, recorded with amalgamated small zinc rods, inserted under the skin; at the bottom: time in 1/10ths sec. Condenser inserted into the circuit.

a small segment of a long curve recorded in this fashion from the same female dog. Having two galvanometers made it possible also to record the electrocardiogram simultaneously. In the figure the latter is written in the middle, whereas the curve of the cerebral oscillations appears at the top. In contrast to the record taken with the string galvanometer, the time signals here indicate tenths of a second. In accordance with *Einthoven's*[1] proposal, the electrocardiogram was recorded with freshly amalgamated small zinc rods which were inserted under the skin of the thorax. It is quite evident that the oscillations recorded from the surface of the two hemispheres do not coincide with those of the electrocardiogram. Thus, it is hardly possible that the cerebral record represents a distorted electrocardiogram, a question to which later in a different context we shall have to return once again.

---

[1] *Einthoven*: Die Aktionsströme des Herzens. Handbuch der normalen und pathologischen Physiologie, Vol. 8, 2nd half, p. 790, 1928.

The deflections of the current oscillations recorded from the brain surface are very much larger when they are derived from the two hemispheres than when one records from two points in the same hemisphere, *e.g.* from the area of the cruciate sulcus in front and from the occipital lobe posteriorly. A bilateral ligation of the common carotid arteries had no influence upon the amplitude of the deflections of the electrical curves recorded from the brain. Certainly, the blood flow in the brain of the dog is thereby, as we know, by no means interrupted, even though the blood supply is at first probably somewhat reduced in its amount. Also, total exsanguination through the opened and incannulated femoral artery in another dog led to no decrease, but to a transient increase in the amplitude of the deflections of the continuous current oscillations recorded from the surface of the cerebral cortex. As shown by *Mosso*[1], it is possible to arouse dogs by an injection of 0.01–0.02 grams of cocaine hydrochloride, even from deep chloral-induced sleep. In one dog, put to sleep by the above described combination of Veronal and morphine, a considerable increase of the current oscillations recorded from the brain surface was obtained by intravenous injection of a large dose of cocaine hydrochloride given into the jugular vein. However, the amplitude of the deflections of the electrocardiogram also increased simultaneously.

I was of the opinion that the procedure which I had devised prevented drying and cooling of the cerebral cortex, but on the other hand I also believed that, owing to the continuous cerebral movements, the fairly large electrodes were certainly not resting uniformly and always under the same pressure on the surface of the cerebral cortex. Since this might give rise to some experimental artefacts[T10], I decided to convince myself in some other way that the oscillations of the curves recorded from the surface of the cerebral cortex were not merely caused by the movements of the brain. It was because of these considerations that I had ligated the carotid arteries, but, as mentioned before, I did not, of course, thereby entirely abolish the circulation within the skull, nor the movements of the brain. Therefore this experiment does not disprove at all that the oscillations of the cerebral curve are caused by the movements of the brain. Furthermore, one may take exception to the experiment involving exsanguination through the femoral artery on the ground that a total exsanguination does not occur and that a certain amount of blood is retained for a fairly long time, precisely to maintain the cerebral circulation. Furthermore, the ensuing cerebral anemia by changing the brain volume and thereby altering the contact areas between the electrodes and brain surface could distort the cerebral record *in such a manner* that it would be impossible to draw reliable conclusions from it. The records which I showed above in Figures 1 and 2 undoubtedly exhibit some distortions of the cerebral current oscillations. This is because the cerebral circulation, which is also greatly influenced by the respiration through the intermediary of the veins, causes the subdurally placed tiny zinc plates to rest on the brain surface at one moment more firmly and at the next less so. This is of course associated with changes in resistance and with changes in the height of the deflections of the current oscillations

---

[1] *Meyer* and *Gottlieb*: Die experimentelle Pharmakologie, p. 28, Berlin, 1920.

which are thereby induced. Although sufficiently incontrovertible observations by other authors already existed, I was nevertheless time and again haunted by the worry that the continuous oscillations, which can be recorded from the brain surface, could perhaps be caused merely by the movements of the brain after all?[T11] I therefore made a transection of the upper cervical cord in the four year old female dog whose curves were shown above in Figures 1 and 2, after first having given an intravenous injection of 0.05 grams of muscarine into the femoral vein. The respiration stopped and shortly thereafter the heart was beating also only between long pauses.

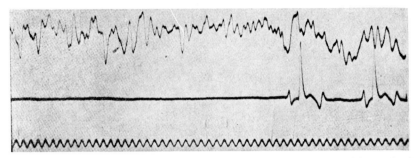

Fig. 3. The same female dog as in Figures 1 and 2 with exactly the same recording conditions as in Figure 2. At the top: the curve recorded from the cerebrum; in the middle: the electrocardiogram; at the bottom: the time in 1/10ths sec.

Figure 3 shows a segment of the record thus obtained. In the middle there is again the electrocardiogram, recorded in the manner indicated above. At the beginning of the strip of record shown here, the heart had already stopped for a fairly long time. Again after a fairly long time two heartbeats occur. These are separated by a brief pause which nevertheless is longer than the normal one; then a prolonged cardiac arrest again sets in. It is evident from the curve that the current oscillations, written at the top and recorded from the two hemispheres of this female dog, continue during the cardiac arrest. They have undergone some changes insofar as they have now become much more regular and also of lesser amplitude. The respiration stops completely and thus its influence upon the cerebral circulation mediated by the venous system is also eliminated. One notices during the two heart beats that the cerebral record at once becomes again more irregular, as in Figure 2. Thus, in spite of the total failure of circulation and respiration and in spite of the fact that the cerebral movements caused by the blood vessels are thereby eliminated, the oscillations of the cerebral record persist. This indicates, as other authors had also emphasized, that the cerebral current oscillations cannot be merely the mechanical consequence of the movements of the brain and more generally of the cerebral circulation. The form of the cerebral record obtained in Figure 3 is in all likelihood the more accurate one, whereas the curves in Figures 1 and 2 are distorted by just those cerebral movements to which the filling of the arteries and the veins, and thus the respiration, contribute. As was pointed out, the contact area between brain surface and electrodes is altered by the movements of the brain. It is true that the oscillations of the cerebral record are not produced by these, but they are distorted by them. In my opinion one can, *e.g.* in Figure 2, scarcely fail to recognize the similarity existing between the oscillations of the curve recorded from the surface of the cerebral cortex and a venous pressure curve. Later we must return to this question again. In any case, the experiment illustrated in Figure 3 proves that even after the arrest of respiration and the elimination of the cerebral circulation, it is possible to record from the surface of the brain regular current oscillation which therefore can neither be caused merely by movements of the brain, nor by the friction of the blood in cerebral vessels. This, therefore, confirms the opinion of the above mentioned authors. Because a condenser was inserted in the circuit[T8] in all cerebral recordings which I made with the string galvanometer and with the double-coil galvanometer, only the rapidly alternating current oscillations appeared in the records. In general these briefer oscillations exhibit two different lengths. One can distinguish between waves of somewhat larger amplitude and greater duration, with an average of 90–100 σ and those of shorter duration and smaller amplitude of 40–50 σ. Therefore these findings also essentially agree with *Pravdich-Neminsky's* reports, who distinguishes between waves of the first order, of which there are 11–15 in one second, and shorter waves, of the second order, of which there are 20–32 in one second. According to my observations, the amplitudes of the current oscillations recorded from the brain surface in the dog reach an average magnitude of 0.0002–0.0006 V for the longer 90–100 σ duration waves, and one of 0.00013 V for the largest of the briefer and essentially smaller second order waves with a duration of only 40–50 σ.

I have not carried out experiments on the influence of peripheral stimuli again, because what mattered to me now was the investigation of the current oscillations present *at all times* that can be recorded from the surface of the cerebral cortex. I need hardly point out that by post-mortem examination of the dogs it was verified that the tiny electrode plates inserted into the subdural space really were placed as intended, and that no alterations visible to the naked eye were produced in the subdural space or on the surface of the arachnoid and pia. In particular, not the slightest hemorrhage could be demonstrated. It goes without saying that the table upon which the dog was lying during each galvanometer recording was insulated from the surroundings by glass legs.

There exist no investigations on electrical events in the brain of *man*, neither do I know of any publication of records which would correspond to those to be reported here. After several fruitless attempts, I was able on July 6, 1924 to make the first pertinent observations in a young man aged 17. This young man had undergone a palliative trepanation over the left cerebral hemisphere performed by *Guleke* because of a suspected brain tumor. Because the signs of increased intracranial pressure after an initial remission recurred, the original trephine opening was enlarged posteriorly, whereupon the signs of increased intracranial pressure receded. About one year after the second operation I attempted to demonstrate currents in the area of the trephine opening, where the bone was missing, by using non-polarizable boot-shaped clay electrodes and the small *Edelmann* string galvanometer. The experiments were initially unsuccessful, and only when the two clay electrodes were placed 4 cm apart in the vicinity of a scar running vertically from above downwards through the middle of the enlarged trephine opening, was it possible with large magnifications[T12] to obtain continuous oscillations of the galvanometer string. This could be achieved either by inserting a platinum thread with a resistance of 5200 Ohms or a quartz thread with a resistance of 3200 Ohms. No oscillations could be demonstrated with the clay electrodes in the region of the trephine opening away from the very firm scar. This was the first result which intimated that probably in man, as in rabbits, dogs and monkeys, continuous electrical currents can be recorded from the surface of the intact cerebral cortex. [See Plate 3.]

Since I had at my disposal only the small *Edelmann* string galvanometer and it was only possible therefore to observe, but not to record, the very small movements of the string, I decided to obtain first of all a large *Edelmann* string galvanometer. Fortunately, after some time, I was successful with this also. But the very first attempt to use it was again unsuccessful. On March 20, 1925, using non-polarizable brush electrodes, I could not obtain current oscillations of any kind from the surface of a fairly markedly protruding cerebral herniation in a young woman aged 20 in whom a large palliative trepanation had been performed in the region of the right frontal and parietal lobes. It is true that the resistance was enormously high; according to the measurements made with the *Edelmann* instruments, it amounted to 44,000 Ohms in the electrode circuit.

Later I succeeded in obtaining a double-coil galvanometer which was brought on the market by Siemens and Halske, and which proved to be of great value for my investigations. I am certainly not sufficiently trained in physics to give an expert opinion on the merits and disadvantages of a Siemens coil galvanometer, but I refer to *Schrumpf's* and *Zöllich's*[1] work which is concerned with the usefulness of the string and coil galvanometers for the recording of cardiac currents. From this work, it seems to me, one can conclude that the coil galvanometer is more sensitive than the string galvanometer and thus quite definitely deserves preference for many physiological investigations. When comparing Figures 1 and 2 above, the different magnitudes of the deflections of the current oscillations which, under otherwise identical conditions, can be picked up from the cortical surface of the dog, are immediately evident. If in the large *Edelmann* string galvanometer the string tension is calibrated at a value of 10 mm = 0.001 V, as is customary for the recording of cardiac currents, the insert[T6] which I used in galvanometer 1 for the recording of cerebral records is, by comparison, several times more sensitive and its deflections are about $7\frac{1}{2}$ times as large as those obtained with the string galvanometer at the indicated string tension. One disadvantage of the coil galvanometer is that with the model put on the market by Siemens and Halske it is impossible to measure simultaneously the resistance in the electrode circuit. However, if, as in my case, one has available an *Edelmann* system at the same time, this resistance measurement can be carried out with ease. [See Plate 5.]

In the investigations in man, to be described next, I used, instead of non-polarizable electrodes, needle electrodes, which were zinc plated according to

---

[1] *Schrumpf* and *Zöllich*: Saiten- und Spulengalvanometer zur Aufzeichnung der Herzströme. Pflügers Arch., **170** (1918).

Trendelenburg's[1] proposal and, except for their tips, were insulated from their surroundings by a coat of varnish. Needle electrodes have also often been used by others for the recording of action currents, thus, *e.g.* by *Straub*, for the recording of cardiac currents, by others for the recording of muscle action currents, etc. Several descriptions of needle electrodes have been made. *Straub* inserted ordinary sewing needles to which copper wires had been soldered, at a flat angle under the skin. *Mann* and *Schleier*[2] used nickel silver electrodes. I have used zinc plated steel needles. According to *Gildemeister's*[3] and *Paul Hoffmann's*[4] explanations, the use of non-polarizable electrodes for the recording of currents from the human body is not required at all in circumstances in which one is concerned with the recording of current oscillations with a rapid time course. These needle electrodes, which of course are by no means completely non-polarizable, have in addition the great advantage of bypassing the skin. The latter, according to the studies carried out by *Einthoven*, and especially by *Gildemeister*, creates very complicated electrical conditions, which are not easily comprehended. These zinc plated electrodes were inserted through the skin into the subcutaneous tissue and whenever a bone defect was present they lay between the dura and the skin, *i.e.* epidurally[5]. It is known from the animal experiments reported in detail above, that one can also record the so-called "cortical currents" from the dura and from the bone shorn of its periosteum. The puncture sites located in the vicinity of the existing bone defects were treated with iodine. The zinc plated needle electrodes, insulated except for their tips, were sterilized by keeping them for several hours in a 10% formalin solution and then transferred into a sterilized physiological saline solution to wash off the last remnants of formalin which would irritate the tissue. Under careful observation of all the rules of asepsis, the needles, just like a hypodermic needle, were inserted in the region of a skin fold elevated from its base and were pushed in, parallel to the skin surface, until the tip was placed securely in the subcutaneous tissue, *i.e.* in the epidural space. The very fine needles could cause no injury with this method of insertion. The double-coil galvanometer was used predominantly for the recording of the current oscillations obtained in this manner from the epidural space with the needle electrodes, firstly because of the larger deflections and the better monitoring of the curves which could always be seen, even during the recording, and secondly, because of the advantage of having these curves written in black on white.

In a 40 year old man in whom 5 months earlier a large gliosarcoma had been removed by *Guleke*, a marked protrusion had again formed in the operative area where the bone had been completely removed. At the same time general signs of increased intracranial pressure had developed again. In this man a record was taken

---

[1] *Trendelenburg, W.*: Zur Methodik der Untersuchung von Aktionsströmen. Z. Biol., **74**, 113 (1922).

[2] *Mann* and *Schleier*: Z. Neur., **91**, 551 (1924).

[3] *Gildemeister*: Passive elektrische Erscheinungen im Tier- und Pflanzenreich. Handbuch der normalen und pathologischen Physiologie, Vol. 8, 2nd half, p. 657.

[4] *Hoffmann, Paul*: Ruhe- und Aktionsströme von Muskeln und Nerven. Handbuch der normalen und pathologischen Physiologie, Vol. 8, 2nd half, p. 703.

[5] In many early postoperative cases there probably remained some remnants of periosteum, which were left behind at the palliative trepanation.

from two points within the bone defect located over the left hemisphere. A double-coil galvanometer and the above mentioned zinc plated electrodes were used; these were inserted subcutaneously and lay 4.5 cm apart. The man lay comfortably on his back on a couch which was insulated from the surroundings by glass legs. He remained completely still during the recording. A curve was recorded of which Figure 4 repre-

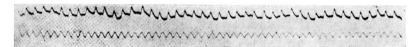

Fig. 4. 40 year old man. Large left-sided bone defect extending from the forehead to the parietal region. Double-coil galvanometer. Condenser inserted into the circuit. Subcutaneous needle electrodes in the area of the bone defect, 4.5 cm apart. Above: oscillations of the curve recorded epidurally; below: time in 1/10ths sec.

sents a small segment. During the recording the condenser was inserted into the circuit and the very sensitive galvanometer 1 of the double-coil galvanometer, connected to the needle electrodes, was set on maximal sensitivity. Galvanometer 2 was also switched on and set on maximal sensitivity in order to exclude with certainty the recording of any currents intruding from outside. In Figure 4 shown here, the completely stable line of galvanometer 2 cannot be seen; to save space the time marking indicating tenths of a second was moved somewhat closer to the curve obtained with the needle electrodes. From Figure 4 it becomes readily evident that the current oscillations recorded from the epidural space are composed of two types of waves alternating regularly with each other. The large waves have an average duration of 90 σ, the smaller ones one of 35 σ. In this record one can furthermore recognize slight pulsatory fluctuations and establish that six large and six small waves of the curve recorded from the dura correspond to *one* pulsatory fluctuation of 0.75 second duration. No influence of respiration is evident in the record, which is several meters long and of which only a small segment is reproduced here. Thus, when recording with needle electrodes placed in the epidural space in the area of a bone defect, we immediately obtain continuous current oscillations, which in their time course also approximately correspond to the two wave types found in the dog. I would like to mention again that, in spite of the large bone defect, a considerable increase in intracranial pressure existed at the time of the recording. A few weeks later the man succumbed to his recurrent brain tumor after displaying signs of increasing brain compression.

In another case, a bilateral temporal *Cushing*-type decompressive trepanation had been carried out by *Guleke* in a 19 year old girl, because of a large tumor in the pituitary region which could be recognized on X-ray plates from shadows caused by calcifications. Six weeks after the operation the two trephine openings, where the bone had been completely removed, were markedly protruding. On both sides, at the upper margins of the right- and left-sided trephine openings, zinc plated needle electrodes were inserted subcutaneously and a record was taken with galvanometer 1 of the double-coil galvanometer. Simultaneously, by means of lead foil electrodes, arranged in a manner to be discussed in more detail later, a record was obtained with galvanometer 2 from both arms and thus the electrocardiogram was also written continuously. Figure 5 represents again a segment from the long record obtained in this manner. In both galvanometers of the double-coil galvanometer a condenser was inserted again. At the top in Figure 5 one sees the current oscillations recorded with

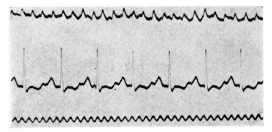

Fig. 5. 19 year old girl. Bilateral bone defect in the temporal area after palliative trepanation. Double-coil galvanometer. Condenser inserted into the circuit. Needle electrodes subcutaneously, right and left, in the upper parts of the bone defects. Electrocardiogram recorded from both arms by means of lead foil electrodes. At the top: curve recorded epidurally; in the middle: electrocardiogram; at the bottom: time in 1/10ths sec.

the needle electrodes epidurally from the bilateral bone defects; in the middle the familiar curve of the electrocardiogram and at the bottom, time recorded in intervals of tenths of a second. Again one is immediately struck by the correspondence between this figure and Figure 4. Here too we see the large and small waves which alternate regularly. The larger waves have a length of 90–100 σ, the smaller ones one of 40–50 σ. In many places one recognizes here also a slight influence of the brain pulsations upon the electrical oscillations, but this is by no means as pronounced as in Figure 4. A relationship between the electrocardiogram and the cerebral record certainly does not exist. There is a pronounced similarity between Figures 4 and 5. In this instance too, in spite of the bilateral decompressive trepanation a considerable increase in intracranial pressure still existed at the time these curves were recorded.

In these epidural recordings with needle electrodes it also depends entirely upon the local conditions whether the curves one obtains are more or less distinct. A small displacement of the needle in the subcutaneous tissue often works wonders. Particularly large deflections and a beautiful display of the waves of the cerebral curve were obtained in the following examination:

In a 15 year old girl a large tumor in the white matter of the left frontal lobe was suspected because of the clinical signs. She underwent an extensive palliative trepanation in the left anterior half of the skull which was performed by *Guleke*. In the course of this operation the bone had been removed. About 8 weeks after the operation needle electrodes were introduced into the subcutaneous tissue at two points 6 cm apart within the large left-sided bone defect. The resistance in the electrode circuit was measured with the *Edelmann* instrument and found to be 1600 Ohms. *Siemens*-type lead band electrodes were attached to both arms for the recording of the electrocardiogram. The needle electrodes in the epidural space were connected to galvanometer 1, set at its maximal sensitivity which wrote on the top of Figure 6; the arm electrodes were connected to galvanometer 2, writing in the middle. The lower curve of Figure 6 indicates time in tenths of a second. A condenser was inserted into the circuit. The curves are brought somewhat closer together to save space, but the time relationships have been strictly preserved. The electrocardiogram written

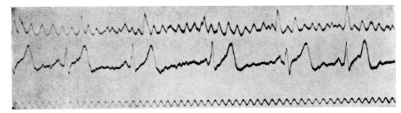

Fig. 6. 15 year old girl. Large palliative trepanation over the left frontal lobe. Double-coil galvanometer. Needle electrodes subcutaneously inserted 6 cm apart in the area of the bone defect. Resistance = 1600 Ohms. Electrocardiogram recorded from both arms by means of Siemens-type lead band electrodes. At the top: curve of the epidurally recorded oscillations; in the middle: pathologically altered electrocardiogram; at the bottom: time in 1/10ths sec.

in the middle is undoubtedly altered pathologically and also shows irregularities in the sequence of heart beats. Even before the operation the patient's pulse rate had been 51; after the operation at the time of this recording it measured 54 beats per minute and thus certainly had considerably slowed down; furthermore, the pulse was markedly irregular. The curve of the epidurally recorded current oscillations, written at the top, shows very large deflections, but also again discloses the regular alternation of large and small waves, exactly as in Figures 4 and 5 discussed previously. The relation between the time course of the first- and that of the second-order waves is also about the same. The larger waves have an average duration of 90 σ, the smaller ones one of 35–40 σ. In the upper curve one is impressed by occasional strikingly large waves; no relationship exists between these and the deflections of the electrocardiogram or with the pulsations in the areas of cerebral protrusion. The time course of the latter can be computed from the electrocardiogram. In this case too there was a considerable increase in intracranial pressure, as is evident from the slowing of the pulse. The trephine opening bulged out markedly.

In the three cases just reported here we have before us the same waves of the cerebral record. What is striking is the regularity with which in all three the large and small waves alternate with each other, a large wave always being followed by a small one, then again a large one, and so forth.

In other cases with epidural recordings I did not obtain curves that were regular *to such a degree.* In a 30 year old woman a tumor in the area of the right precentral convolution was suspected because of the clinical findings. At operation, at the expected site and a depth of 1.5 cm, *Guleke* found a cyst which was emptied of its content. The findings were interpreted as indicating a glioma with cystic degeneration. Because removal of the tumor was impossible and subsequent X-ray irradiation was planned, the bone at the site of trepanation was completely removed. Four weeks

after the operation, by means of subcutaneously inserted needle electrodes, a record
was obtained from two points 6.5 cm apart within the right-sided large bone defect.
The resistance in the needle electrode circuit measured 1500 Ohms. With lead foil
electrodes a record was taken from the arms to galvanometer 2 of the double-coil
galvanometer, while galvanometer 1 was connected to the needle electrodes. A curve

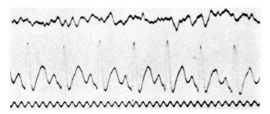

Fig. 7. 38 year old woman with large right-sided bone defect in the region of the motor area. Double-
coil galvanometer. Condenser inserted into the circuit. Subcutaneously inserted needle electrodes
within bone defect, 6.5 cm apart. Resistance = 1500 Ohms. Electrocardiogram recorded from both
arms with lead foil electrodes. At the top: curve recorded from the epidural space; in the middle:
electrocardiogram; at the bottom: time in 1/10ths sec.

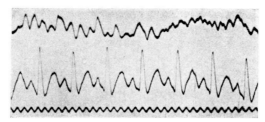

Fig. 8. 38 year old woman. Exactly the same recording conditions as in Figure 7; recorded on the
same day.

was obtained of which a small segment is shown in Figure 7. The current oscillations
recorded from the epidural space with galvanometer 1, set at its maximal sensitivity,
appear at the top; in the middle is the electrocardiogram; at the bottom, time in
tenths of a second. This record, as all the preceding ones, was taken with a condenser
inserted in the circuit. One finds here too the same larger and smaller oscillations,
known from the preceding records, of which the larger ones in this case last for 90–
100 σ, the smaller ones for 40–50 σ. But the consistently regular sequence, characterized
by a large and small wave always following upon each other, is missing here. A little
to the right of the middle of the figure, for instance, there appear seven consecutive
small waves. The curve generally shows much more variety than the strips of records
displayed in the preceding figures.

The same is shown in Figure 8, which reproduces a segment of a curve recorded
in the same patient under the same conditions and on the same day. I would like to
attribute the greater variety of form of the epidurally recorded current oscillations
to the fact that there was no significant increase in intracranial pressure in this case.
This is in agreement with other records obtained in the same manner which are not

shown here. At the time at which these investigations were performed, the site of trepanation was exactly at the same level as the remainder of the skull and was in no way bulging. Neither could any other signs of intracranial pressure be demonstrated in this patient. Yet these investigations also confirm the presence of two wave types, a longer and a shorter one, similar to those also demonstrated by *Neminsky* in his animal experiments.

According to my experience, it would however be an error to assume that these current oscillations, which appear in all the previous curves, could only be obtained with recordings from the dura of the cerebrum. I have been able to record a very similar, although not quite identical, curve from the dura of the cerebellum. A young man, aged 22, had been operated upon six years ago by *Guleke* because of a cyst located in the left half of the cerebellum. At that time the bone had been completely removed. The patient had no further difficulties. In the left occipital region the cerebellar hemisphere, covered only by the dura, protruded under the skin. Needle electrodes were inserted subcutaneously 5 cm apart in the area of the left-sided bone defect and were connected to galvanometer 1 of the double-coil galvanometer. Galvanometer 2 was connected with lead foil electrodes applied to the two arms. A condenser was inserted in the circuit.

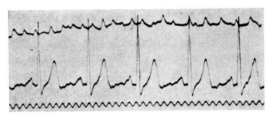

Fig. 9. 22 year old man. Bone defect over the left cerebellar hemisphere. Double-coil galvanometer. Condenser inserted. Subcutaneous needle electrodes, 5 cm apart, within the bone defect. Electrocardiogram with lead foil electrodes from both arms. At the top: curve recorded epidurally from the cerebellum; in the middle: electrocardiogram; at the bottom: time in 1/10ths sec.

Figure 9 shows a small segment of a long curve which was obtained in this manner. At the top are written the current oscillations which were recorded with the needle electrodes from the dura of the cerebellum. In the middle is the electrocardiogram; I retouched its largest deflections in a few places with a pencil. At the bottom the time is recorded in tenths of a second. Again one sees the two types of waves with exactly the same durations as could be recorded from the dura of the cerebrum. The only thing that distinguishes this cerebellar curve from that of the cerebrum is the fact that here, even without any increased intracranial pressure, the curve is again very regular—upon a large wave there always follows a small wave—and that the waves occur somewhat less frequently. I am, however, unable to decide whether this really represents a fundamental difference or whether it is just a fortuitous finding.

By means of subcutaneous needle electrodes placed within the bone defect I recorded the current oscillations from the dura of the cerebrum in still some other cases, without however obtaining anything different from what is evident from the curves reported and discussed here. However, I wish to reiterate what was stated above, that an apparently insignificant displacement of a needle tip in the subcutaneous tissue often greatly influences the quality, *i.e.* the height of deflections, of the curves one obtains. In still other cases, which will not be described here further, I was able to observe several times that the curves recorded with needle electrodes, which a few weeks after the palliative trepanation had been quite well developed, deteriorated with increasing intracranial pressure while the tumor was growing into the trephine openings, as was verified later by post-mortem examination. This fact too, like many others, seems to me to favor the idea that the current oscillations originate locally in the underlying brain tissue.

As a general result of these recordings with epidural needle electrodes I would consequently like to state that it is possible to record continuous current oscillations, among which two kinds of waves can be distinguished, one with an average duration of 90 σ, the other with one of 35 σ. The longer waves of 90 σ are the ones of larger amplitude, the shorter, 35 σ waves are of smaller amplitude. According to my observations there are 10–11 of the larger waves in one second, of the smaller ones, 20–30. The magnitude of the deflections of the larger 90 σ waves can be calculated to be about 0.00007–0.00015 V, that of the smaller 35 σ waves 0.00002–0.00003 V.

Before I carried out the epidural needle recordings from two points within a skull defect, as reported in abridged form above, I had performed a great number of investigations in which I took records by connecting a galvanometer to the skull defect and to the exactly corresponding spot on the contralateral, intact half of the skull. At the beginning of these investigations non-polarizable electrodes were used, and specifically at first boot-shaped clay and brush electrodes which, however, because of their high resistance, turned out to be unsuitable. Conditions were more favorable with the non-polarizable funnel electrodes described by *Piper*[1]. The resistance of these electrodes amounted to 530–2500 Ohms, depending upon the size of the funnel used, the local conditions in the area of the skull defect, and those on the contralateral side of the head. Although very beautiful records were obtained with these electrodes, the greatest misgivings with regard to their use are justified, especially when they are applied to the head, because of the possibility of corroding the skin with the concentrated zinc sulfate solution. There is also the danger that, in spite of the greatest care, small droplets of fluid may happen to come into contact with the conjunctiva of the eye. For this reason these electrodes were only very rarely used and then actually only for the purpose of obtaining curves for comparison. Because one deals with rapidly alternating current oscillations, non-polarizable electrodes, as explained above, were not necessary at all. I therefore changed over to metal electrodes, which can be used much more conveniently and also without any danger[2]. Dry metal surfaces applied to the skin also have a very high resistance. This resistance is much less when a moist pad is used under the electrodes. It is well known that the resistance to be expected decreases with increasing size of the electrode

---

[1] *Piper*: Elektrophysiologie menschlicher Muskeln, p. 20. Berlin: Julius Springer, 1912.
[2] *Schellong*: Über exakte und nichtexakte Registrierung des menschlichen Elektrokardiogramms. Klin. Wschr., **1926**, 541.

surface, with increasing concentration of the salt solution used for moistening, and with increasing temperature of the skin upon which the electrodes rest. I first used round copper plates with an underlying flannel pad of slightly larger size, soaked in a 20% sodium chloride solution. These had a resistance of 240–1200 Ohms when locally applied in such a manner, that, as mentioned, one electrode was placed on the skull defect and the other on the exactly corresponding spot on the other side of the head. Furthermore, I used large thin platinum sheets[1], also together with an underlying flannel pad soaked in 20% sodium chloride solution; these, depending upon local conditions, showed a resistance of 400–1400 Ohms when applied. Silver electrodes were also used with a resistance of 450–3000 Ohms. In spite of the pieces of flannel lying under the electrodes, and even when sometimes cotton wool soaked in 20% sodium chloride solution was added, it was difficult to achieve a close fit of the metal plate electrodes, because of the uneven surface of the skin, especially within the confines of a skull defect. I therefore changed over to lead plate electrodes. Each of these was cut out of a lead plate exactly according to the size of the skull defect, and was fitted to the surface by bending and otherwise manipulating it in the appropriate manner. These electrodes, depending upon the size of the skull defect and the local conditions, had a resistance of 500–7600 Ohms. Lead band electrodes, folded several times in a zig-zag line, applied over the defect and over the exactly corresponding spot of the contralateral half of the skull, had about the same resistance. However, I was really not fully satisfied with any of the arrangements just discussed, because difficulties always arose in attaching the electrodes and one could never be sure that they would be firmly applied to the skin, even when using rubber bands or a rubber swim cap pulled over the head. Finally, the idea occurred to me to use very thin lead foil, similar to the tin foil used for the packaging of chocolate, etc. These pieces of lead foil could always be cut according to the form of the skull defect. A piece of flannel, larger by a few millimeters than the lead foil and soaked in 20% sodium chloride solution, was laid on the skull defect under the lead foil; also the latter was again covered with such a piece of flannel. A lead foil of the same size with the same base and cover was applied to the corresponding spot on the other side of the head. These pieces of lead foil were then fixed with thin rubber bandages of the kind used for other medical purposes. These were wound around the skull several times. This prevented any displacement of the electrodes and pressed them as firmly as possible against the skin over the surface of the cranium and over the skull defect. Drying of the electrodes, which is a factor of utmost importance in the change of resistance, was thereby also completely avoided, and it was possible to obtain perfectly uniform curves over a considerable length of time. The resistance, which in this case could be considerably reduced by the use of lead foil electrodes of the largest possible size, measured only 380–500 Ohms. Moreover, I also wish to mention at this point that I preferred to record the electrocardiogram in the same manner with lead foil electrodes. Instead of the lead band electrode which comes with the Siemens and Halske double-coil galvanometer, a lead foil electrode was used. First, a flannel

---

[1] *Gildemeister*: Über die Polarisation der Elektroden, die zu elektrisch-physiologischen Zwecken gebraucht werden. Z. biol. Techn. u. Meth., **3**, 28 (1915).

band soaked in a 20% sodium chloride solution was wrapped around the forearm, then a lead foil of corresponding size was wound around it once and on top of it was wrapped another moist flannel band. Everything was then covered with a rubber bandage. In this fashion, without any drying, an always uniform electrocardiogram could be obtained for hours. This is an arrangement which modified somewhat the recording conditions of the electrocardiogram described by *Einthoven*[1]. Instead of lead foil he used zinc plated wires. The arrangement proposed here which I used many times is even more convenient than the use of zinc plated wire which has to be wound around the arm in many turns.

I have no desire to report the details of my numerous investigations in people with skull defects, but I do want to discuss two observations somewhat more thoroughly.

In the 19 year old patient of whom before, on page 49, Figure 5 was shown, records were taken from the areas of the bilateral bone defects using lead foil electrodes in the above described manner. A curve was thus obtained of which a small segment is shown in Figure 10. Unfortunately, the record was not entirely perfect.

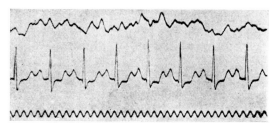

Fig. 10. 19 year old girl. Bilateral bone defect in the temporal region after palliative trepanation. Double-coil galvanometer. Condenser inserted. Recording from the two areas of trepanation with lead foil electrodes. Resistance = 500 Ohms. Electrocardiogram with lead foil electrodes from both arms. At the top: the curve recorded from the skin over the bone defects; in the middle: the electrocardiogram; at the bottom: time in 1/10ths sec (compare with Figure 5).

At the top of the figure is the curve recorded with the lead foil electrodes placed over the bilateral bone defects and connected to galvanometer 1 of the double-coil galvanometer. Below there follows the electrocardiogram which was recorded from both arms to galvanometer 2, also by means of the above described lead foil electrodes. At the bottom, time is indicated again in tenths of a second. The resistance of the lead foil electrodes over the skull defects measured 500 Ohms. When we compare Figures 5 and 10 it is evident that Figure 10 is a somewhat distorted rendering of the curve of Figure 5. But here too one sees again the longer and the shorter waves, even though by far not everything stands out as sharply as in the epidural needle recording from the same girl reproduced in Figure 5. In any case, however, the curve proves that when one records from the skin over skull defects, one can obtain a tolerably good record which also contains the characteristic details of the two wave types.

I shall report here still another observation. It is that of a 43 year old lawyer, who in 1914 had been wounded by a shrapnel fragment in the region of the forehead

[1] *Einthoven: l. c.* p. 790 [see footnote on p. 42].

on the right side of the midline and who presented a markedly pulsating bone defect in this area of about the size of a five mark piece. After the skin in this region and at the occiput had been well scrubbed with alcohol and ether, the somewhat depressed bone defect was filled with a cotton wad soaked in a 20% sodium chloride solution; on the top of it, a layer of flannel, then a thin lead foil and on top of it again a second layer of flannel was laid. Exactly the same type of electrode was placed on the occiput in the midline somewhat above the external occipital protuberance. The two electrodes were fixed by a rubber bandage firmly wound around the skull and further reinforced by a second bandage. The electrodes were thus protected against drying. The record was then taken with galvanometer 1 of the double-coil galvanometer and a curve was thus obtained of which a small segment is represented in Figure 11. The electro-

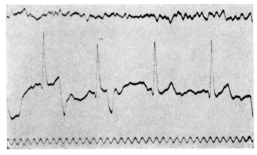

Fig. 11. 43 year old man. Bone defect in the forehead. Double-coil galvanometer, condenser inserted. Record from the bone defect and from the occiput with lead foil electrodes. Electrocardiogram from both arms with lead band electrodes according to Siemens. At the top: the curve recorded from the bone defect and from the occiput; in the middle: the electrocardiogram; at the bottom: time in 1/10ths sec.

cardiogram was also recorded from both forearms, in this case by means of Siemens lead band electrodes. At the bottom, time is indicated in tenths of a second. As always a condenser was inserted in the circuit. Dr. G. remained fairly quiet during the recording. As all other persons in whom records were taken, he lay on his back on a comfortable couch, which was insulated by glass legs against its surroundings. The top curve of Figure 11 again shows exceedingly well the larger and smaller waves, which till now we have observed in all other records.

The two segments of curves shown here, recorded from the skin of skull defects, or from the skin of a skull defect in the frontal region and from an area of skin on the occiput, show a marked similarity with the current oscillations recorded epidurally. In all instances in which such curves were recorded from the defect and from the area contralateral to it, one always obtained the same results. In 101 sessions I recorded in a total of 38 persons with skull defects, 23 men and 15 women, 506 curves, most of them measuring several meters in length. The statements made above are based on the careful analysis of these records. Thus not only with needle electrodes, placed in the epidural space, but also from the skin over a skull defect and the corresponding area of the other side, it is possible to obtain continuous oscilla-

tions of the electrical current with two characteristic wave types, the larger with a
slower time course and the shorter[T13] with a more rapid one.

From the beginning *this* was my hope: that it would become possible to record
from the human scalp with an intact skull the oscillations of the electrical current
which can be obtained in animals from the surface of the brain and in humans
with bone defects from the epidural space, and thus to fulfil what *Fleischl von
Marxow* had said: "It may even become possible by taking records from the scalp
to perceive the currents generated in our own brain by various mental acts", a
statement already referred to above. As early as 1920, in a medical student who had
lost almost all his hair and who, upon my request put himself most obligingly at my
disposal, I had attempted to obtain current oscillations from various places on his
scalp, especially from corresponding areas on the right and left half of the head, but
also from the frontal and parietal regions on one and the same side of the head. I used
Piper's funnel electrodes and subcutaneously inserted needle electrodes, which were
connected to the small *Edelmann* string galvanometer which was then available to
me in addition to the *Lippmann* capillary electrometer. However, I was completely
unsuccessful. Now, of course, I was incomparably better prepared for these investigations. The large *Edelmann* string galvanometer was available to me and especially
also the Siemens and Halske double-coil galvanometer. Above all, however, I had
already recorded many curves from people with skull defects and thus I knew fairly
precisely *what* one had to expect. I pursued right from the start not only purely
scientific, but also practical aims, because I hoped that I might be able to utilize these
observations for diagnostic purposes. I shall return to this point later again. I recorded
curves in a whole series of healthy people with intact skulls and I shall now discuss
the results of these investigations in the light of some characteristic examples.

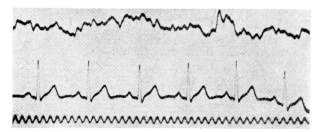

Fig. 12. Klaus at the age of 16. Double-coil galvanometer. Condenser inserted. Subcutaneous needle
electrodes on the forehead and occiput. Resistance = 700 Ohms. Electrocardiogram with lead foil
electrodes from both arms. At the top: the curve recorded from the scalp; in the middle: electrocardiogram; at the bottom: time in 1/10ths sec.

In 14 sessions I have recorded 73 tracings in my son Klaus, who at the time of
these studies was 15 to 17 years old. Whenever these investigations were carried out,
his hair was cut as short as possible. Figure 12 shows such a record obtained from
my son Klaus. Zinc plated needle electrodes were inserted subcutaneously in the
midline of the skull anteriorly within the hair line of the forehead and posteriorly
about two finger breadths above the external occipital protuberance. In this examina-

tion the resistance of the needle electrodes was 700 Ohms when measured with the *Edelmann* instrument. They were connected with galvanometer 1 of the double-coil galvanometer, while the electrocardiogram was being recorded from both arms with lead foil electrodes through galvanometer 2. As in all previous investigations a condenser was inserted in the circuit. In Figure 12, in the top curve, one recognizes immediately and distinctly the already familiar larger waves with an average duration of 90 σ and the smaller oscillations lasting on the average 35–40 σ. The middle curve represents the electrocardiogram. At the bottom, time is indicated in tenths of a second. The amplitude of the deflections of the electrical oscillations recorded with the needle electrodes amounts to 0.00012–0.0002 V when measured in a simultaneously recorded string galvanometer curve.

I also wish to emphasize that curves differing markedly in quality were obtained when recording with needle electrodes from the intact skull, even in the same person, *e.g.* in my son Klaus, and that even the smallest displacements of the needle in the subcutaneous tissue often exert an unexpected and above all unintended effect upon the quality of the curves. Using subcutaneous electrodes records were also taken in Klaus from both parietal regions, as well as crosswise or ipsilaterally from one frontal to one parietal eminence and with various other combinations. However, the fronto-occipital recordings taken with needle electrodes, in which the latter were applied exactly in the midline of the skull, yielded by far the largest deflections.

In Klaus records were taken with every other possible type of electrodes: silver, platinum, lead electrodes, etc.; also, different arrangements of these on the skin surface of the head were used. However, time and again it was found that the best arrangement was that with electrodes placed on the forehead and occiput. Of Klaus' many records, I only want to show in Figure 13 another small segment of a curve obtained in this manner. In this instance lead band electrodes were applied to the forehead and occiput and were fixed with rubber bandages. From these lead band electrodes records were taken with galvanometer 1 of the double-coil galvanometer; galvanometer 2 was set at its maximum sensitivity and was used as a control to make

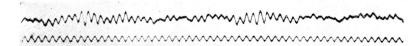

Fig. 13. Klaus at the age of i5. Double-coil galvanometer. Condenser inserted. Recording from fore-head and occiput with lead band electrodes. At the top: the record obtained from the scalp; at the bottom: time in 1/10ths sec.

sure that no outside currents were entering the galvanometer circuit to disturb the examination. At that time I was still very distrustful of the findings I obtained and time and again I applied such precautionary measures. The record of galvanometer 2 ran as a completely straight line, without any oscillation; it is not shown in Figure 13. In the reproduction the second curve indicating time in tenths of a second is moved closer to the cerebral record in order to save space. The curves are recorded with a condenser.

With this type of recording also the larger and smaller waves familiar to us are seen very beautifully, even though the latter are somewhat less distinct than when recorded with needle electrodes.

I also had a whole series of records taken from my own scalp, both with needle electrodes and with other types. In these I used the most diverse placement of electrodes. These curves also confirm essentially what has already been reported here. I have 56 of my own curves. These were recorded by *Hilpert* in 11 sessions. The records from my *scalp* just as those of my son Klaus, were not as beautiful as those of people who had large areas of baldness or, even better, had no hair at all. Taking this into account, I selected a series of people for examination, from whom I then took records.

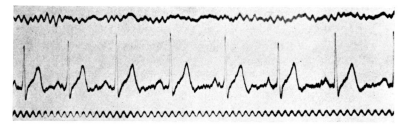

Fig. 14. 36 year old bald-headed man. Double-coil galvanometer. Condenser inserted. Record from forehead and occiput with lead foil electrodes. Resistance = 140 Ohms. Electrocardiogram with lead foils from both arms. At the top: the curve recorded from the scalp; in the middle: the electrocardiogram; at the bottom: time in 1/10ths sec.

Figure 14 is a segment of such a record. It was obtained from a 36 year old healthy man with extensive baldness of the head in whom, especially in the frontal and occipital region, there was a complete lack of hair. In the manner previously described a large lead foil electrode was placed on the forehead and another on the occiput; they were fixed to the head by means of rubber bandages. From these lead foil electrodes on the forehead and occiput a record was taken with galvanometer 1 of the double-coil galvanometer. With this arrangement the resistance for the two fairly large lead foil electrodes measured only 140 Ohms. The top curve of Figure 14 shows the current oscillations recorded in this manner from the forehead and occiput; the middle one shows the electrocardiogram which, as indicated above, was also recorded with lead foil electrodes from both arms through galvanometer 2. At the bottom, time is indicated in tenths of a second. As always a condenser was used. Even though the top curve unfortunately shows a somewhat thick tracing, one nevertheless recognizes in it the characteristic larger and smaller waves of the current oscillations which are sufficiently well known to us from the epidural recordings.

In a 37 year old healthy man without skull defect and with extensive baldness, I took records from the frontal and occipital region successively with *Piper's* non-polarizable funnel electrodes, with subcutaneously inserted zinc plated needle electrodes and finally with the repeatedly described lead foil electrodes. I did this in order to convince myself that, in spite of the differences between these electrodes and the different resistances which they offer, one can nevertheless obtain from the skull curves which in all essential points correspond to each other and readily display the larger and smaller waves which were discussed repeatedly.

In all, I have obtained 231 records in 48 sessions from 13 men, aged 16 to 65, these being predominantly employees of the clinic under my direction, and in one 36 year old woman. The reason why only *one* woman was examined is that the dense hair, especially at the occiput, prevents the attachment of the electrodes or causes such an enormous resistance that successful records can only be obtained by bypassing the skin with subcutaneous needle electrodes. The only woman in whom I performed such investigations had a circumscribed loss of hair and thus the electrodes lay conveniently on the completely hairless surface of the scalp.

I wish to point out again that I tried all conceivable arrangements of electrode positions on the surface of the scalp; thus the electrodes were placed sometimes over both frontal eminences, then again on each side in the planum temporale, a type of recording which is not to be recommended at all because of the subjacent temporalis muscle. Furthermore, the electrodes were placed on both parietal eminences which is a very good type of recording. Moreover, recordings were made from one frontal eminence to the contralateral parietal eminence, but also from one frontal eminence to the ipsilateral parietal eminence and finally from the forehead to the occiput. As already emphasized the latter turned out to be the best recording arrangement, even though it also has many disadvantages to which later we shall have to return once again, when considering the sources of artefacts[T14]. Of the various electrodes, the lead foil electrodes which can remain attached without discomfort for a fairly long time proved to be most satisfactory, along with the subcutaneous needle electrodes which, although somewhat uncomfortable to the subject being examined, can always be used even when there is considerable growth of hair.

In many investigations I also tried to record with one electrode placed on the skull and the other elsewhere on the body, because I believed that perhaps one could in this manner display the current oscillations originating from the skull with that much larger amplitude and all the more beautifully. All these investigations, however, were unsuccessful. In all these experiments the electrocardiogram interfered in a troublesome way. Thus, *e.g.*, when one electrode was located in the midline of the skull on the forehead or at the vertex, and another electrode of equal size was placed on the chest, the back, in the lumbar or sacral region, or was applied as a band around the whole chest, I always obtained the electrocardiogram more or less distinctly. Likewise electrocardiogram curves appeared immediately when a record was taken between the scalp and both palms placed upon the same electrode surface, or both soles of the feet. Also with an arrangement in which one electrode was placed on the vertex and the other on the left leg or foot or on the left arm or hand, the electrocardiogram showed up. Also when recording from the left side of the head and the left arm, the electrocardiogram appeared in a more or less distorted form. Only in a record from the vertex and the right forearm or right hand did I obtain a more composite curve in which, it is true, the presence of the electrocardiogram was clearly recognizable, but in addition other oscillations could also be demonstrated, such as *e.g.* the longer ones of the cerebral current oscillations. In any case, the result was that this curve was not suited for my purposes either. One can actually speak of an *ubiquity* of the electrocardiogram which renders impossible all recordings of this kind. We shall have to point out later that electrocardiogram curves can appear occasionally even when records are taken from various points on the skull. I have therefore, for the time being, abandoned all attempts to find other recording arrangements than those indicated above and I returned time and again to that of recording with lead foil electrodes from the forehead and occiput on the intact skull.

If now I consider the *sources of artefact*[T14] which, under certain circumstances can lead to a distortion of the curves recorded from the skull, I can say that gross experimental errors are easy to avoid, such as those resulting from mutual contact of the electrodes wires, even though they are insulated by some material wrapped around them, or from their contact with or rubbing against areas of the skin on the head. Large movements of the connecting wires too, probably by displacements at the points at which they are screwed in can cause a distortion of the curve by so-called wobbling contacts, owing to the great sensitivity of the galvanometer. These, however, are usually easy to recognize and therefore avoidable.

More important are the movements to which the electrodes placed on the skin surface or in the subcutaneous tissues are subjected. If the electrodes are located in the region of the bone defect, obviously the dura and the skin stretched over it pulsate very vigorously, because of the propagated cerebral movements. Therefore one can often recognize very distinct cerebral pulsations in curves recorded with needle electrodes placed in the epidural space. In Figure 4 such pulsations are apparent and when this curve was discussed, it was already pointed out that pulsatory fluctuations can be recognized, and that in this case six larger and six smaller waves occur for each cerebral pulsation. *Sommer*[1] in particular already drew attention in an excellent way to the origin of these fluctuations. He emphasized that from the changes in the contact areas of the electrodes, caused in turn by differences in pressure, time-related fluctuations of current intensity result. Even with the small needle electrodes used for recording the current oscillations in Figure 4, this can still be clearly recognized, as was emphasized above. Of course, this is much more evident with plate electrodes placed on the skin. This was also the reason why later instead of the metal plates I used pieces of lead foil which by means of a tightly drawn rubber bandage were pressed as firmly as possible upon their base. In the course of successive cerebral pulsations, the influence of respiration also becomes always more or less distinctly apparent, because it determines to a large extent the filling of the cerebral veins. The variations in pressure in a pulsating area of the brain caused by respiration also change the size of the areas of contact of the surface electrodes, or of those introduced into the tissue, and in this manner also alter the deflections of the galvanometer. This is evident in Figures 1 and 2 taken from a dog and reproduced earlier, in which amalgamated tiny zinc plates had been introduced into the subdural space over both cerebral hemispheres. The above mentioned effect of the pressure changes

[1] *Sommer-Fürstenau*: Die elektrischen Vorgänge in der menschlichen Haut. Klin. psych. Krkh., **1**, 197 (1906).

caused by the filling of the arteries and veins, and the concomitant changes in contact areas between electrodes and brain surface, are of course so prominent there that the curve recorded from the brain surface in many places actually resembles a venous curve. Undoubtedly, the current oscillations which were recorded from the brain surface with this arrangement were markedly distorted by the manner of recording, but for the considerations under discussion there this was not disturbing. These oscillations recorded from the brain surface are not generated by the pulse or the respiration, nor by the brain movements caused by these two factors; they are merely markedly altered by these processes in this kind of recording, which of course is something entirely different. But certainly any conscientious investigator will automatically be forced to ask himself the following question: "Are these current oscillations recorded from the brain surface with their two wave types perhaps only distorted pulsations of the brain after all, being thus caused by the movements of the blood in the cerebral vessels, in the arteries, capillaries and veins?"

It is true that each cerebral pulse corresponding to a heart beat does not represent a simple single upward movement of the investigated point on the brain surface, but that it is most often composed of three fairly large individual oscillations. *Mosso* and numerous other investigators have already referred to this. These three oscillations are not all equally pronounced and with accurate recording of the brain movements one can easily demonstrate still a few more, so that one could end up by bringing together the six larger waves of the current oscillations which correspond to each cerebral pulse (page 48). I believe, however, that all theoretical considerations are of no value with regard to such questions and it is better to examine them experimentally.

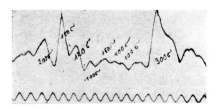

Fig. 15. 43 year old man. Bone defect on the forehead. At the top: oscillating movements of the skin of the bone defect, recorded with a *Marey* capsule and transmitted pneumatically to a *Marey* write-out capsule with an optical recording system. At the bottom: time in 1/10ths sec (compare with Figure 11).

In Figure 11 (page 56) a segment of a curve was shown which had been obtained from a pulsating bone defect and from the occiput in the 43 year old lawyer. The location of his bone defect was such that it was easy to record the movements of the overlying skin with a *Marey* recording capsule which covered the whole extent of the bone defect and was connected through a tube to a write-out capsule with an optical recording system. In this manner a curve was obtained of which Figure 15 represents a segment. At the top the oscillating movements of the skin over the bone defect are recorded by means of pneumatic transmission and optical write-out. At the bottom, as usual, time is indicated in tenths of a second. It is evident that at the onset of every brain pulsation a large wave occurs which rises above all others and which is then followed by a series of smaller oscillations. The magnitudes of the individual oscillations are very different, and so are their lengths. For simplicity's sake I directly entered the time values of these oscillations on the original record. In any event it is clear that the time relationships of these oscillations differ from those of the first and second order waves of the current oscillations recorded from the brain surface. If one compares the record of the pulsations within the bone defect as it is reproduced here with the curve of the current oscillations of the same man, as they were shown in Figure 11, one sees immediately that the pulsatory fluctuations of the bone defect do not at all stand out individually as large high-rising waves above the current oscillations recorded from the area of the defect. On the contrary, this curve of current oscillations is a uniformly continuous one in which large and small waves alternate more or less regularly. From the known delay existing between the movement of the heart and the pulsation of the brain it is easy to calculate the time of onset of each pulsation from the simultaneously recorded electrocardiogram. This applies also to the curve recorded from the skull and one can thus demonstrate unequivocally that the onset of a cerebral pulsation is by no means distinguished by a particularly large wave of the current oscillations.

This method of pneumatic transmission to a rubber membrane upon which a mirror is glued writing out the motions as an optical lever, may nevertheless be criticized with regard to the accurate reproduction of the *time*-relationships, and therefore in the same man I used still another method of recording the timing of the motions of the pulsating skin area. Using an *Edelmann* pulse telephone I recorded these movements with the aid of the galvanometer. The recording head of the pulse telephone was brought to the middle of the pulsating bone defect; the glass cylinder was

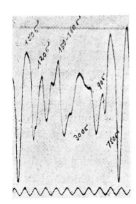

Fig. 16. 43 year old man. Bone defect on the forehead. At the top: recording of the oscillating movements from the middle of the bone defect obtained with the *Edelmann* pulse telephone and galvanometer 2 of the double-coil galvanometer. At the bottom: time in 1/10ths sec.

positioned comfortably upon the rim of the bone defect. The motions of the knob induce oscillations of the microphone plate of a telephone and the currents which are thereby generated are led to a galvanometer. In this particular case the double-coil galvanometer was used. Thus, a record was obtained of which a segment is shown in Figure 16. At the top of the record a single cerebral pulsation is shown which is included between the two deepest points of the curve. Here also, to simplify matters, I have entered into the curves the *time* values of the individual oscillations, *which alone are of importance in this record*. The lower time marker again indicates time in tenths of a second. In any case, however, it is evident from this, that the motions in the region of the defect are much more complex than it appears at first glance. I also believe that under certain circumstances these movements could perhaps exert a modifying influence upon the current oscillations recorded from a defect, even if one were to use a type of electrode such as the described lead foil which may be closely fitted to the shape of the surface to which it is applied. However, I am of the opinion that the current oscillations recorded from the skin over a skull defect cannot be caused *exclusively* by the movements of the brain, *i.e.* only by the degree of filling of the cerebral vessels. The time relationships of the single oscillations *and* the relationships of the magnitudes of the individual fluctuations of the brain movements argue most categorically against it. I can for instance not imagine through what kind of permutations the motions of the dura in an epidural needle recording could cause the regular sequence of the curve as represented in Figure 4 (page 48), such that six large waves of almost equal magnitude and also six small, again completely regular, waves should correspond to each single brain movement. But, when recording from within bone defects, one has to consider the movements of this area and the resultant variable pressure against the electrodes as an important source of artefact.

One could think that the arguments just presented are completely superfluous, since the recording of the current oscillations with the characteristic waves succeeds in people in whom apparently pulsating oscillations of the recording site are out of the question, because at the particular recording site no skull defect exists and thus there are no brain movements. This, however, would be completely wrong. Simple considerations show that the skin everywhere is subject to pulsatory oscillations as is well enough known from plethysmographic investigations. If, however, only fluctuations in the degree of filling of the blood were the cause of the current oscillations that one can record from the skull, with or without a bone defect, then one should actually also be able to record the same curves from other parts of the body, *e.g.* when taking a record from the upper arm and forearm. According to searching investigations carried out to this end by me, this is not at all the case. In fact one also obtains a curve which exhibits current oscillations, but these do not show the characteristic waves of first and second order at all. Nevertheless, one could again take exception to this by saying that the conditions on the scalp are essentially different, insofar as the skin there is stretched over a firm bony base, whereas in the arms, muscles and vessels, etc., lie under the skin. To counter this objection too, I tried to record curves from my right tibia with the double-coil galvanometer and needle electrodes which were placed subcutaneously 6 cm apart after having been inserted as far as the bone. When the galvanometer was set at its highest sensitivity, I could record photographically a few isolated small oscillations, but I did not in the least obtain a curve similar to the one I was able to record from the skull. I also said to myself that if the filling of the blood vessels produces oscillations of the electrical current which can be recorded from the skull, then the oscillations of the curves apparently originating from the brain should surely increase if the vessels of the scalp and brain were to be artificially dilated. With needle electrodes subcutaneously placed over both parietal eminences and recording through galvanometer 1 of the double-coil galvanometer, I was able to record on myself the known current oscillations discussed above. A handkerchief upon which 5 drops of amyl nitrite had just been dropped was brought before my nose. I inhaled the amyl nitrite and shortly there occurred a marked dilatation of the external vessels of the face and of the scalp; I noticed a distinct pounding of the temporal arteries. During all this time the galvanometer curve from the two parietal eminences was being written continuously. No amplitude increase of the current oscillations occurred in spite of the fact that upon inhalation, amyl nitrite causes a dilatation of the vessels of the scalp and of the brain[1]. This observation made on myself also militates against a purely vascular origin of the current oscillations recorded in man from the scalp and from the epidural space.

Then finally still, to leave nothing that occurred to me untried and to reassure myself completely on this point which caused me many worries, I carried out the following investigation on my son Klaus: I used small lead foil electrodes which were placed in the described manner on the two parietal eminences. These were laid on top of a piece of flannel and covered by a similar piece; they were firmly pressed to the skull by a rubber bandage. I thus recorded from the scalp to galvanometer 1 of the double-coil galvanometer. Exactly in the midline between the two parietal eminences the recording pin of the *Edelmann* pulse telephone was placed which, as reported above, had already been used for displaying the pulse in the area of defect

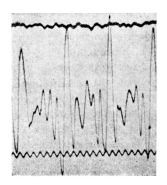

Fig. 17. Klaus at the age of 16 years. Double-coil galvanometer. Condenser inserted. Recording from both parietal eminences with small lead foil electrodes. Oscillations of the scalp between the two parietal eminences are recorded with the *Edelmann* pulse telephone. At the top: the current oscillations recorded from the scalp; in the middle: the mechanical oscillations of the scalp; at the bottom: time in 1/10ths sec.

in Dr. G. The pulse telephone was connected with galvanometer 2. Thus was obtained the curve of which a segment is shown in Figure 17. On the top is written the familiar curve of the current oscillations, as they can be recorded from the scalp; the deflections certainly are not very large, because only a small electrode surface could be used, and in addition the electrodes were lying on hair which even though it had been cropped fairly short, nevertheless did not provide a hairless scalp. However, in the top curve one can distinguish clearly enough, for our purposes at least, the waves of the first order. In the middle, the time relationships of the scalp movements are recorded by means of the pulse telephone. At the bottom, time is indicated in tenths of a second. It is immediately apparent that the mechanical oscillations of the scalp, which of course are caused by the changing degree of filling of the vessels, do not coincide *in time* with the cerebral waves. On the other hand I was nevertheless very amazed at

---

[1] *Meyer* and *Gottlieb*: *l. c.*, p. 308 [see footnote on p. 43].

the considerable oscillations which the scalp exhibits, even over an intact skull. One recognizes from this how advisable it is to carry out such investigations in order to guard oneself against serious errors.

I believe that in view of the results of these investigations I must reject the criticism that the current oscillations which can be recorded from the skull over bone defects or also from the intact skull and from the epidural space, and which were described in detail above, are merely the expression of movements of the brain or only of the scalp caused by variations in the degree of filling of the vessels, arteries, capillaries and veins. As I already once emphasized before, with such an assumption one could by no means explain such a regular curve, displaying oscillations which essentially are always of the same size within *one* heart beat, as *e.g.* shown in Figures 4 and 5. Neither, on the other hand, would it be easy to explain merely on the basis of fluctuations in the filling of blood vessels *such* irregular curves as those reproduced in Figures 7 and 8.

By disproving the assumption that the current oscillations recorded from the scalp or from the epidural space are caused by a changing degree of filling of the blood vessels of the scalp or brain, one has, of course, not yet refuted the other objection to which *Tcheriev* referred, that the electrical phenomena originate through friction of the blood on the blood vessel walls. Certainly, however, one could then expect a somewhat different course of the electrical oscillations and surely also a certain parallelism with the pulse wave. But in my opinion the animal experiment too militates against such an assumption. Exsanguination causes a transient increase in the amplitude of the current oscillations recorded from the brain surface of the dog; likewise the bilateral ligation of the carotid arteries does not influence their magnitude and, finally, it can be observed that in spite of the cessation of the heart beat and of respiration, as shown in Figure 3, the current oscillations persist. Just like *Kaufmann*, *Cybulski* and *Pravdich-Neminsky*, I also believe that *Tcheriev's* objection is incorrect.

But as far as man is concerned one may still have to ponder the question whether, *e.g.* with needle electrodes inserted subcutaneously into the tissue, one records streaming currents[1]. As streaming currents one designates those electrical currents which appear when a fluid in which the electrodes are placed is made to flow, starting from a state of rest. These streaming currents, however, appear also whenever in an already flowing liquid the velocity of flow changes. Thus, for example, in every artery the velocity of flow is enhanced with each systole and therefore an oscillation coincident with the pulse occurs at an electrode introduced into the artery. These streaming currents in my opinion could only be relevant to our considerations if by chance the tip of the subcutaneously introduced needle lay in a larger blood vessel of the kind that may indeed be found in the subcutaneous tissue. But certainly this could only be an exceptional situation and would be recognized because of a considerable local hemorrhage. Furthermore these currents would also again have to coincide in time with the pulse wave.

---

[1] *Gollwitzer-Meier* and *Steinhausen*: Pflügers Arch., **220**, 551 (1928).

Likewise the electrical phenomena described by *Helmholtz*[1] as vibration currents are in my opinion of no importance for the question under consideration. If the vibrations caused by the blood flow, or the flowing of the blood in the subcutaneous connective tissue by transmission to the electrodes were sufficient to cause these current oscillations, why then do they also not appear when one records from the tibia? Why does one not find exactly the same current oscillations consisting of waves of first and second order on the forearm, etc.? All these arguments appear to me to militate against the assumption of an exclusively vascular origin of the above described current oscillations.

I have, however, to discuss yet another source of artefact which under certain conditions could cause distortions of the current oscillations recorded from the scalp or from the epidural space. This is muscular movement. One might think that movements in the area of the M. frontalis, M. occipitalis, M. corrugator supercilii, Mm. ciliares, M. orbicularis oculi and of the other eye muscles, the muscles of the external ear and finally of the very powerful M. temporalis and M. masseter and perhaps also of the muscles of expression could be involved in the generation of these current oscillations recorded from the skull. Anyone who ever recorded muscle currents with the string or the coil galvanometer will immediately discard the notion that the curve of the presumed cerebral current oscillations, repeatedly shown above, merely represents transmitted muscle currents. Muscle currents look quite different. One could, however, be dealing with a displacement of the electrodes on the scalp. Or, in the case of needle electrodes, there could be displacements of the electrodes within the scalp or subcutaneous tissue, caused by the pulling of these various muscles. *Sommer*, in the above cited paper, demonstrated in an excellent way that in fact the area of contact between the skin and an electrode placed on it can be considerably influenced by muscle contractions, *e.g.* by contraction of the frontalis muscle, and that oscillations of an existing current can thereby be elicited. But here too, all theoretical considerations do not lead to our objective and what matters is testing by experiment.

In a series of investigations I therefore examined the effect of voluntary movements of the above muscle groups on the curves recorded from the scalp. The result was that the influence of these active muscle movements can be demonstrated both upon needle electrodes in the subcutaneous tissue and upon lead foil electrodes which are firmly pressed against the skin. With the insertion of a condenser into the circuit, this influence manifests itself mainly in a simple upward or downward displacement of the level of the galvanometer line. If however the same movements are performed several times as rapidly as possible in a repetitive manner, then in fact wave-like oscillations may appear. But they still differ markedly from the first and second order waves of the curves recorded from the scalp. Chewing movements performed rapidly in a repetitive fashion cause current oscillations of a duration averaging 400 σ; frowning causes oscillations of 450 σ. The shortest oscillations are seen with repetitive eye blinking, performed as rapidly as possible; wave-like oscillations of a duration

---

[1] *Wiedemanns* Annalen der Physik. **11**, 737 (1880).

of 160–180 σ then appear. Other movements, *e.g.* movements of the entire head, can also elicit wave-like oscillations; with very rapidly performed forward and backward head nodding movements these oscillations measure 250 σ, with head rotation 200 σ, etc. Speaking, tongue movements, mouth movements such as puckering of the lips, pulling the mouth to the side and other similar movements did not influence the deflections of the curve recorded from the skull, if these movements were not associated with others, *e.g.* speaking with head rotation, eye movements, etc. Naturally, the influence of these movements was most marked when metal plate electrodes were attached to the scalp; but, as mentioned before, they appeared also with the frequently used lead foil electrodes and even with needle electrodes! If one knows these effects they are easy to interpret. With lead foil electrodes placed on the forehead and occiput the influence of these movements was much more pronounced than when the lead foil electrodes were placed upon the two parietal eminences; in the latter case the influence of all the above movements could hardly be demonstrated anymore. Undoubtedly, this greater susceptibility to movements of the muscles is a disadvantage of the recording arrangement with lead foil electrodes placed on the forehead and occiput. The interpretation of the records, however, hardly ever seriously suffers because of this. I believe it to be completely impossible that the above reported current oscillations and their first and second order waves could be caused merely by these muscle movements. However, the muscle movements can under certain circumstances markedly change the current oscillations of first and second order by altering the areas of contact between electrodes and skin surface, or those between the needle electrodes and the surrounding subcutaneous tissue. They may thereby influence the form of the curve and lead to distortions. If perchance the current oscillations of apparent cerebral origin were to represent unperceived movements, then surely one should be able to record these over a bone defect just as well or as poorly as on the opposite side. Investigations in people with skull defects, however, have shown unequivocally that *e.g.* on the left side with epidural needle electrodes placed in the area of the defect, one obtains the known curve, but that on the right side with needle electrodes inserted subcutaneously against the intact skull, one does not obtain as pronounced oscillations as in the area of the bone defect, even though they are present. If these oscillations were only the result of transmitted movements, then surely they would show up equally on both sides, perhaps even better on the intact than on the other side, where at operation the fibers of the frontalis muscle, etc., had been severed or damaged in some other way. Certainly one must take muscular movements into consideration as a source of artefact when recording current oscillations from the skull. I do not, however, believe that these current oscillations are caused solely by the movements of the external muscles of the head or even by the movements of the eye muscles.

Finally, one might still consider whether the currents could originate in the human skin. Perhaps the smooth musculature, the piloerector muscle, but also the skin glands, *i.e.* the sebaceous and the sweat glands, might play a part in this[1]. Gland

---

[1] See *Stöhr*: Lehrbuch der Histologie, 15th ed., p. 379, Fig. 330, 1912.

currents, however, have a different course and therefore we are probably justified in excluding them from our considerations without further ado. But the situation is different for the piloerector muscles which belong to the smooth musculature. I recorded the current oscillations in the subcutaneous tissue in the area of the bone defect and thus bypassed the skin. Yet, currents originating in the skin could surely also be conducted downwards, exactly as the currents presumably originating from the cortical surface by going through the dura and also through the periosteum reach the needles in the subcutaneous tissue. I therefore coated subcutaneously inserted straight surgical needles including their tips with varnish. This covered their entire surface as far as the latter penetrated below the skin, except for a small area left bare of varnish on the undersurface of the tip. With these needles the current oscillations showed up in the same fashion. Yet, even so a conduction of the currents from the skin downwards was not excluded. But if these were really currents originating from the skin, it would be strange that they should only appear on the scalp, but not also for instance on the leg, on the calf or over the tibia, where surely piloerector muscles are also present in abundance. From the arm too where, as is well known, the skin contains hair and therefore piloerector muscles, such records cannot be obtained. This, in my opinion, militates quite categorically against the cutaneous origin of the above described current oscillations. But I believe that on two occasions, when recording with lead foil electrodes from the skin surface, I saw current oscillations which perhaps could be attributed to the influence of the piloerector muscles. In a man, who on a cold day in spite of adequate heating of the examination room felt fairly chilly, goose pimples developed; short oscillations of 17–20 σ, in addition to the usual ones of 90 and 35 σ, appeared simultaneously in the electrocardiogram *and* in the curve recorded from the surface of the skull in the area of a bone defect, as well as in that recorded from the opposite side. These short oscillations, as I said, could be demonstrated in the electrocardiogram as well as in the curve recorded from the skull, and this not only with the double-coil galvanometer, but also with the string galvanometer. I presume that these short oscillations were related to the goose pimples and that they were perhaps caused by the contraction of the piloerector muscles. Of course I am not able to prove this.

In the course of the investigations, another not insignificant source of artefact became apparent which has to be considered in detail. This is a fact which I already mentioned once before, namely the ubiquity of the electrocardiogram. I already explained above that recordings from the head and the back, the head and the chest, etc., always yielded an electrocardiogram. I even saw the electrocardiogram with a lead foil recording from the skull in which the lead foil electrodes were lying on the forehead and occiput. The main deflections of the electrocardiogram could be recognized without difficulty in this curve. I therefore, at least temporarily, arrived at the somewhat peculiar notion that the curve supposedly recorded from the dura was actually only a distorted electrocardiogram, an electrocardiogram altered by changes in the area of contact of the electrodes caused by the changing blood content of the skin and brain and, perhaps also by associated changes caused by polarization and capacitative phenomena of the skin. With needle electrodes one bypasses the skin, of course, and thus the latter with its electrical fluctuations could not induce any changes; but the objections with regard to the changes in the area of contact between electrode and tissue and to polarization remained[1]. Figure 3 obtained in the animal experiment in which current oscillations recorded from the brain surface continue in spite of the arrest of the electrocardiogram, decisively argues against the notion that the supposedly cerebral curves may only represent an altered electrocardiogram. In any case, however, the fact that a distorted electrocardiogram appeared in the course of a scalp recording, led me later to record an electrocardiogram simultaneously and in addition to the current oscillations derived from the skull in all these investigations. This circumstance was also the reason why I set such particularly great value on the possession of a double-coil galvanometer. The simultaneous recording of the electrocardiogram also has the great advantage that, from the known delay of the pulse in its propagation to the brain, one can by calculation approximately determine the time of onset of each cerebral pulsation in the curves recorded from the skull, even when these pulsations are not recognizable in the curves.

I therefore believe I have discussed all the principal arguments *against* the cerebral origin of the curves reported here which in all their details have time and again preoccupied me, and in doing so I have laid to rest my own numerous misgivings. Moreover I refer to the results of the animal experiments in dogs and monkeys, performed from *Caton* to *Pravdich-Neminsky*, which for this very reason I reported in somewhat greater detail above. I believe indeed that the cerebral curve which I have described here in great detail originates in the brain and corresponds to *Neminsky's* electrocerebrogram of mammals. Because for linguistic reasons I hold the word "electrocerebrogram" to be a barbarism, compounded as it is of Greek and Latin components, I would like to propose, in analogy to the name "electrocardiogram", the name "*electroencephalogram*" for the curve which here for the first time was demonstrated by me *in man*.

I therefore, indeed, believe that I have discovered the electroencephalogram of man and that I have published it here for the first time.

The electroencephalogram represents a continuous curve with continuous oscillations in which, as already emphasized repeatedly, one can distinguish larger first order waves with an average duration of 90 σ and smaller second order waves of an average duration of 35 σ. The larger deflections measure at the most 0.00015–0.0002 V.

To begin with I only investigated those continuous oscillations which correspond to the continuous oscillations recorded by *Cybulski*, *Kaufmann* and *Neminsky* from the cerebral cortex of the dog and the monkey. In man, as I said, such investigations have up to now been unknown. It is true that *Bissky*[2] claimed "he had discovered the physiological rhythm of the human nervous system" and had established that

---

[1] *Note added to proofs*: Meanwhile I obtained in the area of skull defects in several cases exactly the same curves as those reported above by using chlorided silver needles which according to *Proebster* (Über Muskelaktionsströme am gesunden und kranken Menschen, Stuttgart, 1928, p. 10) can be considered as practically non-polarizable.

[2] *Friedländer*: Die *Bissky*sche Diagnostoskopie. Umschau, **1926**, 1053.

"our nervous system and brain only reacts to a special alternating current with a certain number of oscillations per second". The frequency of this alternating current is, however, several times greater than the one that corresponds to the oscillations of first and second order found by me in man. I gather from a paper by *Schulte*[1] concerning this method of *Bissky* that the current that was used exhibited 335 interruptions per second. It is in any case evident from this that these investigations by *Bissky* bear no relationship to our findings. For, of the larger waves of the human electroencephalogram there are 10–11 in one second, of the smaller ones 20–30 in one second and therefore if one adds both together, there are about 10–30 in one second.

In contrast to *Bissky*'s vagaries serious investigators showed evidence suggesting an entirely different rhythm of the human central nervous system. Of many investigations I select only those of *P. Hoffmann* and *H. Strughold*[2]. They studied in man by means of action currents the voluntary innervation in movements at the elbow joint and found that a double rhythm of the action currents can be demonstrated. They distinguish between a rhythm A and a rhythm B. Rhythm A shows 10–50, rhythm B 150–180 current pulses per second. These investigators express the opinion that rhythm A probably originates from higher centers, whereas rhythm B may be caused by the activity of the last motor neuron. This rhythm A of 10–50 current pulses per second which is attributed to the higher centers of the central nervous system would correspond well to our 10–30 per second waves of the electroencephalogram. But in any case these objective findings by *Hoffmann* and *Strughold* already show that it is really wrong to speak of a rhythm of the human central nervous system in general. The various subdivisions of the central nervous system have different rhythms.

If we now consider the question of how the electroencephalogram originates, I would like to point out again that it is not only possible to record these current oscillations from the dura of the cerebrum, but also from that covering the cerebellum. The electroencephalogram therefore certainly does not represent a particular characteristic of the cerebrum, even though perhaps the electroencephalogram of the cerebellum may show a somewhat different form and more infrequent large current pulses. But we are completely unable to determine whether the current originates in the cortex of the cerebrum and cerebellum or in deeper parts, and I wish once more to refer to *Garten*'s[3] above quoted view. It is, however, certain that the oscillations of the electroencephalogram do not, in the strict meaning of the word, represent resting currents, but they are action currents, *i.e.* bioelectric phenomena which accompany the continuous nervous processes taking place in the central nervous system. For we have to assume that the central nervous system is always, and not only during wakefulness, in a state of considerable activity. This is, *e.g.*, true for the cortex in

---

[1] *Schulte*: Über Elektrodiagnose seelischer Eigenschaften. Psychol. u. Med., **1**, 62 (1925), especially p. 66.

[2] *Hoffmann, P.* and *H. Strughold*: Ein Beitrag zur Oszillationsfrequenz der willkürlichen Innervation. Z. Biol., **85**, 599 (1927). Abstract: Zbl. Neur., **47**, 614 (1927).

[3] *Garten*: *l. c.* [see footnote 1 on p. 37].

which, in addition to those events connected with consciousness, a whole series of other activities take place. Indeed, one can say that the processes connected with conscious phenomena probably only represent a small part of the total cortical work. It goes without saying that the electrical manifestations which continuously appear in the electroencephalogram are only concomitant phenomena of the true nervous processes. For one has long abandoned the old notion that the electrical phenomena in themselves are of special importance for the functions of the central nervous system. Such views were still held by *Rolando* who saw in the lamellar arrangement of the cerebellum evidence that the latter had a particular significance for the development of electricity, and also by *Baillarger*, when he compared the six-layered structure of the cerebral cortex observed by him with the arrangement of individual plates in a *Voltaic* pile[1].

We see in the electroencephalogram a concomitant phenomenon of the continuous nerve processes which take place in the brain, exactly as the electrocardiogram represents a concomitant phenomenon of the contractions of the individual segments of the heart.

Naturally, in the course of the investigations various questions quite spontaneously forced themselves upon my mind, *e.g.* whether in the human electroencephalogram too, as has been found in the animal experiment, changes occur under the influence of peripheral stimuli; furthermore, the question whether one would be able to demonstrate a difference of the electroencephalogram in wakefulness from that of sleep, how it would behave in narcosis and others of this kind. Above all, however, what about the question which already preoccupied *Fleischl von Marxow* when he wrote that under certain circumstances one would perhaps be able to go so far as to observe the electrical concomitants of the events in one's own brain? Is it possible to demonstrate the influence of intellectual work upon the human electroencephalogram, insofar as it has been reported here? Of course, one should not at first entertain too high hopes with regard to this, because mental work, as I explained elsewhere, adds only a small increment to the cortical work which is going on continuously and not only in the waking state. But it is entirely conceivable that this increment might be detectable in the electroencephalogram which accompanies the continuous activity of the brain. Naturally, I have performed numerous such experiments, but I did not arrive at an *unequivocal* answer. I am inclined to believe that with strenuous mental work the larger waves of first order with an average duration of 90 σ are reduced and the smaller 35 σ waves of second order become more numerous. With complete mental rest, in the dark, with the eyes closed, one obtains the best electroencephalograms showing both types of waves in a fairly regular pattern. This information is based primarily upon investigations in healthy human individuals who had no skull defects and in whom therefore records were taken from the scalp with lead foil electrodes. In this type of investigation, *i.e.* when recording from the skin, the interference especially by the *Tarkhanov* phenomenon[2] must however be

---

[1] *Soury, J.*: Système nerveux central. **1**, 570 (Paris 1899).

[2] *M. Gildemeister*: Die Elektrizitätserzeugung der Haut und der Drüsen. Handbuch der normalen und pathologischen Physiologie, VIII, p. 776, 1928.

considered. The *Tarkhanov* phenomenon, which can be demonstrated particularly during the performance of intellectual tasks, can level out the larger deflections of the electroencephalogram by a compensating action, so that the amplitude of the waves of first order decreases and one gains the impression that the small waves stand out more prominently. Of course one can avoid being deceived in this manner by measuring the length of the individual wave types, but for this purpose one naturally needs very well written curves. Especially in experiments on my son Klaus I gained the impression that with exacting intellectual work, even with just a high level of attention, the smaller and shorter waves predominate. However, this can by no means be regarded as a conclusive finding, but still requires many follow-up investigations so that I would not like to commit myself to a definite answer here. I hope, however, to be able to report later on this particular question. Naturally the investigation of the influence of drugs and stimulants upon the electroencephalogram would also be of great interest so that really an abundance of problems is presented, for here in the electroencephalogram we may possess at last an objective method of investigating the events occurring at the higher levels of the central nervous system. Predominantly practical considerations were those which repeatedly for many years induced me to work on this task, especially the specific question whether, as is the case for the electrocardiogram in heart diseases, one could discover an objective method of investigating *pathological* alterations of the activity of the central nervous system. This, of course, could then also become of utmost importance from the diagnostic point of view. I already carried out a series of investigations in this direction. Here too, I cannot make any definite statements because unequivocal results are not yet available. But these studies as well as those of the problems indicated above will be continued as far as time will allow me, and I hope to be able to report on them later. In the pursuit of these questions and investigations it would of course be desirable if one could use still more sensitive instruments of the type which technology is in fact able to provide[1].

---

[1] Siemens and Halske, upon my inquiry, offered me such an apparatus as early as 1927; however, I had to forego its acquisition because of the costs.

II

On the Electroencephalogram of Man

Second Report

by H. Berger, Jena

(With 7 figures)

(Received February 18, 1930)

[Published in the *Journal für Psychologie und Neurologie*, **1930**, *40*: 160–179]

In an earlier study[1], published in the year 1929 in the "Archiv für Psychiatrie", Vol. 87, No. 4, p. 527 [this book p. 37], I have reported in detail on the demonstration of the human electroencephalogram. In that paper I published a series of curves which in part represent recordings taken with needle electrodes from the area of the skull defect in patients with palliative trepanations. For these recordings the zinc plated needles described by *Trendelenburg*[2] were used. These are insulated from their surroundings by a coat of varnish except for their tips. However, these needles proved to be not completely free of polarization. After prolonged recordings the curves became increasingly smaller in amplitude and the recognition of details was no longer possible. In these investigations[3] I therefore subsequently made exclusive use of the chlorided silver needles described by *Proebster*[4], as I reported in a footnote added in the proof of my earlier paper on page 70. These needles, made of pure silver, having been suitably shaped and coated with varnish, received a silver chloride coating on their bare tips by exposure to newly formed chlorine gas. If certain precautions were taken, this coating remained intact, even after insertion of the needles. I always inserted them in the following manner: The hollow needle of a *Pravaz* syringe which had been changed into a hollow trough by grinding, was pushed through the skin into the subcutaneous tissue in the area of the skull defect and within this hollow trough the chlorided silver needle was carefully introduced. Before each new use the needles were again freshly prepared, *i.e.*, cleaned, coated with varnish and then

---

[1] I also spoke about the results of this earlier work at the 31st Meeting of the Middle German Psychiatrists and Neurologists on November 3, 1929 in Jena; furthermore I reported in detail on the earlier findings and on those published here on February 5, 1930 at a meeting of the Medical Society in Jena.

[2] *W. Trendelenburg*: Zur Methodik der Untersuchung von Aktionsströmen. Z. Biol., **74**, 113 (1922).

[3] Privatdozent[T15] Dr. *Hilpert* helped me in the performance of these, as well as of the earlier investigations, for which here too I express my thanks to him.

[4] *Proebster*: Über Muskelaktionsströme am gesunden und kranken Menschen, p. 10. Stuttgart, 1928.

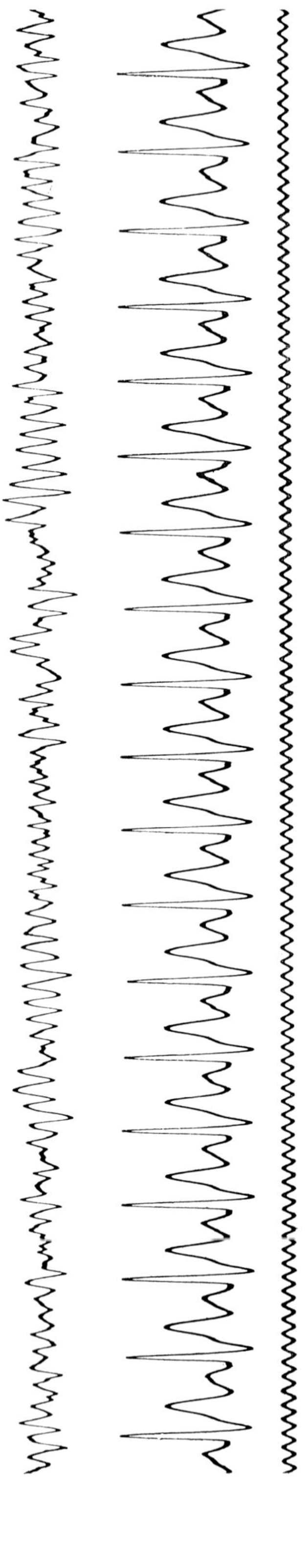

Fig. 1. 39 year old woman. Large bone defect in the left parietal and temporal region after palliative trepanation. Double-coil galvanometer. Condenser inserted. Chlorided silver needle electrodes, 6 cm apart, within the bone defect. Electrocardiogram recorded with lead foil electrodes from both arms. At the top: the curve recorded from the epidural space; in the middle: the electrocardiogram; at the bottom: time in 1/10ths sec.

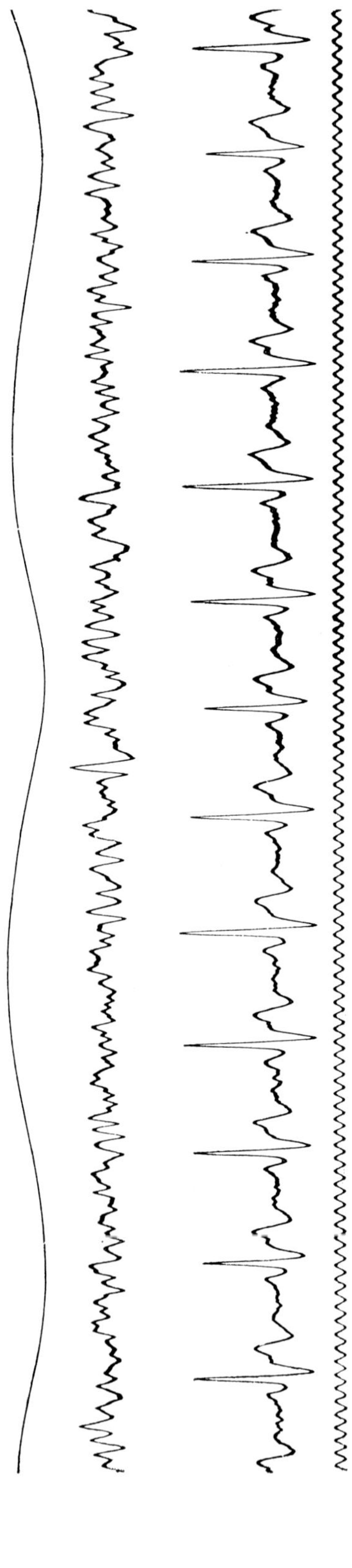

Fig. 2. 30 year old lady. Bone defect in the right parietal and temporal region after palliative trepanation. Double-coil galvanometer. Condenser inserted. Chlorided silver needle electrodes subcutaneously in the area of the bone defect, 7 cm apart. Electrocardiogram with lead foil electrodes from both arms. At the top: the curve of respiration; second line: the electroencephalogram; third line: the electrocardiogram; at the bottom: time in 1/10ths sec.

exposed to the action of the newly formed chlorine gas. In this manner I obtained very excellent curves, because as *Proebster* also emphasized in his studies, these needles in fact can be considered as practically free of polarization. This is shown by the observation that with these electrodes recordings can be carried on for as long as one wishes, without the appearance of any change in the curve. Also a polarity reversal exerts no influence upon the form of the curve. As I explained in detail in my earlier report, these investigations were carried out predominantly with the double-coil galvanometer, but they were also repeatedly checked by corresponding recordings with the large *Edelmann* string galvanometer.

Figure 1 shows such a record at a somewhat reduced scale. At the top one sees the electroencephalogram recorded with the double-coil galvanometer; in the middle the electrocardiogram, and at the bottom, time is indicated in tenths of a second. The record was obtained from a 39 year old woman who had a large left-sided palliative trepanation because of a basal tumor. The bone defect extended from the left parietal to the left temporal region. Chlorided silver needles were inserted and advanced as far as the subcutaneous tissue, so that they lay in the epidural space. These needles were 6 cm apart. A condenser was used both for the recording of the electroencephalogram and for that of the electrocardiogram. The electrocardiogram was recorded with lead foil electrodes from both arms (*Einthoven*: lead I) in the manner described in my earlier paper. One sees very clearly how in the electroencephalogram the larger waves, the waves of first order, appear besides the smaller ones, the waves of second order. Polarity reversal has no influence upon a curve recorded in this manner.

For the sake of brevity I shall subsequently designate the waves of first order as alpha waves = α-w, the waves of second order as beta waves = β-w, just as I shall use "E.E.G." as the abbreviation for the electroencephalogram and "E.C.G." for the electrocardiogram.

The average duration of the waves reproduced in Figure 1 is for the α-w = 120 σ and for the β-w = 30–40 σ.

Since my earlier report I had the opportunity to make a series of further recordings of this kind and I always obtained excellent curves, unless perchance small hemorrhages occurred at the points at which the needle electrodes were placed. This disturbs the recording considerably. In several cases, probably because of local pathological conditions, only curves of small amplitude could be obtained; most of the time, however, it was possible to record the curves in a perfect manner.

Figure 2 also shows a recording with chlorided silver needles. The curve was recorded from a 30 year old lady who had a large right-sided palliative trepanation in the temporal and parietal region because of a tumor close to the hypophysis. As mentioned, records were taken with chlorided silver needles which had been inserted into the subcutaneous tissue in the area of the bone defect and thus in essence lay in the epidural space. The silver needles were 7 cm apart. The E.C.G. was recorded from both arms by means of lead foil electrodes. The top line represents the curve of respiration. It is again evident that no relationships whatsoever exist between the respiratory oscillations or the deflections of the E.C.G. and the E.E.G. which again exhibits large waves.

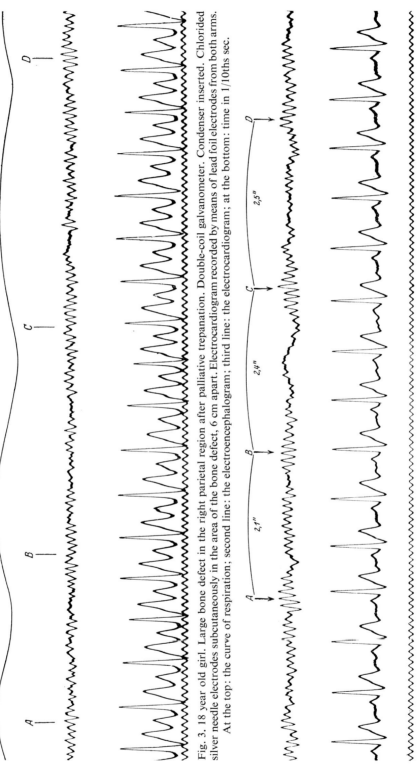

Fig. 3. 18 year old girl. Large bone defect in the right parietal region after palliative trepanation. Double-coil galvanometer. Condenser inserted. Chlorided silver needle electrodes subcutaneously in the area of the bone defect, 6 cm apart. Electrocardiogram recorded by means of lead foil electrodes from both arms. At the top: the curve of respiration; second line: the electroencephalogram; third line: the electrocardiogram; at the bottom: time in 1/10ths sec.

Fig. 4. Dr. G., 34 year old physician. Double-coil galvanometer. Condenser inserted. Recording from forehead and occiput with silver foil electrodes; resistance = 200 Ohms. Electrocardiogram recorded with lead foil electrodes from both arms. At the top: the electroencephalogram; in the middle: the electrocardiogram; at the bottom: time in 1/10ths sec.

I carried out a series of investigations on the influence of respiration upon the E.E.G. Arrest of respiration for as long as possible, which usually cannot be performed by untrained subjects for longer than 15–17 seconds, has no significant influence, just as little as deep breathing, as long as the latter remains within the usual limits and is not accompanied by the performance of all kinds of associated movements or by particular focussing of attention upon breathing; about this latter point more will have to be said. Figure 1 shows a distinct waxing and waning which manifests itself by an increasing and decreasing amplitude of the α-w. In longer segments of records which cannot be reproduced here, this becomes even more evident. For years already I have been repeatedly struck by this phenomenon, particularly in records taken with the string galvanometer in which only the larger deflections become barely perceptible. I had already performed a series of investigations on the duration of the periods of such waxing and waning in string galvanometer curves, and already at that time I became aware of the fact that they show a striking correspondence with the phenomena which had been designated as fluctuations of attention, or by *Wundt*, as waves of apperception.

Figure 3 which exhibits an E.E.G., written with a somewhat smaller amplitude, shows this waxing and waning very clearly. This curve was obtained from an 18 year old girl in whom there was a large palliative trepanation in the right parietal region. Chlorided silver needles lay 6 cm apart in the subcutaneous tissue in the area of the bone defect. The curve of respiration is entered into the figure. The peaks of the waves are indicated approximately by the letters *A*, *B*, *C* and *D*. From measurements it follows that the distance $A-B=2.3$ seconds, $B-C=3.1$ seconds and $C-D=3.6$ seconds.

A comparison of the time course of respiration with the location of the peak amplitudes of the waves of the E.E.G. shows that these peaks do not coincide with respiration or with any particular phase of the latter. The duration of the fluctuations indicated above measures 2.3–3.6 seconds in the segment of record reproduced here and agrees very well with the duration of the waves of attention, as established by several investigators.

Meanwhile I have also improved somewhat the method of recording from the intact skull. Instead of the lead foil used previously, I changed to 5 μ thick foil made of pure silver, laid upon a piece of flannel soaked in a sodium chloride solution, and covered with another such piece of flannel. These electrodes, chosen to be as large as possible, are attached to the forehead and the occiput and are fixed to the head with a rubber bandage which covers them completely. In doing so one has to exercise great care that the two electrodes do not touch each other, not even with their flannel base or covering. With this type of recording one obtains very excellent curves.

Figure 4 shows such a record. It was obtained from a 34 year old physician of my clinic, Dr. G., who kindly put himself at my disposal for these investigations. The amplitude[T16] fluctuations of the E.E.G. are clearly evident. In the course of these the α-w are particularly prominent at *A*, *B*, *C* and *D*. The duration of these fluctuations measures for *A–B*, 2.1 seconds, for *B–C*, 2.4 seconds and for *C–D*, 2.5 seconds. I made numerous measurements of the duration of these fluctuations in Dr. G.

and these agree with the results of the measurements in other curves. I cite only the following numbers from a curve recorded in Dr. G. on August 27, 1929. For these fluctuations the following values were found: 2.35 sec; 1.5 sec; 1.35 sec; 1.8 sec; 1.6 sec; 1.3 sec; 2.4 sec; 1.5 sec; 1.55 sec; 2.15 sec; 2.35 sec; 1.5 sec; 1.75 sec; 1.75 sec; 2.25 sec; 1.4 sec; 1.85 sec; 1.5 sec; 2.05 sec; 2.3 sec; 2.55 sec; 2.2 sec; 2.65 sec, etc., thus a length of 1.3 to 2.65 seconds. In the 18 year old girl from whom Figure 3 was obtained, I found with local recording from the skull defect durations of fluctuation of 2.3 sec; 3.1 sec; 3.6 sec; 3.3 sec; 4.7 sec; 4.2 sec; 4.1 sec; 4.2 sec; 4.5 sec; 4.3 sec; 3.3 sec; 4.5 sec, etc. In the 39 year old woman (Fig. 1) I found values of 3.9 sec; 3.1 sec; 1.9 sec; 3.6 sec; 2.1 sec; 3.9 sec; 3.3 sec; 3.5 sec; 4.3 sec; 2.7 sec; 3.2 sec; 1.5 sec; 3.1 sec; 2.4 sec; 2.5 sec; 2.2 sec; 2.9 sec; 3.2 sec; 3.2 sec; 3.8 sec; 2.9 sec; 2.1 sec, etc. If one compares with these numbers those of the duration of the fluctuations of attention recorded in the literature, *e.g.* the older accounts of *Lange*[1], one finds that he mentions values of 3.5–4 seconds for light stimuli, 3–3.4 seconds for sound stimuli and 2.5–3.0 seconds for touch stimuli as the durations of the fluctuations of attention. Other investigators found somewhat larger values. Important, however, are the studies carried out by *von Voss*[2]. He found that periodic fluctuations of efficiency can also be demonstrated for mental work, *e.g.* for the performance of calculations. He considers this demonstration as proof for the central origin of the fluctuations of attention. He found that most frequently the duration of the fluctuations measured 2.6 seconds; then in order of frequency there followed periods of fluctuations of 2.0 sec; 1.4 sec; 3.2 sec; 3.8 sec; 4.2 sec and 5.0 sec. *Von Voss* also pointed out that a similar period plays a special role for other central processes as well, *e.g.* for estimating time. It is evident that the durations of these periodic fluctuations of the E.E.G. correspond very well with those of the fluctuations of attention reported by various investigators, for which *Wundt* assumed a central origin and which therefore he named waves of apperception. Furthermore *Mosso*[3] had already drawn attention to the fact that the energy of the nerve centers is not released continuously in a uniform way, but that it tends to appear alternately with a stronger or weaker force. He thought it likely that fatigue of a nerve cell of the brain already sets in after 3–4 seconds of activity. We know of numerous phenomena exhibiting such a short periodicity, *e.g.* the oscillating fluctuations of memory images and other psychological processes to which I merely wish to allude here.

I did not specifically emphasize above, but would like to do so now, that the segments of curves reproduced in Figures 1–4 were recorded while the experimental subject was lying in a darkened room with eyes closed at complete bodily and also, if at all possible, mental rest. In this manner one obtains the largest deflections of the E.E.G., a fact to which I had referred before in my earlier report. In that earlier account I only reported on the continuous current oscillations which can be recorded

---

[1] *A. Lange*: Beiträge zur Theorie der sinnlichen Aufmerksamkeit und der aktiven Apperzeption. Philosophische Studien, **4**, 390.

[2] *von Voss*: Über die Schwankungen der geistigen Arbeitsleistungen. Kraepelins psychologische Arbeiten, **2**, 399.

[3] *Mosso*: Die Ermüdung, p. 186. Leipzig, 1892.

from the dura of man at rest, without as yet considering the influence of stimuli upon the E.E.G. Although I already referred to the results obtained in animal experiments by earlier investigators, I wish to mention again briefly the following:

Caton, who first saw these current oscillations recorded from the cerebral cortex of animals and who designated them as cortical currents, was already able to establish that large current oscillations occurred upon exposure of the eye to light. He speculated even then that perhaps these cortical currents could be used for purposes of localization within the cerebral cortex. *Fleischl von Marxow*, who recorded from two symmetrically located points on the surface of the cerebral hemispheres of the dog, found that deflections were obtained upon exposure of the eyes to light when the electrodes were located in the region of *Munk's* visual area. *Beck* reported that a strong current oscillation occurred in the contralateral occipital lobe of the dog upon stimulation of the eye with magnesium light and that with the aid of these current oscillations one can delineate the dog's visual area. *Beck* and *Cybulski* found that large current oscillations occurred in the region of the cruciate sulcus of the dog upon stimulation of the foreleg, and in the occipital lobe upon exposure of the eye to light; they also found these localized electrical phenomena in the cerebral cortex of monkeys. *Gotch* and *Horsley*, *Danilevsky* and *Trivus* and furthermore *Kaufmann* and *Pravdich-Neminsky* also were able with peripheral stimulation to demonstrate these cortical currents in sharply circumscribed localized areas[1]. So far I have not reported on corresponding investigations in man and wish to do so at this time. According to the available references in the literature on the results of stimulations in the animal, it was to be expected that upon peripheral stimulation one would obtain larger deflections of the human E.E.G. The results, however, were different and did not correspond to my expectations at all!

Because these were indeed fairly difficult psychological investigations, these studies were carried out at first in intelligent, completely healthy subjects and several of my assistants put themselves at my disposal, for which they deserve my thanks. In these investigations the E.E.G. was recorded with silver foil electrodes placed on the forehead and occiput, as well as with chlorided silver needles, which were inserted as far as the bone, either at the frontal hairline and above the external occipital protuberance, or on the right and left side below the parietal eminence. In comparison with the recording from the skull with silver foil, the recording with chlorided silver needles, which are best pushed as far as the periosteum of the bone, has the one great advantage of circumventing the skin with its very variable electrical conditions to which *Gildemeister* especially called attention. Of course the recording with needles also has many disadvantages. Small hemorrhages may occur at the site of insertion and these may disturb the recording. Also the fact that sometimes the needle may cause pain and that the latter may persist throughout the whole recording can profoundly alter the E.E.G. When the skull was intact, I introduced the needles most of the time under light local anesthesia and only made use of absolutely perfect curves which, in addition, were always rechecked by recordings taken from the skull surface

---

[1] Concerning the bibliographic references to the authors cited here, see my earlier report in Archiv für Psychiatrie, **87**, 527. [See this book p. 37–39]

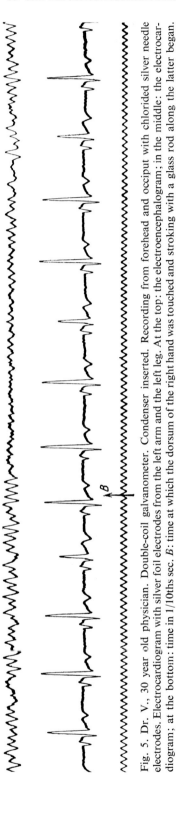

Fig. 5. Dr. V., 30 year old physician. Double-coil galvanometer. Condenser inserted. Recording from forehead and occiput with chlorided silver needle electrodes. Electrocardiogram with silver foil electrodes from the left arm and the left leg. At the top: the electroencephalogram; in the middle: the electrocardiogram; at the bottom: time in 1/10ths sec. B: time at which the dorsum of the right hand was touched and stroking with a glass rod along the latter began.

with silver foil electrodes. For these investigations it was necessary that the room in which the galvanometer stands and the photographic recording of the curve takes place, be separated from the other in which the experimental subject stays. I used two adjacent rooms, separated from each other by padded soundproof double doors. The room in which the experimental subject stayed was darkened; in this room there were only the experimental subject and the person conducting the experiment. Communication with the recording room took place by means of electrically triggered light signals. The experimental subject lay comfortably and with eyes closed on a couch which was insulated from the surroundings by glass feet. Cables lead from the experimental subject to the recording room.

I had been struck early by the fact that in many experimental subjects opening of the eyes, while recording the curve from the skull surface, caused an immediate change in the E.E.G. and that during mental tasks, *e.g.* when solving a problem of arithmetic, the mere naming of the task sometimes caused the same change of the E.E.G. It was therefore urgently necessary to first carry out more precise investigations, because these findings seemed to indicate that the E.E.G. was very sensitive to external stimuli. I performed many experiments and rechecked the results time and again. I want to report here only on results that are firmly established. I shall start by referring to Figure 5! It was obtained in 30 year old Dr. V., an assistant physician[17] of my clinic. The recording was carried out with chlorided silver needles inserted anteriorly at the frontal hair line, somewhat to the left of the midline, and posteriorly over the external occipital protuberance, a little on the right of the midline. The needles were pushed in as far as the bone. The E.C.G. was recorded from the left arm and left leg by means of silver foil electrodes (*Einthoven*: lead III). At *B* the dorsum of the right hand of the experimental subject, who was sitting with his eyes closed, is being touched with a glass rod; 0.27 second later a striking change in the E.E.G. sets in which cannot be overlooked. The letter *B* was transferred to the time curve from the signal curve, omitted from the reproduction.

This experiment has been repeated many times and also with another arrangement of the needle electrodes in which the chlorided silver needles were applied bilaterally on the right and left somewhat below the parietal eminence; the deflections occurred in exactly the same manner. When recording with silver foil electrodes from forehead and occiput, the same results were obtained. A condition for the occurrence of this change in the E.E.G. is, however, that other simultaneous stimuli be excluded. As emphasized above, the subject was touched by means of a glass rod, in order to avoid any transmission of electricity.

If we look at this change of the E.E.G. more closely, we find that the α-w, which in the present case have an average duration of 110 σ, disappear, and in their place there appear β-w with a duration of 35 σ. In all experiments the result is the same. Always the same change of the E.E.G. occurs. These experiments were also repeatedly checked in another experimental subject and the result was the same. This result at first appears very strange, if one considers the findings obtained for example by *Beck* and *Cybulski* in their experiments on monkeys, and my own single positive experiment in the dog in the year 1902, which I described in my earlier report. One should expect that in man too a larger deflection of the E.E.G. would appear under the influence of a sensory stimulus, whereas in this case one unequivocally observes a decrease in the amplitude of the curve.

Next a series of further experiments was carried out. Pricking with a sharply pointed glass rod the dorsum of the hand of an experimental subject sitting in the darkened room with his eyes closed, elicited the same rapidly transient change. Sound stimuli had the same effect. For sound stimulation the instrument described by *Wundt* for the measurement of the reaction time was used. It consists of a ball which is made to fall from any arbitrarily chosen height upon a plate, causing a simultaneous closure of an electrical contact. The height of the fall was chosen to be low, in order to prevent any startle of the experimental subject. All experiments were performed several times. Time and again the change in the E.E.G. clearly appeared under the influence of this sound stimulus. When a cap pistol was suddenly fired, it had the same effect; here, of course, the experimental subject's emotional responses were also involved, because the unexpected sudden bang acted as a startling stimulus. Otherwise, for all other sensory stimuli used, the element of surprise was eliminated as far as possible by informing the experimental subject beforehand about the stimulus to be applied, by repeated application of the same stimulus during the same sitting and by the repetition of similar sessions. The aim was to minimize as far as possible the influence of emotional factors which, of course, can never be completely excluded in such experiments.

It has already been mentioned above that the most beautiful E.E.G.s could be obtained in experimental subjects who were sitting with closed eyes and were completely relaxed. Opening of the eyes was sufficient to elicit a change in the record. This fact caused me many worries and led to a whole series of investigations on just this problem. Consequently I would now like to report the following.

One succeeds in obtaining exactly the same E.E.G.s with ample deflections from experimental subjects also when their eyes are open, if they sit in a completely darkened room. This observation made it likely that the diversion of attention by visual impressions after opening of the eyes caused the change of the E.E.G. This could also be confirmed experimentally. If to an experimental subject sitting in a completely darkened room with open eyes and receiving no visual impressions, such an impression[T18] is suddenly presented by turning on a flashlight, there occurs immediately the same change as shown in Figure 5 following a touch stimulus. These experiments were checked many times, also with various methods of recording, namely with needle recording from forehead and occiput, with needle recording laterally from the region of the parietal eminence and with recording by means of silver foil electrodes. The result was always the same, just as it had been with sound stimuli, for which also various recording methods had been employed. To me, therefore, there seemed to be no doubt that directing the attention to a stimulus causes this change in the E.E.G.

The problem now was to prove this by showing that a stimulus which does not elicit a sensation, though it affects the experimental subject, also fails to evoke a change in the E.E.G. Dr. V. submitted to the following experiment. A fairly large area on the dorsum of his hand was made anesthetic and analgesic by an intradermal and subcutaneous injection of a 0.5% Novocaine–adrenalin solution. Dr. V. sat with his eyes closed in a darkened room and if now the dorsum of his right hand was touched in the anesthetized area, the change in the E.E.G. shown above only occurred when, in spite of the local insensitivity, the touch happened to be perceived because of some fairly pronounced movement of the neighboring skin. If even the slightest movement was carefully avoided when the touch was applied and if the latter remained strictly confined to the anesthetized area, no change occurred in the E.E.G.! This is probably proof that only a stimulus which penetrates into consciousness and becomes a perception, is capable of producing this change of the E.E.G.

Simultaneously with these investigations I made measurements in which I determined how much time elapses between the application of the stimulus and the change in the E.E.G. Of course, only well written curves could be used for this purpose. The experiments were carried out in such a manner that the previously mentioned stimuli were applied to Dr. V. and Dr. G. by observing the appropriate precautionary measures (dark room, closed eyes, avoidance of all sounds, etc.). One galvanometer of the double-coil galvanometer was used to record time, because a separate recording of the E.C.G. did not appear necessary. The time of touching or pricking was determined by having the touch applied by means of the *Edelmann* pulse telephone enclosed in an insulating cover. The sound stimuli were also recorded with the pulse telephone, which was simply placed on the base of *Wundt's* instrument operated by the falling ball. The firing of a cap pistol too could be recorded in this fashion. The time when words or orders were called was recorded with a telephone connected to a galvanometer. It could thus be demonstrated that in most experiments carried out on Dr. V. 0.275–0.5 second elapsed between a touch and the change of the E.E.G.; when pricking the dorsum of the hand, the distinct change once occurred only after 0.675 second. With sounds (using *Wundt's* instrument) the change appeared after 0.425 second; after the firing of a cap pistol, however, it occurred as early as 0.09 second after the stimulus. These measurements demonstrate clearly that vascular processes, as *e.g.* those in brain vessels, do not play a significant role in these changes of the E.E.G. Earlier I had found[1] that following a shot which acts as a violent startling stimulus, a change in the cerebral curve[T19] can be demonstrated only after 2.3 seconds, *i.e.* after 2300 σ, whereas here the values for a startling stimulus may go down to as low as 90 σ. It was not possible to determine precisely at which time the effect of a light stimulus occurred, because the only selenium cell available to me had too great a latent time to permit accurate measurements. Even if a stimulus acts only for a brief period of time, the change of the E.E.G. lasts for 0.5–2 seconds, and only then does the curve appear again in the same form as before the influence of the stimulus.

I also performed many experiments in which the experimental person received the order to carry out a particular movement, *e.g.* with the fingers, the arm, the leg, the toes, or the eye muscles. It becomes evident from these experiments that the order

---

H. Berger: Über die körperlichen Äusserungen psychischer Zustände. Table 10, curves 18 and 19 in the atlas. Jena, 1904.

to execute such a movement causes a change in the curve which occurs after 0.24, 0.3 or 0.35 to 0.55 second. I believe, however, that I have to attribute this change merely to the direction of attention consequent to the order, for in itself the perform- ance of the movements, which ought to be frequently repeated, is not accompanied by any change in the E.E.G., as long as these are simple and do not necessitate a particular direction of attention. Also in experiments on reaction time in which the subject is required to respond as fast as possible to a sound signal, more specifically to *Wundt's* one-tone signal, if one adopts the procedure of warning the experimental subject of the impending bell signal by a preceding signal, *e.g.* calling out the word "now", a change in the E.E.G. occurs immediately after the latter. I was able to demonstrate this in many experiments performed in a great variety of people. Mental work also, *e.g.* strenuous mental arithmetic when performed in a dark room, with eyes closed and with the exclusion of all external stimuli, is accompanied by those changes in the E.E.G. which transiently appear upon the influence of a sensory stimulus. These changes are most striking when in the course of mental work the direction of attention to external stimuli and the simultaneous mental work coincide, as *e.g.* when reading a difficult essay. During the time of reading, the E.E.G. exhibits almost exclusively β-w. Thus, the result is exactly the same as shown in Figure 5 as a transient phenomenon. I carried out three experiments in Dr. G. on the influence of sleep upon the E.E.G. which lead to the result that in *deep* sleep a considerable decrease in the height of the deflections of the E.E.G. occurs. This is essentially caused by a diminution in the amplitude of the α-w, the pattern[T20] of the curve, especially with regard to the length of the α-w, showing no changes in comparison with the waking state.

These observations also indicate why sometimes with needle recordings only curves with small deflections are obtained, namely when one of the inserted needles causes pain and thus the experimental subject's attention is continuously diverted by the painful stimulus. The fact that opening and closing the eyes is associated in many experimental subjects with such profound changes of the E.E.G., probably points to the close relationship existing particularly between this sense organ and the phenomena of attention. Moreover, I also observed that under the influence of sensory stimuli, *e.g.* that of sound stimuli, when the same stimulus is repeatedly applied in one and the same session, the changes of the E.E.G. appear less and less distinctly; also the time intervals before the onset of the change become longer. It seems as if the experimental person had lost interest in the stimulus and that correspondingly the changes also occur more slowly and less distinctly. This could probably be interpreted as indicating an involvement of emotional processes, in spite of all precautions (compare p. 84).

After I had observed this change in the E.E.G. under the influence of sensory stimuli, I investigated whether these changes could also be demonstrated in people with skull defects when recording in the region of the circumscribed area of trepana- tion. In suitable patients the result of these experiments was that this is in fact the case. All sensory stimuli, most clearly and with the greatest ease touch stimuli, cause this change also in the locally recorded E.E.G. In a 41 year old man, who had a skull defect in the right parietal and temporal region, touching the right hand with a glass rod elicited a clear-cut change of the E.E.G. recorded from the skull defect by means of chlorided silver needles placed 4 cm apart. In a 16 year old girl with a defect localized to the same area on the right side, touching the right hand also caused a change in the E.E.G.; in this patient pricking, sound stimuli and light stimuli applied in the dark with eyes open had the same effect. The needles in this case were placed 7 cm apart. When recording from a defect the changes in the E.E.G. which are elicited by the influence of sensory stimuli are, however, not as marked as in records taken from the whole skull. They nevertheless appear distinctly: the α-w diminish or disappear completely and the β-w emerge more clearly, and this when a condenser is used, as well as when one has compensated for the local current. This result therefore demonstrates that with this kind of recording too the same change of the E.E.G. appears under the influence of sensory stimuli. In any event, however, this finding, as I have emphasized, differs completely from what I had anticipated. The results in animal experiments cited above led one to expect that the deflections of the human E.E.G. would increase in magnitude under the influence of a stimulus. The question, naturally, arises whether and how such observations on the human E.E.G. can be reconciled with the findings obtained time and again by reliable investigators in the animal experiments?

The following explanation seems probable to me. When in man one records from the area of a skull defect or from the skull as a whole, one does not record from a circumscribed sensory center as was the case in the animal experiments. Furthermore, the human sensory centers, such as the auditory and visual areas, are certainly not located on the brain surface which is accessible to recording. The visual area lies on the mesial surface, the auditory convolution is located in the depth of the Sylvian fossa and only the touch area reaches the surface. With regard to the latter, however, one has to consider that the part of the postcentral convolution which lies in the depth of the Rolandic sulcus represents a substantial portion of the touch area. Cytoarchitectonic studies demonstrate that the boundary between the motor cortex of the precentral and the sensory cortex of the postcentral convolution lies in the depth of the Rolandic sulcus. These locations of the human sensory centers make it very improbable that one could record from them, even when a record is taken from the area of a skull defect, all the more so as the dura extends as a continuous sheet over the surface of the convexity[1]. Yet, we have to assume that with every sensory perception there occurs in the sensory center itself an event, whose concomitant phenomena in the form of a cortical current were demonstrated in the animal experiments by the above named investigators. *Beritov*[2] emphasized that the whole central nervous system is in a state of mobile equilibrium; each time a new activity originates in a center, the existing equilibrium is said to be disturbed and

---

[1] Moreover *C. v. Economo* claims that in the human brain the receptive functions are localized in the depth of the sulci and on the lateral surfaces of the convolutions, and efferent function on their crests. Allg. Zeitsch. f. Psychiat., **84**, 123 (1926).

[2] *Beritoff*: Allgemeine Charakteristik der Tätigkeit des Zentralnervensystems. Ergebnisse der Physiologie, **1922**, 407, especially 424.

the whole central nervous system brought into a new equilibrium. He rightly refers to the pervading interconnection of all processes within the central nervous system. *Pavlov*[1] expresses a similar opinion concerning the cerebral cortex when he says: "When an area (of the cerebral cortex) is in a state of optimal excitability, the entire remaining part of the cerebral cortex is at the same moment in a state of more or less reduced excitability". In the case under consideration here, the conditions seem to me to be the same. During sensory perception vigorous activity occurs in the area of the involved sensory center by which other processes taking place simultaneously in the cerebrum are influenced. This manifests itself in an alteration of the E.E.G. The alteration of the E.E.G. is not caused by vascular changes such as a vasodilatation which may occur in the sensory centers with consequent contraction of the vessels in the other parts of the brain. The change occurs far too quickly to even suggest the likelihood of such a vascular reflex. It is highly probable that neurodynamic influences are involved. From the focus of activity which is formed in the sensory center, inhibitory influences spread to all other parts of the cerebrum. This general inhibition arising from the local excitation causes a cessation of those nervous processes whose concomitant phenomena appear in the E.E.G. as α-w. The α-w disappear and only the β-w remain. One could also imagine that the energy required for the genesis of the nervous processes which are associated with α-w is used up elsewhere, *i.e.* precisely in the active sensory center, and that therefore this would cause the energy to flow off to this area. But in earlier publications, especially in a lengthy discussion with *Alfred Lehmann*, I already maintained that in the cerebrum the locally available energy is also used up locally and that it would be impossible to consider a transport of energy. Thus, I am now also of the opinion that because of an inhibitory influence, originating from a local center of activity, those processes whose visible manifestations appear in the E.E.G. as α-w are arrested everywhere. When recording from a skull defect one is surely always concerned only with a relatively small part of the cerebrum. It is for this reason that the change in the E.E.G. which occurs under the influence of a stimulus appears less distinctly in a locally recorded curve than when one records from the entire skull in an antero-posterior direction or between the two sides. These observations therefore by no means militate against the concept of localization of function[T21]. They indicate, however, that a local event influences the whole of the cerebral processes. They confirm what moreover we assume to be true for other reasons also, namely that the cerebrum from the functional point of view represents an undivided whole. These observations thus complement and extend the principle of localization. That such changes were not observed in animal experiments may perhaps be due to the fact that the galvanometers used did not have the kind of sensitivity which would make it possible to recognize the small and very fleeting changes of the electrical processes in recordings outside of a sensory center.

Let us discuss in more detail the form of the waves of the E.E.G. by basing our considerations on the diagram reproduced in Figure 6. A closer scrutiny of

---

[1] *Pawlow*: Die höchste Nerventätigkeit von Tieren, p. 202. Munich, 1926.

many E.E.G.s recorded from areas of defects or from the intact skull demonstrates
in fact that the α-w do not at all exhibit such a smooth[T22] course as appears on first
glance. As becomes evident upon closer inspection, they display without exception
on their descending limb notches, usually two, which are easily recognizable as β-w,
superimposed upon the α-w. Thus, there are usually three β-w for each α-w. From

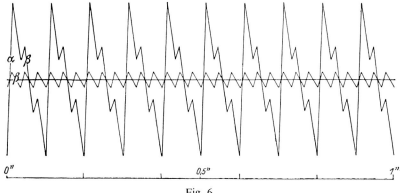

Fig. 6.

all curves it also follows that the α-w never occur alone; even if at first this may sometimes appear to be the case, one nevertheless observes in the photograph two slight
kinks or thickenings of the descending limb, thus barely indicating the β-notches. If in
recordings from the forehead and occiput of the intact skull one carries out a polarity
reversal by interchanging the connections to the galvanometer, or if one does the
same in a needle recording from a defect, the form of the E.E.G., as mentioned, is
in no way altered. One can turn Figure 6 shown above upside down and obtain the
same picture of the curve. Because the length of one second has been indicated on
the lowermost line, the time relationships can be read from the curve. Wherever
α-w occur, β-w are also superimposed upon them. The α-w on the other hand can
drop out temporarily, e.g. in Figure 5, and only β-w appear, which are also indicated
here in the diagram[T23]. These β-w are always present.

In a 15 year old child on whom two years earlier a large palliative trepanation
had been carried out in the region of the right frontal lobe, only β-w were found with
needle recordings carried out in the area of a large cerebral herniation which protruded far above the area of trepanation. The autopsy later showed that brain
substance still remained at both recording points where the needles had been inserted
into the epidural space; this brain substance, however, lay above an enormous
tumor with cystic degeneration and at one of the recording points was still 29 mm,
but at the other only 9 mm thick! It is to be assumed, especially also in the light of
the clinical manifestations, that the cerebral mass bulging over the tumor which
emerged from the depth was no longer normally active. In spite of this, however,
β-w were found in the record and therefore precisely on the basis of this observation
I came to the conclusion that the β-w correspond to the vital processes[T24] of the
cerebral tissue and thus are always present wherever one records from live cerebral

tissue. The α-w, however, seem to me to represent concomitant phenomena of the special function of this tissue. I shall presently return again to this question, but before doing so I first wish to discuss Figure 7 which elucidates the relationship between the α-w and β-w, and a cerebral pulsation, the latter being schematically represented here as a sinusoidal line.

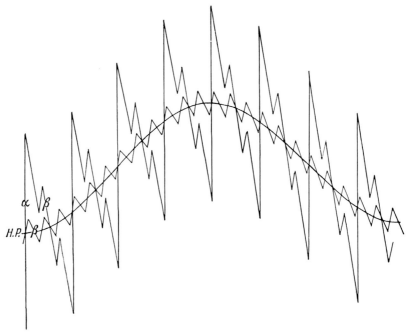

Fig. 7.

Many investigations actually have shown that whenever cerebral pulsations were recorded simultaneously with the E.E.G., a very definite number of α-w correspond to each cerebral pulsation. In the case shown here diagrammatically, the number is 8 α-w or, respectively, 24 β-w. It can be shown that the beginning of a pulsation and its end also coincide with the onset or the end of an E.E.G. wave. This indicates, of course, that the blood supply plays a determinant role for the processes which become apparent in these electrical phenomena. This in itself is nothing new, because we know that the functions of the human central nervous system are "slavishly dependent" upon the blood supply.

Above I expressed the supposition that the α-w are the manifestations of those nervous processes which constitute the specific activity of nervous tissue. I shall offer no opinion as to where the waves originate; that they arise in the central nervous system appears to me certain from all the evidence at hand. I hold it to be extremely likely that the cerebral cortex is involved in this to a very prominent degree. One can hardly go any further than this, however, as I have pointed out before in my first report, in connection with *Garten's* statements. I am nevertheless attracted by the view that the α-w probably represent concomitant phenomena of those nervous processes which have been termed psychophysical, *i.e.* of those material cortical processes which under certain circumstances can also be associated with phenomena of consciousness. Among the psychophysical processes one does not only include those which in fact are associated with conscious phenomena, but also those which perform the so-called unconscious cortical activity. Frequently only the results of the latter enter consciousness.

If now I ask myself the question how I have been led to ascribe to the α-w in particular this important role, it is first of all because of the circumstance that they exhibit the same periodic fluctuations as conscious processes, as was explained above with regard to the fluctuations of attention. But we know that these periodic fluctuations also occur in numerous other mental processes, which exhibit periods of the same approximate length. Furthermore, we know from our psychic life that there exists a narrowness of consciousness. When our attention is fully directed towards a particular sensory impression, all other mental processes are simultaneously shut off for a brief period of time. We can see something similar here in the E.E.G. Directing attention to a sensory stimulus, *e.g.* towards a touch, causes an immediate extinction of the α-w of the E.E.G., whether the latter is recorded from the frontal and occipital regions or from both parietal eminences, or even from a circumscribed skull defect. Furthermore, we observed that strenuous mental work, *e.g.* solving mentally a difficult problem of arithmetic, or reading and mentally assimilating a difficult text, is accompanied by a distinct change of the E.E.G. recorded from the skull. This observation, in conjunction with the interpretation given above that the α-w are concomitant phenomena of psychophysical processes and that a local center of activity exerts an inhibitory effect upon all simultaneous psychophysical cortical processes, would easily explain why, in spite of the most exhaustive investigations, it could never be demonstrated that mental work is associated with an important increase of the total energy turnover[1]. In a beautiful piece of work *von Liebermann*[2] explained that cerebral work and the expenditure of energy necessary for it is an invariable quantity, regardless of whether actual intensive (oriented) or extensive (dispersed) mental work is performed. What we call true mental work is said to differ from the other, dispersed, kind only insofar as in the former attention is concentrated upon a particular object or group of ideas and that the energy expenditure in the corresponding parts of the cortex is increased at the expense of others. In extensive or dispersed cerebral work, many cortical areas are said to become excited, if only fleetingly so, whereas in intensive or oriented activity only certain circumscribed parts of the cortex become involved, but all the more intensely. The interpretation of the findings obtained which was given above would very well support this view expressed by *von Liebermann*. Of course the assumption that the α-w represent concomitant phenomena of psychological processes is, for the present, only a working

---

[1] *Grafe*: Der Stoffwechsel bei psychischen Vorgängen. Handbuch der normalen und pathologischen Physiologie, **5**, 199 (1928).

[2] *L. von Liebermann*: Energiebedarf und mechanisches Äquivalent der geistigen Arbeit. Biochem. Ztschr., **173**, 181 (1926).

hypothesis which in the course of further investigations may either have to be extended and improved, or on the contrary may have to be abandoned again.

As an argument against such an assumption of the significance of the α-w one could cite the fact, already emphasized in my first report, that one obtains a similar E.E.G. when recording from the cerebellum to which surely so far no psychological functions have been attributed and to which I do not wish to ascribe any either. Meanwhile I had again the opportunity on two occasions to take records from bone defects located over the cerebellum. In a 33 year old woman in whom a few months earlier a cyst in the right cerebellar hemisphere had been opened, a record was taken with chlorided silver needles from the skin of the bone defect. In spite of all efforts it was impossible to obtain a curve, although everything was in good order, as was evident upon rechecking. The woman was well and had merely come to the clinic for a follow-up examination. It was thus unlikely that there were new pathological lesions in the right cerebellum, although, of course, these cannot be excluded. It goes without saying that this lack of success could also have been caused by some local peculiarities. — In a 24 year old girl in whom the year before a fairly large tumor had been removed from the cerebellum, a record was taken with chlorided silver needles in the area of the bone defect which extended across the whole cerebellum; one needle was placed over the right, the other over the left cerebellar hemisphere. Only very small deflections of the curve could be obtained. The autopsy performed a few weeks later demonstrated a recurrence of the tumor and showed that tumor masses were present in both cerebellar hemispheres and that necroses had developed around these masses. Thus one cannot make use of this examination either. Therefore only the curves remain of which one was published as Figure 9 in my earlier paper[1]. I then expressed the opinion that the curve was essentially the same as the E.E.G. of the cerebrum; the only difference was said to consist in the single fact that the α-w occurred somewhat less frequently. Nevertheless I now wish to assume that this altered frequency of occurrence of the α-w in particular represents a significant difference, especially when I compare these curves with those, for example, published in this paper in Figures 1, 2 and 3. I once before[2] expressed the opinion that it is probably not necessary to assume that fundamental differences exist between nervous processes and psychophysical events. In the light of phylogenetic evolution the more likely assumption seemed to be that there were no qualitative differences between nerve processes and the psychophysical events, but merely quantitative or time differences in the speed and intensity of dissimilation[T25]. Only such nervous processes in which the amount of substance breaking down in the unit of time exceeds a certain minimum, can be psychophysical, whereas those breakdown processes in the central nervous substance in which the dissimilation takes place more slowly, represent simple nervous processes. This idea would therefore agree very well with the views developed here and would surely imply that the less frequent occurrence of the α-w constitutes a significant difference between the curve recorded from the cerebrum and that

---

[1] Archiv für Psychiatrie, **87**, 545. [This book p. 52]

[2] *Hans Berger*: Über die körperlichen Äusserungen psychischer Zustände, 2nd part, p. 205. Jena 1907.

obtained from the cerebellum. Thus to me the possibility of recording a similar curve from the cerebellum is not an argument against the working hypothesis which I advanced above, according to which the α-w are diphasic action currents of the central nervous system, representing concomitant phenomena of the psychophysical processes.

I have now recorded in all 1,133 records, most of them several meters long, from a total of 76 persons, among whom there were 51 people with skull defects mostly because of palliative trepanations[1], so that by this time I have gained some experience concerning the pattern[20] of the normal E.E.G. Among these experimental subjects there were 25 completely healthy persons with intact skulls in whom recordings were taken from the surface of the head with foil electrodes or needles. Although without the recordings in people with skull defects I would probably not have discovered the human E.E.G. at all, and even though still now such E.E.G.s are for me of decisive importance for settling certain problems, I have nevertheless gained the impression that the E.E.G.s of healthy people are of the greatest importance for defining the normal patterns, because with recordings from skull defects one obtains E.E.G.s which exhibit abnormal patterns. This is the case in brain tumor patients in whom, in spite of palliative trepanations, a considerable increase in intracranial pressure still exists. Therefore in Figures 1, 2 and 3 above only three E.E.G.s were shown which had been taken in subjects in whom at the time of recording no signs of raised intracranial pressure existed. If I survey my best observations on highly intelligent, healthy people in whom records were taken from the intact skull, I find for the α-w values of 90, 100, 110 and 120 σ with a maximal amplitude of 0.2 mV, for the β-w values of 30, 35, 40 and 45 σ and a maximum amplitude of 0.1 mV. It is apparent that values in one and the same experimental subject in several sessions and under different conditions of recording usually are found to be the same. I therefore believe that through these investigations in normal individuals I am sufficiently prepared to approach the question of the pathological changes of the E.E.G. on which I shall report later.

---

[1] which in all cases had been carried out by my colleague *Guleke*.

III

On the Electroencephalogram of Man

Third Report

by HANS BERGER, Jena

(With 31 figures)

(Received January 19, 1931)

[Published in *Archiv für Psychiatrie und Nervenkrankheiten*, **1931**, *94*: 16–60]

In my earlier reports[1] I gave a detailed account of my investigations which were designed to demonstrate the relationship existing between the curve, which I called the electroencephalogram (= E.E.G.), and the cerebral circulation. On the basis of my studies I came to the conclusion that, although in general a definite number of E.E.G. oscillations occur for each single cerebral pulsation, no relationship exists between the individual oscillations of the E.E.G., which I divided into α-waves and β-waves (= α-w and β-w), and the individual peaks of the cerebral pulse. Neither therefore are there any relationships with the blood content of the brain. Thus I was able to confirm the results previously obtained in animal experiments by earlier authors. In my earlier studies, however, I did not succeed in recording the plethysmogram of the brain and the E.E.G. simultaneously, although the curves from people with skull defects reproduced in my first report show plethysmograms and E.E.G.s recorded from the same area, but one after the other. In these I was able to observe time and again the profound influence of a single deep breath upon the cerebral plethysmogram, a fact which has been known for a long time and had been documented with excellent curves especially by *Mosso*. In Figure 53 of his monograph *Mosso*[2] shows a curve in which, as a consequence of a single breath, the amplitude of the pulsatory oscillations of the brain is changed in a proportion of 1:30. Although I repeatedly investigated people with skull defects of very similar location to that exhibited by *Mosso's* subject Bertino, and also observed similarly large fluctuations

---

[1] Über das E.E.G. des Menschen, Arch. f. Psychiatr., **87**, 527 (1929), especially p. 557 [This book p. 62] and following pages; 2nd report: J. Psychol. u. Neur., **40**, 160 (1930), especially p. 175 [This book p. 90], Fig. 7. Med. Welt, No. 26 (1930). In response to a kind invitation by the editors of "Medizinische Welt", I briefly reported there on my results to a larger group of physicians. My investigations thus became better known; unfortunately, soon afterwards there appeared in the daily papers some sensationally exaggerated and also misleading news reports, from which I would like to dissociate myself completely and which I very much deplore.

[2] *Mosso, G.*: Über den Kreislauf des Blutes im menschlichen Gehirn, p. 137, Fig. 53. Leipzig, 1881.

of the cerebral plethysmogram in these cases, I was nevertheless unable to detect any noticeable effect of a single deep breath upon the E.E.G., a further argument which strengthened my conviction that the E.E.G. certainly does not owe its origin merely to the movement of the blood within the brain. In spite of this I decided to obtain further uncontrovertible evidence, should the opportunity present itself to me.

The simultaneous recording of the cerebral plethysmogram and of the E.E.G. is in fact technically somewhat difficult, inasmuch as, according to the technique proposed by *Mosso* which I tested many times, the pulsating area of the brain must be hermetically sealed by a gutta-percha cap firmly resting on the margins of the bone defect. One records from the inside of the cap to a *Marey* drum through an inserted glass tube connected to a flexible tube. Anyone who has had much experience in this knows how difficult it is to seal the cap tightly around the rim where it touches the skin. With some patience and care one nevertheless usually succeeds. In the present investigations, however, an additional difficulty arises because the connecting wires of the needle electrodes, inserted in the area of the skull defect, have to be led out of the cap through openings which have to be hermetically closed again. After much effort I succeeded in obtaining faultless records in a man A.K., now 56 years old, whom I had known from my earlier investigations on cerebral circulation. As I reported in detail elsewhere[1] K.'s frontal bone had been extensively destroyed 30 years ago by the kick of a horse's hoof. A bone defect therefore exists, somewhat to the left of the midline in the frontal region, measuring 4×7 cm. After the silver needles, coated with silver chloride, had been inserted subcutaneously in the area of the skull defect with their tips 4 cm apart, I obtained good E.E.G.s. The gutta-percha cap which had been fitted before and provided with holes through which the wires could be passed, was now slightly heated at the rim and placed on the margins of the bone defect. The holes through which the wires passed were then closed with heated gutta-percha and, by suction through the flexible tube leading out of the inside of the cap, it was verified whether the cap really fitted in an airtight manner. After prolonged efforts it became possible to seal off the cap hermetically by softening with a heated metal spatula those areas which let the air pass through and then pressing them down firmly. The electrocardiogram ($=$E.C.G.) was recorded simultaneously from both arms with a double-coil galvanometer of *Siemens* and *Halske*. I obtained a curve as shown in Figure 1. To simplify matters, a condenser was always used[2].

It is apparent that there are no relationships of any kind between the E.E.G. recorded at the top and the cerebral plethysmogram appearing in the second line, especially with regard to individual oscillations of the two curves. In the short segment of curve shown here, it is important and of interest that during the recording a ventricular extrasystole with a compensatory pause occurs at the time indicated by an " × "; this, incidentally, was frequently the case in A.K. One can see that the amplitude of the cerebral pulsation is immediately reduced from 8 to 4 mm, *i.e.* by half. The peak of the smaller cerebral pulsation, which otherwise occurs on the average 0.17

---

[1] *Berger, H.*: Über die körperlichen Äusserungen psychischer Zustände. II, p. 19. Jena, 1907.
[2] All figures are reproductions of original curves at a reduced size.

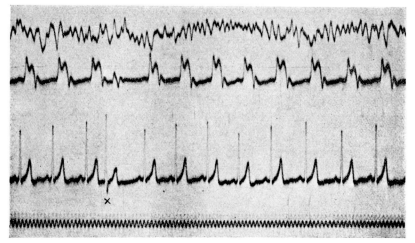

Fig. 1. 56 year old man. Bone defect caused by the kick of a horse's hoof to the forehead. Double-coil galvanometer: condenser inserted. Subcutaneous needle electrodes within the bone defect, 4 cm apart. Recording from both arms with lead foil electrodes. At the top: E.E.G.; below it: plethysmographic cerebral curve; below it: E.C.G.; at the bottom: time in 1/10ths sec. ×: ventricular extrasystole.

second after the peak of *Einthoven's* R wave, as shown by a large number of measurements, is reached later because of the lesser amount of blood being pumped in with a lesser force. Whereas in this curve the interval between the R wave and the highest peak of the cerebral pulsation is 0.15 second, the interval at this particular point is 0.20 second, and thus a delay of 50 σ occurs. An average delay of 45 σ was found in six measurements taken in A.K., when the ventricular extrasystoles occurred at a similar time within the cardiac cycle.

At the approximate time of the ventricular extrasystole and of the corresponding cerebral pulsation which is thereby reduced, the E.E.G. does not show a decrease in amplitude. Rather one could even speak here of an increase in the amplitude of the E.E.G. oscillations. But because such an increase cannot be demonstrated in other similar E.E.G.s with extrasystoles, this is probably a fortuitous finding. This result, obtained with simultaneous recording of the cerebral plethysmogram and of the E.E.G., like earlier observations, supports the view that the E.E.G. in all likelihood is not caused by the movements of the blood in the areas of the brain located within the confines of the bone defect. In my earlier reports, especially in my second one, I referred to the fact that very frequent and more or less regular fluctuations occur in the E.E.G. which are caused by a temporary waning of the larger and longer waves, which I called α-w, while the quicker and smaller waves, which I called β-w, persist alone.

In Figure 2, also obtained in A.K., one sees such a segment with a temporary lack of the α-w at "×", but without any demonstrable changes in the cerebral plethysmogram. The figure only shows the E.E.G. at the top and the cerebral plethysmographic curve below. Thus changes in the blood supply to the brain, as they become apparent in Figure 1, are not associated with alterations of the E.E.G. and changes in the E.E.G. occur without simultaneous alterations of the cerebral plethysmogram.

Whereas the findings of several investigators are not yet in complete agreement with regard to the changes in cerebral circulation in affective states, there is, however, unanimity that very definite changes regularly appear during mental work. These have been confirmed by several authors. Mental work is associated with an increase in systemic blood pressure, a slight acceleration of the pulse, an increase in blood flow to the brain, dilatation of its vessels and simultaneous contraction of the skin vessels of the extremities and the head.

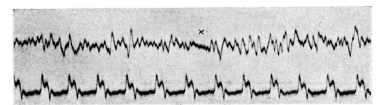

Fig. 2. From the same man as Figure 1. The same recording conditions. At the top the E.E.G.; below the curve of the cerebral plethysmogram.

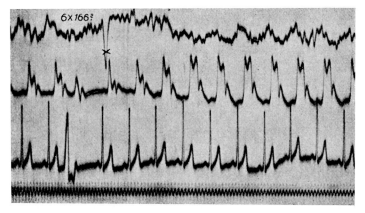

Fig. 3. From the same man as Figures 1 and 2. The same recording conditions. At the top: the E.E.G.; below it: plethysmographic cerebral record; below it: E.C.G.; at the bottom: time in 1/10ths sec. The problem (6 × 166?) was given; its correct solution was given beyond the segment of the curve reproduced here.

Figure 3 demonstrates the changes in A. K. associated with the successful solution of the problem "6 × 166". By chance, or perhaps because of emotional excitement caused by the arithmetic problem which is somewhat difficult for him, A.K. again exhibits an extrasystole very soon after the task has been stated. This again causes a drop in the amplitude of the cerebral pulsation to half its former value. Simultaneously the interval between the appearance of *Einthoven's* R wave of the E.C.G. and the highest peak of the cerebral curve is prolonged; it increases from 0.23 second to 0.27 second. Thus a delay of 40 σ occurs, very similar to that after the extrasystole of Figure 1. The pulse is slightly accelerated, as can be recognized from a comparison of the illustrated segment of the curve with the preceding ones. The cerebral plethysmogram shows considerably higher deflections during the mental work; the pulsations increase in amplitude from 9 mm to 14 mm. Thus the ratio between the pulsations during the preceding period of rest and those during the period of calculation is 1:1.55. Simultaneously the form of the cerebral plethysmogram undergoes a change, the second notch, to be regarded as a dicrotic wave, moving up higher along the catacrotic limb and simultaneously increasing in amplitude, so that the cerebral curve at times appears double peaked. *Frédericq*, in his analysis of the plethysmographic curve of the brain, distinguished in it venous and arterial components and attributed the first steep rise as well as the immediately following second peak to the arterial component. He also interpreted the second peak as the well known dicrotic wave[1]. In his very careful investigations on the cerebral pulse *E. Becher*[2] finds that, even though the pulsatory oscillation of the brain owes its origin primarily to the arterial pulse, it can also be modified by the venous pulse. He suggests that the diastolic wave of the venous pulse may have some importance especially for the second deflection, interpreted as the dicrotic wave. A systemic increase in blood pressure, which one must assume is taking place during mental work, usually leads to a decrease in the size of the dicrotic wave. But in this instance the dicrotic wave appears more distinctly in the cerebral pulse. Therefore one can probably assume, in accordance with other observations, that the more prominent dicrotic wave points to a decreased cerebral vascular resistance and thus to a dilatation of the cerebral vessels[3]. Unfortunately the E.E.G. at the point marked " $\times$ " is somewhat distorted, because at this moment the wires leading to the electrodes were rubbing on the cap or on the skin. (Appropriate investigations established that under such circumstances deflections of this kind do occur.) However, the amplitude of the deflections of the E.E.G. does not increase in proportion to the larger deflections of the cerebral plethysmogram, but rather decreases. The smaller β-w appear more often, replacing the α-w, as is usually the case with mental work. During the increased pulsation of the brain which is being more profusely supplied with blood, some pulsatory oscillations appear more distinctly in the E.E.G. This can be understood from a purely mechanical point of view and has nothing to do with the true E.E.G. waves. In spite of a dilatation of the cerebral vessels and larger pulsations of the brain, the amplitude of the deflections of the E.E.G. rather decreases.

To the three segments of records reported here I could add a series of others which show the same features, namely that the amplitude of the deflections and the

---

[1] *Berger, H.*: Zur Lehre von der Blutzirkulation in der Schädelhöhle, p. 43, Fig. B. Jena, 1901.

[2] *Becher, Erwin*: Über photographisch registrierte Gehirnbewegungen. Mitt. Grenzgeb. Med. u. Chir., **35**, 329 (1922), especially p. 336 and 341.

[3] *Tigerstedt, Robert*: Die Physiologie des Kreislaufes. Vol. 3, p. 253, 2nd edition. Berlin and Leipzig, 1922.

whole pattern[T20] of the E.E.G. is independent of the cerebral plethysmogram obtained simultaneously at the recording site of the needle electrodes. In yet another man I made a simultaneous record of the cerebral pulsations and of the E.E.G., which also demonstrated the relative independence of the two curves. As emphasized above and in my earlier reports, a certain relationship between the cerebral circulation and the deflections of the E.E.G. nevertheless exists, insofar as most often to every cerebral pulsation there corresponds a very definite number of α-w. Thus, a certain linkage of the two phenomena can be demonstrated after all, a relationship which appears self-evident, considering the great amount of blood the brain needs to fulfil its functions.

I already related in my first report that the E.E.G. can also be recorded from the intact skull, and, in my first as well as in my second report, I reproduced several such curves. In the further pursuit of these investigations, I changed over completely to recording with chlorided silver needles inserted as far as the periosteum of the skull, and have hardly used any more the method of recording from the skin with silver foil which I had employed earlier, because of the artefacts[T26] which result from it. I reported earlier on multiple recordings from the scalp carried out simultaneously, but I have not so far published any such curves which allow one to make important observations.

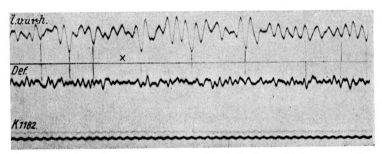

Fig. 4. 20 year old student. Large left-sided bone defect following palliative trepanation, extending from the forehead to the parietal region. Condenser. At the top: E.E.G. recorded with needle electrodes from the left frontal and the right occipital quadrants of the head. In the middle: E.E.G. recorded with needle electrodes, placed 5.5 cm apart in the area of the skull defect. At the bottom: time in 1/10ths sec.

Figure 4 shows such a double recording from the scalp. It is the E.E.G. of a 20 year old student in whom a palliative trepanation had been carried out in the area of the left frontal and parietal lobes by Mr. *Guleke*, because of a deep lying tumor of the cerebrum. Records were taken with chlorided silver needles which were placed anteriorly on the left at the hairline, 2 cm from the midline, and posteriorly on the right at the same distance from the midline over the occiput in the region of the lambdoid suture. Records were taken with these needles through the first, somewhat more sensitive galvanometer of the double-coil galvanometer. A record was taken through the second galvanometer with two additional silver needles inserted under the skin in the area of the skull defect and placed 5.5 cm apart. In order to save space and to facilitate inspection, the curves were brought closer together and a few lines were entered in pencil connecting simultaneous points of the two curves. At the top, the E.E.G. recorded from the skull as a whole is shown and below it that recorded from the bone defect. The subject is lying in a supine position on a comfortable couch; his head rests on a pillow; the eyes are closed. The needles are connected to link the two anterior needles to the equivalent poles of their respective galvanometers. It is easy to see that the two curves exhibit a certain degree of correspondence and that simultaneous points on the two curves fall into the same phase; but on the other hand it is also evident that the two curves are not identical. At " × ", for instance the record from the forehead and occiput displays large α-w, whereas in the simultaneous record from the area of the defect α-w are missing. This observation, which could be confirmed by a great number of additional records, is of particular importance. *Löwenstein*[1] in his beautiful studies pointed out that the head of a person sitting upright continuously exhibits fine oscillations. Under the influence of stimuli, thus with each increase in attention, these oscillations cease for a short period of time. For the large oscillations of the α-w of the E.E.G. one could well have considered the possibility of such an extracranial origin. Even though in my investigations the head was lying on a support, one cannot entirely exclude the possibility that, even in the recumbent position, fine trembling movements could occur, which through some experimental error could be transmitted to the galvanometer curve. But first of all, my whole experimental design argues against such explanation; furthermore still, the time relations of these head oscillations also are different from those of my α-w[T27]. According to *Löwenstein* there are 4–6 oscillations in one second, whereas I found 10 or more α-w in one second. The pauses in the E.E.G.s, *i.e.* the segments in which the α-w are missing, would also have to correspond to pauses in the trembling movements of the head. However, because in these the entire head would be set in motion, naturally the curves with double recordings from the skull would have to become congruent, or at least the times of the presumed pauses in the trembling movement would have to coincide. One of these would be present at " × ", according to this supposition. I have examined a great number of curves with regard to this possibility and can only report that neither congruence of two simultaneous records, nor coincidence of the segments which are free of α-w can be demonstrated in the simultaneously recorded E.E.G.s. Thus, an extracranial origin for the oscillations of the E.E.G. described by me[T28] is completely out of the question.

For the same reason I have to reject the explanation that the eye muscles could be involved in the E.E.G. oscillations. The single fact that one obtains the E.E.G. in more regular form and with larger deflections from an area of skull defect, wherever it may be located, than with a recording from the intact skull, argues against this. In the latter case, one records by preference from the forehead and the occiput, so

---

[1] *Löwenstein, O.*: Über den Nachweis psychischer Vorgänge und der Suggestibilität für Gefühlsvorgänge im Stupor. Z. Neur., **41**, 304 (1920). Schwierigere Fragen aus dem Gebiet der experimentellen Hörfähigkeitsbestimmung bei psychogener Schwerhörigkeit und Taubheit. Arch. f. Psychiatr., **68**, 363 (1923).

that precisely with this method a region is involved which lies in immediate proximity to the eye muscles. Admittedly *P. Hoffmann*[1] observed that with a sensitive galvanometer continuous current oscillations can be recorded from the eye muscles. The frequency of these oscillations, as with all muscle currents, is, however, an entirely different one and displays 60–100 oscillations per second. Furthermore, *even* if one were to accept this explanation, the segments which are free of α-w in the two simultaneously recorded E.E.G.s again ought to coincide. I have recorded simultaneously from skull defects and intact parts of the skull in several people, and the results reported here are based upon a whole series of such investigations.

Furthermore, on the intact skull I have used seven different recording methods, each time two together, in all combinations that had to be considered. Essentially the same results were always obtained in these studies. Both simultaneous E.E.G.s show the large and small oscillations. Certain correspondences between them can be demonstrated, but by no means a congruence. The individual segments of the record occurring between corresponding segments can be patterned quite differently. This appears most clearly in longer segments of records, which for practical reasons I cannot reproduce here.

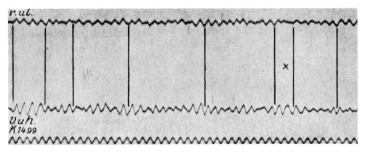

Fig. 5. 18 year old young man. Recordings from the intact skull. Double-coil galvanometer. Condenser. At the top: E.E.G. recorded with needle electrodes from both parietal eminences; below: the E.E.G. recorded with needle electrodes from the left frontal and the right occipital quadrants of the head. At the bottom: time in 1/10ths sec.

Figure 5 shows such a double recording. These are the E.E.G.s of a young man aged 18. The upper record shows the E.E.G., recorded from both parietal eminences with chlorided silver needles, the middle line represents the recording from forehead and occiput. The lines connect simultaneous points of the two curves. It is evident that the E.E.G. recorded from the parietal eminences displays deflections of lesser height than the other curve, even though the needle electrodes are connected to the more sensitive galvanometer[T29]. This is a fact which I have repeatedly observed. The small segments of curves reproduced here show much correspondence, but also distinct discrepancies, *e.g.* at " × ". During this recording the experimental subject

[1] *Hoffmann, P.*: Aktionsströme der Augenmuskeln; in: Handbuch der normalen und pathologischen Physiologie, Vol. 8, 2nd part, p. 731, and
Köllner and *Hoffmann*: Der Einfluss des Vestibularapparates auf die Innervation der Augenmuskeln. Arch. Augenheilk., **90**, 173 (1922).

was lying with eyes closed, the head resting on a comfortable pillow. Everything said above *against* a possible extracranial origin of the oscillations, or their causation by innervation of the eye muscles, is also confirmed by this record. The many other recordings show the same picture. In the E.E.G.s recorded from very different regions of the skull, a certain general rhythm of the oscillations is certainly discernible, nevertheless, the pattern is often quite different between those segments of curves which are similar and which coincide in time. I would like to say: a general melody is prescribed, but the elaboration of the single voices within the composition is an independent one.

In my second report I gave a detailed account of the changes of the E.E.G. occurring upon the influence of sensory stimuli and the focussing of attention caused thereby. Since then, I have carried out investigations concerned with this question in an additional seventeen persons and I can only confirm the results reported at that time. For instance, the following change of the E.E.G. occurs 0.2–0.3 second after the influence of a touch stimulus to the hand: the α-w disappear for 1–2 seconds and only β-w can be demonstrated. After the influence of a touch stimulus to the foot, the change in the E.E.G. occurs with a considerable delay, a finding which is in complete agreement with observations concerning the reaction time to touch stimuli applied to various locations[1]. I also stressed in my second report that during a mental effort, *e.g.* when solving an arithmetic problem, a decrease of the α-w becomes evident in the E.E.G., just as was observed here in A.K. in Figure 3, p. 98. In addition I was able to determine that a combination of sensory attention and mental work especially, as when reading a difficult text, causes a very pronounced change of the E.E.G. The attempt of holding a fine needle mounted on a long rod within the aperture of a steel spring, without touching its edges, is a task which also demands a high degree of sensory attention. I satisfied myself that with this task very distinct changes occur in the E.E.G. which are of the kind appearing with any focussing of attention. One can probably say that the degree of change in the E.E.G. is proportionate to that of the intensity of attention. Especially as an explanation for this peculiar change of the E.E.G., *Löwenstein's* observations could well be considered. However, in these experiments too, the head of my experimental subjects was resting on a support. Furthermore, the time relations argue against such an explanation, as was mentioned above. One could, however, think of still another explanation. As I stated above, mental work is associated with a dilatation of the cerebral vessels and a constriction of the skin vessels, especially those of the scalp. The same applies to sensory attention; it shows the same bodily concomitants. Thus, if the E.E.G., entirely contrary to my supposition, were related to the circulation and, let us assume, to that of the skin, then the changes in the E.E.G. with sensory attention could be related to a contraction of the skin vessels and to the changes in caliber caused thereby. However, the rapid onset of the change which occurs after 0.2–0.3 second, even in some cases as early as after 90 σ, argues against an explanation which invokes vascular processes, as I already emphasized once before in my second report[2]. Likewise against vascular

---

[1] *Ziehen*: Physiologische Psychologie. 12th edition, p. 539. Jena, 1924.

[2] According to *Fano*, vascular reflexes occur only after 2–7 seconds.

processes is the fleeting character of the change which is frequently over after 1, or at the latest after 2 seconds. In my first report I pointed out that the impossibility of recording a curve with similar oscillations from the subcutaneous tissue of a limb, *e.g.* from the tibia, militates against the assumption of a vascular origin of the α-w of the E.E.G. In spite of this, and even though this view is also supported by the fact that the E.E.G. is not changed by amyl nitrite, I wanted to discuss this objection here briefly once again, because for *this* question too the result obtained when one records the E.E.G. from a skull defect and simultaneously from the skull as a whole is of particularly great importance. In three people with skull defects I performed a total of 28 experiments in which a simultaneous recording from the defect, and from forehead and occiput was taken when a precisely timed stimulus was applied. In these experiments differences in the time of onset of the reaction of the E.E.G. were found. Figure 6 shows such an experiment.

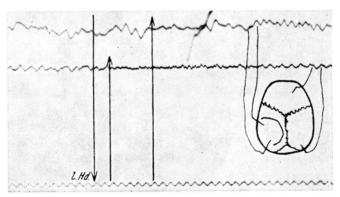

Fig. 6. 48 year old man. Large left-sided skull defect in the parietal region after palliative trepanation. Double-coil galvanometer. Condenser. At the top: E.E.G. recorded with needle electrodes, 9 cm apart, in the area of the skull defect; below: E.E.G. recorded with needle electrodes from the right frontal and the right occipital quadrants of the head. At the bottom: time in 1/10ths sec. *l.HD.*: touching and stroking the left hand.

In a 48 year old man Th. a large palliative trepanation had been carried out by Mr. *Guleke* because of a tumor in the depth of the left hemisphere. Through one galvanometer a record was taken from the patient's skull defect in the left parietal region with chlorided silver needles placed 9 cm apart. Through a second galvanometer a record was taken with chlorided silver needles from the forehead and occiput on the right side. Upon touching the left hand the familiar change in the E.E.G. recorded from the forehead and occiput takes place after 0.25 second, whereas the corresponding change in the E.E.G. recorded from the skull defect takes place only after 0.75 second, thus 0.5 second later. As in all simultaneous recordings, the needles were arranged in the same fashion, so that those placed anteriorly were connected with the corresponding poles of their respective galvanometers. Th. had his eyes closed and was lying in a comfortable supine position on the couch. As already emphasized before, the difference in time, as well as the non-congruence of the segment of the record marked with a cross in Figure 5, argues, of course, against an extracranial cause of its origin[T30], such as *e.g.* tremor movements and so forth. The difference in time also militates against the possibility that the stimulus might have caused a change in the skin vessels. Obviously such a change would have to manifest itself simultaneously on the two sides of the skull and under these circumstances there would be no reason why such a considerable time difference of 0.5 second should appear. Such time differences were observed repeatedly when recording simultaneously from a defect and from the entire skull. They argue unequivocally against any extracranial causes of the change in the E.E.G. and confirm its cerebral origin. With a different location of the defect and the application of other stimuli, the change in the E.E.G. recorded from the defect may occur earlier than in the E.E.G. recorded from forehead and occiput. For the time being I do not want to discuss this matter in more detail and only wish to emphasize strongly that time differences were found and that this fact prohibits any explanation that would attribute these differences to extracranial causes, head movements and the like or to changes in the skin vessels of the head. The considerable time difference observed in the present case can probably be explained by the fact that in Th., in spite of the extensive palliative trepanation, a considerable increase in intracranial pressure existed at the time of recording of the curves. In another of the cases studied, there also existed a certain increase in intracranial pressure at the time when the measurements were made, whereas in the third this was not the case. Perhaps I would have missed the only very small time difference existing under normal conditions had my attention not been drawn to this delay in these pathologically altered cases which therefore made it possible for me to recognize its great significance for the problems which interest us here.

In my second report I proposed the working hypothesis that the α-w represent concomitant phenomena of those material processes in the cerebrum which one calls psychophysical, because they can be associated with conscious phenomena. I do not wish to discuss once again the reasons which prompted me to make such an assumption. Furthermore, in that paper I came to the conclusion that the changes of the E.E.G. which occur under the influence of sensory stimuli that focus the attention, have to be attributed to inhibitory effects. Of course, one could also consider whether peripheral innervations, stimulated by the processes of attention, could perhaps cause these changes of the E.E.G. Through *Allers'* and *Scheminzky's*[1] studies it is known that the mere imagining of a movement leads to current oscillations in the involved muscles. These oscillations can be observed with suitable methods of investigation. *Ottfried Foerster* pointed out as early as 1929[2] that the hitherto accepted notion that only afferent excitations are involved in sensations, needs to be amended. According to him, the central nervous system intervenes by means of efferent pathways in these excitatory processes and this especially then, when attention is focussed on a

[1] *Allers* and *Scheminzky*: Über Aktionsströme der Muskeln bei mot. Vorstellungen und verwandten Vorgängen. Pflügers Arch., **212**, 169 (1926).

[2] *Foerster, Ottfried*: Verh. Ges. dtsch. Nervenärzte. Discussion of *Altenburger's* and *Kroll's* report, p. 268. Würzburg, 1929.

sensory event. Thus, besides the processes of adjustment in the corresponding sense organ, one would have to assume the operation of additional efferent excitatory processes when attention is focussed upon a sensory impression. For instance, corticofugal pathways of this kind, which connect the visual cortex of the calcarine fissure with the lateral geniculate body, were demonstrated experimentally by *Biemand*[1]. On the basis of the earlier and the present observations, I imagine that the changes in the E.E.G., which *e.g.* occur when a visual stimulus affects an experimental subject who lies in a dark room with open eyes, originate in the manner schematically represented in Figure 7.

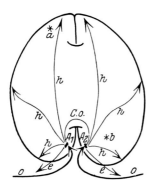

Fig. 7. Schema. *o*, corticopetal visual pathways; *e*, corticofugal pathways originating from the visual area. A_1 and A_2, regions excited within the visual area; *C.o.*, fibers interconnecting the two visual areas; *h*, fiber connections between the visual area and other cortical regions through which inhibitory effects can be mediated. *a* and *b*, areas over which needle electrodes lie on the skull.

Through the corticopetal visual pathway *o* an excitatory process is conveyed to the two visual centers in the calcarine fissures, which are interconnected by commissural fibers (*C.o.*). Thus, the centers of activity A_1 and A_2 are formed in the visual area, from which, through the efferent pathways *e*, influences are transmitted to the lateral geniculate body. The excitatory process in the centers of activity is, however, associated with an inhibitory influence exerted upon the entire cortex, which, it is assumed, is transmitted by the pathways labelled *h* in the diagram. When the E.E.G. is recorded from the areas of the skull lying above *a* and *b*, an inhibitory process will become apparent at the recording points shortly after the influence of the visual stimulus; the α-w disappear transiently to return after 1–2 seconds. As I had emphasized in my second report, such an explanation would confirm the assumption that the cerebrum reacts as a whole to every sensory stimulus and thus in fact represents a unified entity. I likewise emphasized that by making such an assumption there may be a simple explanation for the negative results of metabolic investigations on mental work obtained so far. I do not wish to repeat this here, but I would like to discuss the observation reported above and illustrated in Figure 6, because meanwhile the result of the autopsy carried out in our Pathological Institute (Prof. *Berblinger*) has also become available. As had been suspected, a large, fairly sharply circumscribed tumor, which because of its location could not have been removed, was found deep in the left cerebral hemisphere in the region of the palliative trepanation. The

[1] *Biemand, A.*: Experimentell-anatomische Untersuchungen über die corticofugalen optischen Verbindungen bei Kaninchen und Affen. Z. Neur., **129**, 65 (1930).

conditions in this case were approximately as represented schematically in Figure 8.

The touch stimulus to the left hand is conveyed through the lemniscal fibers S to the postcentral gyrus (c=central sulcus). There a center of activity A arises, from which probably efferent excitations are projected centrifugally along pathway e, when attention has been aroused. The excitatory process itself, in A, generates an

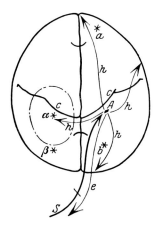

Fig. 8. Schema. S, lemniscal pathway; c, central sulcus; A excited area in Cp[T31]; e, corticofugal pathways originating from there; h, fiber connections from Cp with other cortical areas of the ipsilateral and the contralateral hemisphere through which inhibitory effects could be transmitted. Oval-shaped area outlined by the interrupted line: localization of the tumor in the 48 year old man (Figure 6); a and b, location of the needle electrodes over the right hemicranium; α and β, location of the needle electrodes in the area of the left-sided skull defect.

inhibitory influence which is conveyed through pathways h to the various regions of the ipsilateral and the contralateral hemisphere. If one now records from the areas on the right side of the skull, overlying a and b, and in addition with the second galvanometer from points α and β in the region of the skull defect, one finds that the inhibitory effect at electrodes α and β occurs 0.5 second later than at points a and b. In the light of the post-mortem[T32] findings, this appears quite understandable. For in the depth of the left hemisphere there is the large tumor which, in spite of the palliative trepanation, exerts pressure upon the neighboring area. A slowing of conduction in the connecting pathways subjected to the effects of the pressure, or, alternatively, a slow response of the cortex over the tumor to the inhibitory influence, transmitted from A, offers a likely explanation for the delay. This delayed reaction, in the present case, argues in favor of an explanation invoking an inhibitory process originating from the center of activity and against any influence upon the E.E.G. exerted by the efferent excitation simultaneously emanating from this center. Because, as previously mentioned, this is not an isolated observation, and the time differences found in other investigations with simultaneous recordings also easily fit this explanation, there is a certain probability that it is correct. As had been mentioned above, in another case where there was no increase in intracranial pressure, the differences in time were much less and amounted to only 0.1–0.15 second. Together with the other arguments set forth above, these results of measuring the time of the response to sensory stimuli[T33] carried out in records taken simultaneously from a skull defect and from the skull as a whole, seem to me to argue unequivocally in favor of a central origin of the E.E.G. These results are more easily understood in the light of the explanation just given, but further investigations are still necessary to determine whether it is entirely correct. However, according to the material available so far this interpretation seems to me the most natural one. For us, the fact that in the two different simultaneous recordings a difference in the time of the reaction can be demonstrated, is sufficient for the present. It renders improbable explanations invoking extracranial and also extracerebral causes for the occurrence of the E.E.G. changes appearing under the influence of sensory stimuli. In conjunction with the reasons cited above, the responsiveness of the E.E.G. to all processes which focus attention argues in favor of its central origin.

If therefore it is correct — and in view of the above argument there can hardly be any further doubt about this — that the E.E.G. does in fact originate in the brain, one would expect that it should be possible to influence it by poisons known to affect the central nervous system. Cocaine is such a poison and is unfortunately often abused precisely because of its stimulating action upon psychic processes[1]. In my first report I gave an account of an animal experiment in which a distinct increase in the amplitude of the curve recorded from the cerebral cortex occurred under the influence of cocaine. Simultaneously, however, in the animal subjected to the pharmacological influence of cocaine, the amplitude of the deflections of the E.C.G.[T34] also considerably increased.

I have two observations on the influence of cocaine upon the human E.E.G. Both were obtained in persons in whom recordings were taken with chlorided silver needles from the intact skull. In a 24 year old man, after a dose of 0.03 gram of cocaine hydrochloride was given subcutaneously, dilatation of the pupils, striking pallor of the face, acceleration of the pulse and a distinct stimulating action upon psychic processes could be noted. Under the influence of cocaine the amplitude of the α-w of the E.E.G. had increased several times in spite of a diminution in the height of the R wave of the E.C.G.[T35] from 33 mm to 22 mm which corresponded to the acceleration of the pulse.

In a second observation on the influence of cocaine upon the E.E.G., this change was not so pronounced, but still distinctly recognizable. Figure 9 is taken from this observation.

This is a 21 year old young man in whom a record was taken with chlorided silver needles from forehead and occiput. Simultaneously an E.C.G. was recorded from the left arm and left leg (*Einthoven*: lead III).

Figure 10 is recorded 20 minutes after subcutaneous administration of 0.03 gram of cocaine hydrochloride, the young man remaining in the same position, resting comfortably on a couch with his eyes closed. The pupils have become distinctly dilated, the face of this man, who normally has a very fresh complexion, shows the characteristic pallor and the length of the pulse has diminished from 0.85 to 0.65 second. If one compares Figures 9 and 10, one sees the amplitude increase

---

[1] A clear compilation and critical discussion of the literature concerning the effect of cocaine on psychic functions is given by *A. Offermann*: Über die zentrale Wirkung des Cocains und einiger neuen Ersatzpräparate. Arch. f. Psychiatr., **76**, 600 (1926), especially p. 606 and subsequent pages; compare also: *R. Allers* and *O. Hochstädt*: Über die Angriffsorte des Cocains im Zentralnervensystem. Z. exper. Med., **59**, 359 (1928).

of the α-w of the E.E.G. The highest α-w found in Figure 10 measure 9.1 mm, whereas before administration of cocaine only exceptionally an α-w amplitude of 8 mm was reached. I also wish to stress that the numerous measurements in this and the previous observation indicated that the length of the α-w does not change under the influence of cocaine; their length remains the same, the deflections, however, become higher,

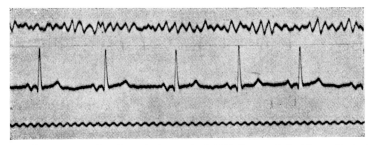

Fig. 9. 21 year old man. Recording from the intact skull. E.E.G. recorded with needle electrodes from the left frontal and right occipital quadrants of the head. E.C.G. from the left arm and left leg with lead foil electrodes. Time in 1/10ths sec.

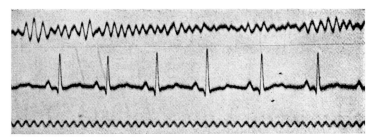

Fig. 10. From the same young man as Figure 9 and with the same recording conditions; 20 min after subcutaneous administration of 0.03 gram of cocaine hydrochloride.

whereas the β-w remain unaltered. The stimulating action of cocaine upon psychic processes is thus associated with a distinct increase in amplitude of the E.E.G., which is exclusively attributable to an amplitude increase of the α-w.

Among the poisons which in therapeutic doses exert an action predominantly confined to the central nervous system are the sleep-inducing drugs[T36]. I need not discuss here the profound difference which exists between sleep and narcosis and can refer to the extensive literature on this question. — In psychiatric clinics it is sometimes necessary to make use of scopolamine in extremely agitated patients who may become dangerous to themselves and to others. The action of scopolamine, in the doses used, is predominantly confined to the cerebrum. The paralyzing influence exerted upon the motor cortex by this drug becomes manifest by the appearance of *Babinski's* sign. In clinical practice scopolamine is usually given together with morphine, in order to attenuate some of the disagreeable side effects which scopolamine exerts upon the mucous membranes, etc. Thus, the psychiatrist not infrequently has the opportunity to observe the action of this drug. In a 38 year old engineer, suffering from manic-depressive psychosis and who exhibited states of extreme motor agitation, the administration of scopolamine had become necessary on repeated occasions, so that with the rapid habituation to the drug an increase in dosage was required.

Figure 11 shows the effect of scopolamine upon the E.E.G.: 0.001 gram of scopolamine hydrobromide+0.02 gram of morphine had been given because of a

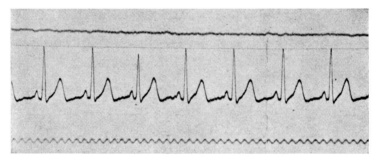

Fig. 11. 38 year old man, F. Recording from the intact skull. E.E.G. with needle electrodes recorded from the left frontal and the right occipital quadrants of the head. E.C.G. from both arms with lead foil electrodes. Time in 1/10ths sec. — F. had received 1.75 hours before 0.001 gram of scopolamine hydrobromide + 0.02 gram of morphine hydrochloride subcutaneously.

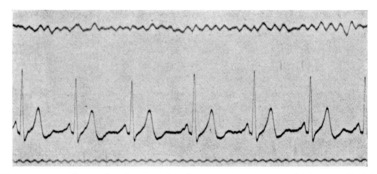

Fig. 12. The same recordings taken in F., as in Figure 11, but three weeks later and without drugs.

state of extreme agitation. The E.E.G. was recorded during deep scopolamine sleep 1.75 hours after the injection. The scopolamine effect was clearly pronounced: the pupils were maximally dilated, there was striking pallor of the face and the reaction to stimuli was almost completely abolished. The E.E.G. barely shows some small oscillations and in many places discloses only suggestions of α-w; most of the time it runs as a horizontal line. In the same engineer, the curve shown in Figure 12 was recorded three weeks later under exactly the same conditions, after the agitation had abated to some extent. This enabled one to establish some rapport with the patient and therefore made it possible to perform such an investigation without hesitation. F. was lying on a couch in a supine position with his eyes closed. The record was taken with chlorided silver needles from forehead and occiput. The great differences of the E.E.G.s in the two recordings are unmistakable and demonstrate a very powerful action of the scopolamine upon the E.E.G. That this change of the E.E.G. only occurs when the scopolamine actually exerts a paralyzing action upon the central nervous system becomes apparent from the following observation. With a 22 year old patient, who also suffered from manic agitation and had also received scopolamine on repeated occasions, I was forced to give scopolamine during the examination, the 0.0005 gram dose in her case being too small in view of her state of habituation to the drug. There was no effect of the scopolamine upon psychic functions, nor was there any alteration of the E.E.G., although the pupils became distinctly dilated and the face paler. A change in the α-w of the E.E.G. could thus not be demonstrated in this case.

One could, of course, object that the change in the scopolamine curve could be related to the fact that F. had been deeply asleep, in other words that sleep in itself, including physiological sleep, may be associated with such changes of the E.E.G. As I already emphasized in my second report, this is definitely not the case.

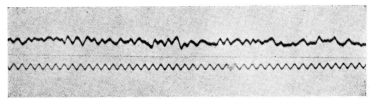

Fig. 13. 35 year old physician. E.E.G. recorded with silver foil electrodes from forehead and occiput. Time in 1/10ths sec. In deep sleep, 1.5 hours after falling asleep.

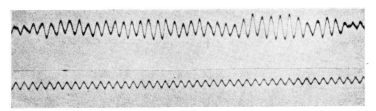

Fig. 14. From the same gentleman as Figure 13 with the same recording method. Following arousal from 2 hours of sleep.

Figure 13 shows the curve of one of my assistants, Dr. G. He is deeply asleep; 1.5 hours have elapsed since he fell asleep. The record from the skull in this case is taken with silver foil electrodes attached to the forehead and the occiput, in the manner described earlier. Needle electrodes could not be used, because G. could have injured himself, had he suddenly turned his head at the beginning of sleep. Also, it was decided to omit the recording of an E.C.G. from the arms, because undoubtedly the electrodes would have hindered the onset of sleep. In the curve the α-w of the E.E.G. are very distinctly visible, however, the difference in comparison with Figure 14 is very striking.

It was obtained from the same Dr. G., on the same day. He was gently awakened after 2 hours of sleep. He lies comfortably on the couch, exactly in the same position as during the preceding sleep, completely awake and with his eyes closed. One sees how much higher are the α-w of the E.E.G. Whereas in deep sleep the maximal amplitude of the α-w measures 5.5 mm, their amplitude after arousal is 10 mm and is thus almost twice as large. The length of the α-w undergoes no change during sleep, as many measurements have demonstrated. Thus, even though in deep sleep a flattening of the E.E.G. also occurs, the record shown in Figure 13 is nevertheless not comparable with the altered curve appearing in the narcotic sleep induced by scopolamine. Therefore the objection that the state of sleep in itself is associated with a disappearance of the α-w is rendered untenable. Of course, a very cautious interpreter could raise the objection against the scopolamine curve that three weeks had elapsed between the two recordings and meanwhile the local conditions at the sites of recording on the skull could have become altered to such an extent that the larger amplitude E.E.G. of the later curve could be related to this. I hold such an objection to be entirely incorrect.

Nevertheless, the only completely convincing changes are those which occur and, when circumstances permit it, also disappear again in one and the same examination. This can be observed during a narcosis as it is performed for the purpose of carrying out surgical interventions. Over the years I had the opportunity to make such observations three times. In 1927 I made such an observation in a 40 year old man who had a large bone defect in the left temporoparietal region following a palliative trepanation carried out by Mr. *Guleke* because of a basal tumor. Records were taken by means of a galvanometer with the zinc plated steel needles described by *Trendelenburg* and a curve was recorded before narcosis; the recording was taken from the skull defect. For reasons irrelevant to the present discussion, the needles were then removed and were reinserted only during deep narcosis, and this, as much as possible, at the same sites used before narcosis. The E.E.G. recorded now showed a profound change; α-w were hardly recognizable any longer, while in the record before narcosis they had been very distinct and of large amplitude. One can of course criticize this result, which appeared at first convincing to me, on the ground that the needles described by *Trendelenburg* are not entirely free of polarization and also, that during the second recording they may not have been lying at exactly the same spot in the tissue. I must admit that in fact even small displacements of the needle tips in the tissue have exerted a completely unexpected influence upon the quality of the E.E.G., especially when recordings were taken from bone defects. I therefore convinced myself, on the basis of further observations, that the observation just described cannot be considered as conclusive because of these objections.

The second observation concerns a 56 year old man who had a large skull defect over the forehead. Before the planned narcosis he remained fasting and received 0.02 gram of Pantopon + 0.05 gram of ephedrine subcutaneously. Thirty minutes later the E.E.G. was recorded with chlorided silver needles which were placed 4 cm apart in the area of the skull defect, and the E.C.G. was recorded from both arms with lead foil electrodes.

Figure 15 shows the record which was written at a somewhat slower speed of the recording instrument. Shortly after this recording a drop chloroform narcosis was started, while the two curves were continuously observed on the galvanometer.

Very soon after the chloroform application was begun, the amplitude of the deflections of the E.E.G. clearly increased in this man, who at that time was still lying completely quiet with his eyes closed. Very soon thereafter an unmistakable stage of excitation began during which, by a sudden movement of the head, he pulled out the silver needles which had been placed subcutaneously in the area of the defect,

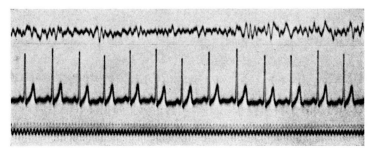

Fig. 15. 56 year old man. Bone defect on the forehead. E.E.G. from the area of the defect with needle electrodes 4 cm apart; E.C.G.[T37] recorded from both arms. Time in 1/10ths sec.

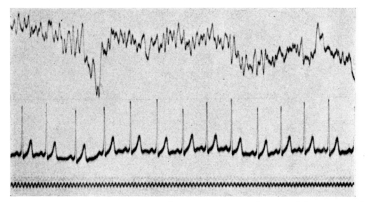

Fig. 16. From the same man as Figure 15, under the same recording conditions, but during the stage of excitation of chloroform narcosis.

so that they had to be reinserted. Figure 16 shows a record taken immediately thereafter, which is somewhat distorted by head movements.

One nevertheless recognizes the considerable increase in amplitude of the α-w of the E.E.G., which grew from 4 to 11 mm, *i.e.* almost three times and whose amplitude increase had been observed already before the pulled out needles had been reinserted[T38]. Because of the continuous restlessness of the man who, as it turned out later, was quite addicted to drink, it was impossible to obtain a satisfactory narcosis without using excessive amounts of chloroform, and therefore the attempt was given up. Yet this second observation yielded the important result that in the stage of excitation of narcosis, just as one would have expected, the amplitude of the deflections of the E.E.G. augments, the α-w alone being involved in this amplitude increase.

Only the third observation, which I wish to report here, may be considered successful and perfect in every way. It is that of a 21 year old healthy man who once before in his 17th year, after an injury, had undergone a narcosis, which he had tolerated well. I particularly made sure that he was a complete abstainer, so that I did not have to expect a stage of marked excitation. Two hours before the planned narcosis he received 0.02 gram of Pantopon + 0.05 gram of ephedrine. A biparietal needle recording from the skull was chosen to make it possible for him to lie with complete comfort in a supine position during the narcosis and to ensure that the results would not be prejudiced by changes in position or movements. As was explained above (see Figure 5), the deflections of the E.E.G. in such a recording are in general somewhat smaller, but the E.E.G. nevertheless exhibits all characteristic details. The E.C.G. was recorded from both arms with lead foil electrodes.

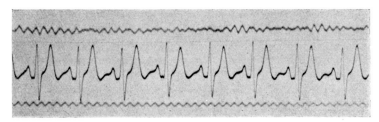

Fig. 17. Young man, aged 21 years. Recording from the intact skull. E.E.G. with needles from both parietal eminences; E.C.G. recorded from both arms. Time in 1/10ths sec.

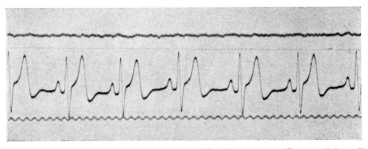

Fig. 18. From the same young man as Figure 17 and under the same recording conditions. During light chloroform narcosis.

Figure 17 reproduces a record taken in this man shortly before beginning of the narcosis, while he lay with his eyes closed in a comfortable supine position. In the E.E.G. curve recorded with a rather low amplitude, the α-w are clearly visible. After recording several meters of the curve, the drop chloroform narcosis is started. A light narcosis with a completely quiet onset and without a stage of excitation sets in; the two needle electrodes attached to the skull remain in place and the heart is observed simultaneously in the E.C.G. curve. After a pronounced anesthetic effect of chloroform has taken place and the corneal reflex has just been extinguished, several additional meters of the curve are recorded, of which Figure 18 represents a small segment.

It is evident that the E.E.G. now more or less approaches a straight line and in many places discloses only flattened α-w in the form of insignificant deflections. It was now possible to observe very beautifully how every time the narcosis subsided, the E.E.G. curve increased in amplitude; when it was deepened by renewed dropping of chloroform, the E.E.G. again approached more closely a straight line. The chloroform mask was now removed and while the needle electrodes remained in place, the

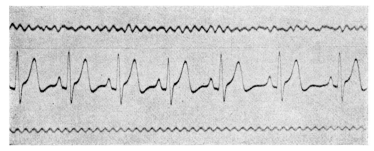

Fig. 19. From the same young man as Figures 17 and 18, and under the same recording conditions; 30 minutes after removal of the chloroform mask.

man's awakening was awaited. Thirty minutes after removing the chloroform mask a third series of curves was recorded in the fully awake man who also, upon questioning, denied any headaches, nausea and other such symptoms. At that time he lay exactly in the same position as during the narcosis and kept his eyes closed. Figure 19 shows such a record.

It is evident that the E.E.G. has changed in comparison with Figure 18 and has again assumed the same form as before induction of the narcosis. The third observation therefore confirms the alteration of the E.E.G. during narcosis, which I had already observed in 1927. The second, otherwise incomplete observation, established that the stage of excitation of narcosis causes an increase in the amplitude of the α-w. During the narcosis itself a decrease in amplitude or, respectively, a disappearance of the α-w of the E.E.G. occurs. This observation is in excellent agreement with the observations made with scopolamine administration and confirms the results obtained there. Above all, the third observation demonstrates very well how a steady amplitude increase of the α-w of the E.E.G. takes place, as the cerebrum increasingly takes up its functions during awakening from narcosis. An objection which I already discussed above could, however, also be raised here. During narcosis a relaxation of the musculature occurs and certain tremor movements, which perhaps are present in the waking state and disappear during narcosis, could be the cause of the change of the E.E.G. during narcosis. Upon return of consciousness the innervation of the muscles would be reestablished and then the tremor movements could again become manifest. With regard to the simultaneous recordings from two areas of the intact skull, or from a bone defect and from the skull as a whole, I have already adequately refuted the explanation that the α-w of the E.E.G. are caused by extracranial factors, and thus, I believe, I need not go into this here again.

The demonstration of the alteration of the E.E.G. under the influence of centrally acting poisons seems to me to be of utmost importance for the evaluation of the E.E.G. We know that chloroform in doses used during narcosis, as administered also in these cases, does not produce any alteration of the circulation in the sub-cutaneous tissue and in the bone, in whose immediate proximity the chlorided silver needles lie, and that therefore the disappearance of the α-w of the E.E.G. could not be explained on this basis. Also the influence of chloroform upon the cerebral circulation is not such as to cause an interruption of the latter. Thus the change of the E.E.G. could not be explained by such an effect[1]. With the customary dosage of chloroform indeed one wants to avoid precisely any damage to the heart and circula-tion. These reasons unequivocally argue in favor of the view that the change of the E.E.G. in narcosis can only be related to the altered state of activity of the central nervous system, and particularly, I presume, to that of the cerebral cortex, which is the first to be rendered inactive by the narcosis. This observation certainly indicates that the E.E.G. must be intimately connected with the function of the brain and especially with that of the cerebral cortex. Also, the observations on the change of the E.E.G. in the excitatory stage of narcosis, those concerning the changes under the influence of cocaine and, finally, the alterations in deep scopolamine sleep, together with the changes of the E.E.G. observed during natural sleep, point in the same direction. I therefore believe that by these observations on centrally acting poisons my working hypothesis advanced in the second report, which postulates that the α-w of the E.E.G. are concomitant phenomena of those material processes which one calls psychophysical, has received very substantial support. Thus, I am of the opinion that the α-w indeed originate from the cerebral cortex and that they represent concomitant phenomena of the material processes in the cerebral cortex which are connected with processes of consciousness.

If centrally acting poisons which elicit clear alterations in the course of psychical events produce such evident findings in the E.E.G., then one also ought to expect that those diseases of the brain which are associated with disturbances of psycho-physical processes should produce similar changes. In investigating such patients the physiological changes of the E.E.G. caused by an increase in attention or move-ments etc., of course had to be taken into consideration. Also, it was necessary that the subjects investigated should not be under the influence of potent drugs, which by themselves could change the E.E.G. All patients in whom states of motor agitation were present, whether these were the urge to move of a manic, the movements of fear of a melancholic, or the stereotyped movements of a schizophrenic, were of course unsuited for my investigations, for satisfactory E.E.G.s could not be recorded because of such behavior exhibited by the patients. In addition, all hallucinating patients, who because of their perceptual illusions exhibit an increase in attention, are not suited for such investigations. Anxious agitation elicited by the impending recording of an E.E.G. in patients with whom rapport is otherwise easy to establish, equally falsifies the results; any physical pain acts in the same way. Thus, *e.g.* an other-wise successful record in a completely quiet patient whose thinking was well organized,

---

[1] According to *Yamakita's* excellent animal experiments the blood supply to the brain even increases during narcosis!

was distorted because during the recording he suffered from a toothache, a fact which at first he had concealed.

As always, the records were taken with the patient lying in a comfortable, supine position, the head resting on a pillow which was somewhat raised. The needles were inserted under local anesthesia so that no painful stimulus was produced. During the recording the eyes of the experimental subject were closed; also, all external stimuli were, as far as possible, excluded, as already stressed in my second report. These dispositions could, however, not be put into effect in all patients who appeared suitable for the examination, even after exclusion of those mentioned above; for this reason the examination sometimes had to be terminated before its completion. Nevertheless in 70 patients good E.E.G.s could be recorded and I would like to report now on some of the results obtained in them.

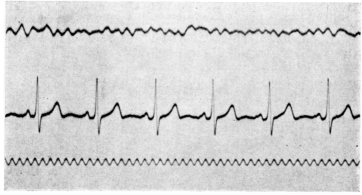

Fig. 20. 19 year old man with cerebellar tumor. E.E.G. with needle electrodes from the left frontal and the right occipital quadrants of the head. E.C.G. recorded from both arms. Time in 1/10ths sec.

Progressive increase in intracranial pressure, as is well known, is associated with increasing stupor. Finally, somnolence sets in. At this stage the patients at first can still be aroused for a short time by energetic stimuli and be made to respond. When left to themselves they continue to doze on again. It was this marked alteration in the course of the psychophysical processes which I decided to investigate first. In a 19 year old farmer F., in whom headaches, vomiting, visual and gait disturbances had allegedly appeared only five weeks before, a high degree of bilateral papilloedema and unequivocal neurological signs were found which pointed to a tumor in the posterior fossa, most likely in the left cerebellar hemisphere. F., it is true, was clear in his mind and not confused, but nevertheless markedly stuporous and, for instance, ate only when coaxed to do so. The E.E.G. of this patient F. is shown in Figure 20.

As in all figures shown here, only a small segment taken from a curve of several meters length is reproduced; in every case at least six separate recordings of the curve, each at least 1 m in length, were written in order to exclude dubious results. In contrast to the E.E.G. of a healthy individual, of which I illustrated examples in my earlier reports, one is struck by the length of the α-w which exhibit a duration of 140–250 σ, whereas in a healthy person they do not exceed an upper limit of 120 σ. This change is found not only in the very small segment of the curve reproduced here, but in all six curves, and these longer α-w do not appear in an isolated fashion but regularly in trains, one after another, whereas between them waves of normal length of 115–120 σ are also found. Even though in the numerous E.E.G.s which I have now recorded in 158 persons in the course of six years, I have, in isolated instances, also noted a few α-w prolonged beyond the average length, these nevertheless occur only sporadically as isolated waves in normals, and not as trains of waves, one after another, as is the case here. Measurements in the curves recorded in F. show that the length of the pulse has changed in correspondence with the more or less distinctly apparent general signs of increased intracranial pressure, the somnolence being at times deeper, at others lighter. Sporadically the periods of relative slowing of the pulse, measured in the E.C.G., coincide with the appearance of trains of longer α-w in the E.E.G., but this is by no means consistently the case. I regard the alteration of the E.E.G. reproduced in Figure 20 to be pathological. Only a few days after the record which is reproduced here had been obtained, the patient expired very suddenly, after having exhibited severe signs of increased intracranial pressure. The autopsy carried out at the Pathological Institute (Prof. *Berblinger*) revealed a tumor in the left cerebellar hemisphere. I hardly need to point out that the curves of this patient, who had been rendered somnolent by increased intracranial pressure, differ fundamentally from those of a healthy sleeping subject as shown in Figure 13, *insofar* as in normal sleep, in spite of a diminution in amplitude, no change of the length of the α-w, as seen here, takes place. It is precisely this change of the E.E.G. which I have very frequently observed in raised intracranial pressure and had already established in a series of string galvanometer curves dating from the year 1925. At that time I did not correctly recognize that they were pathologically altered. Also in patients with palliative trepanations, when the general signs of increased pressure persist in spite of the decompression, because of rapid growth of the neoplasm, the prolonged α-w appear very clearly in E.E.G.s recorded with needles locally from the skull defect. For this reason, as was stressed in my second report, one can by no means consider as normal all E.E.G.s recorded from skull defects in patients with palliative trepanations[T39].

An acute hydrocephalus as well, whether caused by a small tumor obstructing the pathways of flow of the cerebrospinal fluid or by other factors, is accompanied by a marked increase in intracranial pressure and can therefore lead to somnolence and mental changes.

Figure 21 shows the record from a 33 year old woman who, after a head injury, fell acutely ill with very severe signs of increased intracranial pressure. The encephalogram[T40] disclosed an enormous internal hydrocephalus involving predominantly the lateral ventricles. In Figure 21 one again sees the very distinct changes of the E.E.G. which consist of the appearance of strikingly long α-w exhibiting a length of 160–200 σ; in addition, however, normal α-w of 100–105 σ are also found. During the recording the somnolent, usually completely disoriented and frequently incontinent patient lay with her eyes closed and was completely listless, so that distortions by movements, which incidentally were carefully looked for, are out of the question. This recording further confirms the statements made previously, that an increase in intracranial pressure is associated with a change in the E.E.G. In the present case the autopsy (Pathological Institute, Prof. *Berblinger*) revealed a small tumor in the

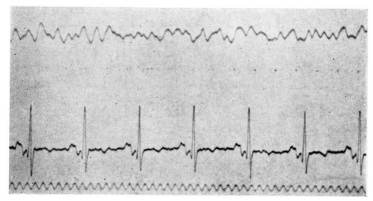

Fig. 21. 33 year old woman with extensive internal hydrocephalus, associated with tumor of the 4th ventricle. E.E.G. with needle electrodes from the left frontal and the right occipital quadrants of the head; E.C.G. recorded from both arms. Time in 1/10ths sec.

floor of the 4th ventricle which obstructed the flow of cerebral spinal fluid, but by itself had not produced any significant focal signs. In other cases of brain tumor, in patients who did not present general signs of increased pressure, I obtained normal curves when recording the E.E.G. with chlorided silver needles from forehead and occiput. Thus, I am indeed of the opinion that the increase in intracranial pressure, quite independently of the location of the tumor, leads to the changes of the E.E.G.

Intracranial hemorrhages too, which most often are associated with increased intracranial pressure, lead to alterations of the E.E.G. Figure 22 comes from a 29 year old man who, 14 days previously, while apparently in perfect health, had suffered a "stroke".

At the time of recording clear signs of increased intracranial pressure still persisted; at lumbar puncture the intracranial pressure measured 310 mm of water. The patient was slightly somnolent. Certain signs, not to be discussed further here, as well as the results of the cerebrospinal fluid examination, indicated an intracranial subarachnoid hemorrhage the sequels of which receded in the course of subsequent months. The alteration of the E.E.G. as compared with a normal record again manifested itself by an increased duration and fusion of the α-w, resulting in wave lengths of 140–180 σ, and occasionally even of 210 σ. Such prolonged fused α-w did not just appear singly, but they frequently occurred several times one after the other.

In another patient, a 30 year old civil servant, a hemorrhage from a small aneurysm of the anterior cerebral artery had occurred 14 days before the recording reproduced here was obtained; subsequently, the bleeding recurred and led to a clinical state of severe stupor and disorientation, but with only transient signs of increased intracranial pressure. At the time of the recording of the E.E.G. the pressure, measured at lumbar puncture, was 260 mm of water.

The findings are shown in Figure 23. Again there are clear alterations of the E.E.G. There were 166–230 σ α-w which could be demonstrated time and again in records taken several days apart. The autopsy (Pathological Institute, Prof. *Berblinger*) showed old and fresh hemorrhages from an aneurysm of the anterior cerebral artery with softening of the medial portions of the orbital gyri on both sides.

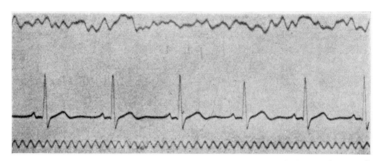

Fig. 22. 29 year old man. 14 days after a subarachnoid hemorrhage. E.E.G. with needle electrodes from the left frontal and the right occipital quadrants of the head; E.C.G. recorded from both arms. Time in 1/10ths sec.

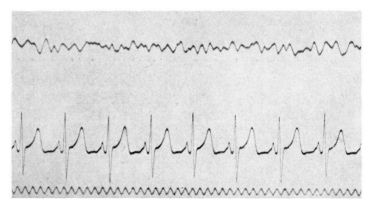

Fig. 23. 30 year old man. Repeated hemorrhages from aneurysm of the anterior cerebral artery. E.E.G. with needle electrodes from the left frontal and the right occipital quadrants of the head; E.C.G. recorded from both arms. Time in 1/10ths sec.

Very severe and striking changes of the E.E.G. were found in a 38 year old woman who three weeks prior to the examination had sustained a skull fracture with cerebral contusion in a motorcycle accident. She was conscious on admission, yet completely disoriented and when left alone repeatedly lapsed into a somnolent state and was incontinent, but did not exhibit any signs of raised intracranial pressure.

Figure 24 shows the record obtained from her. In this patient who was lying completely still, with eyes closed, and was not paying the slightest attention to any of the events in her surroundings, nor to the recording of the curves, the α-w show a length of 150–290 σ; these prolonged or fused α-w in this case too are not isolated, but occur one after another for prolonged periods of time.

In cases of severe traumatic dementia after skull fracture in which, at the time of recording, signs of increased intracranial pressure were absent, I also found clear alterations of the E.E.G. These findings indicate that alterations of the E.E.G.

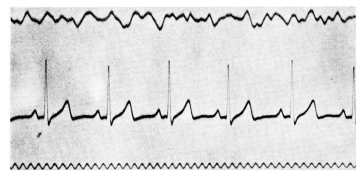

Fig. 24. 38 year old woman. Skull fracture with cerebral contusion three weeks earlier. E.E.G. with needle electrodes from the left frontal and the right occipital quadrants of the head; E.C.G. recorded from both arms. Time in 1/10ths sec.

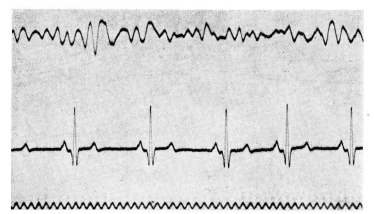

Fig. 25. 22 year old girl with genuine epilepsy. E.E.G. with needle electrodes from the left frontal and right occipital quadrants of the head; E.C.G. recorded from both arms. Time in 1/10ths sec.

certainly do not occur only with increased intracranial pressure, or with intracranial disturbances of circulation, as we had to assume from the cases reported before. Very early I was also struck by the observation that genuine epilepsy frequently — eleven times among fourteen investigated patients — reveals distinct alterations of the E.E.G. In almost all cases of genuine epilepsy surprisingly large amplitude deflections of the E.E.G. were found and this quite independently of whether the cranial vault was found to be relatively thin or thick at fluoroscopy.

Figure 25 shows the E.E.G. of a 22 year old housemaid who has suffered from seizures since the 5th year of her life. That this is indeed a case of genuine epilepsy follows from the fact that her mother is also an epileptic. Prior to the recording of the E.E.G. this patient had never received any drugs and thus, as I wish to emphasize, was not under the influence of bromide or Luminal. Mentally she exhibited distinct slowing. This is a case of pronounced epileptic dementia; she also repeatedly exhibited twilight states. One is first struck by the height of the deflections of the curves, essentially to be attributed to high voltage α-w; but in addition the α-w also show a length of 135–200 σ. During the recording the patient was lying completely still with her eyes closed. In ten additional cases of genuine epilepsy I made the same observation. The changes are most pronounced in cases of epileptic dementia which usually develops on a background of genuine epilepsy when seizures persist for a considerable length of time. I reproduce in Figure 26 the E.E.G. of a 35 year old woman with genuine epilepsy, in whom the epileptic seizures have been present since adolescence.

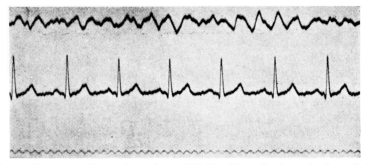

Fig. 26. 35 year old woman with genuine epilepsy. E.E.G. with needle electrodes from the left frontal and the right occipital quadrants of the head; E.C.G. recorded from both arms. Time in 1/10ths sec.

Her father was an epileptic and was known to us in the clinic; the patient's sister also suffers from genuine epilepsy. She has developed the well known epileptic personality changes with irritability and angry disposition. There is a considerable slowing of mental processes, a marked tendency to cling to certain ideas, some tendency to shallow religiosity and a striking weakness of judgement; thus there is a clear epileptic dementia. In Figure 26 a pervading change of the α-w is apparent. They exhibit a length of 170–250 σ. A change in technique with the record being taken from both parietal eminences, instead of from forehead and occiput, resulted in exactly the same curve. In three cases of genuine epilepsy, besides the strikingly high voltage of the E.E.G., one could only sporadically demonstrate very long α-w of the kind occasionally also occurring in normal individuals. In all three cases the illness was recent, only a few seizures had occurred and significant mental changes could not be demonstrated. I consider the alteration of the E.E.G. in epileptic dementia which develops on a background of genuine epilepsy to be of such great importance, because in this case, of course, there can hardly be any question of a disturbance of the general or even of the cerebral circulation. When there is increased intracranial pressure such a disturbance obviously would have to be expected.

I have recorded E.E.G.s in many other patients, as *e.g.* in a case of very severe

Alzheimer's disease, which was confirmed by microscopic examinations and in which the whole cortex was riddled with innumerable lesions. I found in this case an E.E.G. with clear pathological alterations. In another patient with the same disease who is still in hospital, I was, however, not successful in demonstrating deviations of the E.E.G. from normal. The results were similar with patients suffering from multiple sclerosis. In a very severe case with marked mental changes, impaired judgement, disturbances of recent memory and intense euphoria, the E.E.G. is pathological; in several other cases in which mental defects could not be demonstrated the E.E.G. was normal. Also in manic-depressive patients, whenever a satisfactory examination was possible, I was unable to demonstrate any changes in either the manic or the depressive phase. A case of melancholia with most severe inhibitory phenomena[T41] exhibited a normal E.E.G. Cases of schizophrenia too, as far as they could be examined (hallucinating patients, as explained above, were excluded from the investigation) showed no deviations of the E.E.G. from normal.

The study of several cases of congenital mental deficiency which, according to the severity of the defect of intellect and moral sense had to be classified as imbeciles, also caused me a great disappointment. I could not demonstrate any deviations of the E.E.G. from normal. However, I would like to emphasize particularly that it is only possible for the time being to compare the *time* course of the waves of the E.E.G., because the amplitude differences of its waves in different people are essentially dependent upon the local resistance. In this respect the bony skull, the variable thickness of the dura, etc., play a very considerable role. Thus, if one finds a low amplitude E.E.G. in an imbecile, one cannot by any means regard this as obviously pathological, for a very low amplitude E.E.G. may likewise be found in a normal human subject in whom because of anatomical conditions, such as the thickness of the skull etc., a greater resistance in the electrode circuit exists. In the comparisons made above on the actions of poisons, of narcosis etc., it was always the E.E.G. of *one and the same* person in various states that was being compared. Here, however, the comparison would be between the amplitudes of the E.E.G.s of *different* persons. The difference of resistances in various people can have no influence upon the *time* course of the curves, so that the arguments just presented are irrelevant with regard to the temporal alteration of the α-w, yet are applicable to the *amplitude* of the deflections. Besides, up to now I have only studied adults with congenital mental retardation; the investigations are being continued and combined with suitable resistance measurements.

In residual states after epidemic encephalitis I could not find pathological E.E.G.s when the clinical signs indicated the presence, not of the more rarely occurring lesions in the cerebrum, but of the more typical changes in the midbrain.

Also very striking were the findings in the ten cases of dementia paralytica examined to date. In patients with general paresis in whom the disease process had become arrested after malaria treatment, I could not demonstrate definite pathological changes of the E.E.G., even when a considerable mental defect remained. On the other hand, in cases of general paresis which were admitted to the clinic because of mental symptoms of acute onset, I usually found pathological E.E.G.s. As I just explained, no reliance can be placed upon the amplitude of the E.E.G. waves as compared to that of normal ones, although I very definitely had the impression that in general paresis the E.E.G. curves were strikingly low in amplitude. Perhaps this is related to the alterations in the leptomeninges which are so common in general paresis, and to an external hydrocephalus, which, of course, is bound to increase the resistance considerably. These are, however, only conjectures to which I cannot attribute any particular importance. Even if we disregard on principle the amplitude of the deflections of the E.E.G. for the moment, the records in general paresis nevertheless remarkably often exhibit a pattern as shown in Figure 27. This curve was

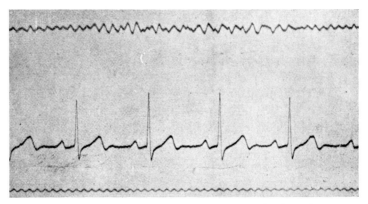

Fig. 27. 44 year old man with dementia paralytica. E.E.G. with needle electrodes from the left frontal and the right occipital quadrants of the head; E.C.G. recorded from both arms. Time in 1/10ths sec.

obtained in a 44 year old farmer, K., in whom dementia paralytica apparently had developed very insiduously, for only three weeks before this recording signs of illness appeared, which drew the attention of his relatives to his condition and led to his admission to the clinic. The neurological findings were those of typical general paresis with marked posterior column signs. The patient was obtunded, apathetic, exhibited a severe intellectual defect and was incontinent. The E.E.G. recorded in the usual fashion in K. who was lying completely still with eyes closed, shows a strikingly irregular pattern[20] of the curve. First, in the segment reproduced here, there appeared α-w of 105 σ; then they became longer, reaching a value of 120 σ, to lengthen still further after a short while to 170 and 200 σ. In cases of general paresis characterized by clinical symptoms of recent onset I have repeatedly found this irregularity of the curves and the marked changes in the length and amplitude of the α-w within a short period of time. I would like to consider this a pathological finding.

The cases of cerebral arteriosclerosis with massive focal manifestations, *e.g.* a sensory aphasia or similar signs, again caused me disappointment. With a recording from forehead and occiput I found a completely normal E.E.G., *provided* a sufficiently long time had elapsed between the onset of the deficits and the recording of the E.E.G.! This is a finding which is in accord with the ones reported above, that *e.g.* a tumor of the temporal lobe which had evolved without general signs of increased pressure, whose location could be verified at operation and which could be removed, had also not caused any alterations in the curves when the E.E.G. was recorded from forehead and occiput. It is precisely on the basis of such observations that I came to believe that with recordings from forehead and occiput in the intact skull, changes of the E.E.G. can only be demonstrated when there exist *general disturbances of function of the cerebrum*[T42] — if for the time being I may be allowed to express myself briefly in this manner. If the function of the entire cerebrum is more or less impaired by a rise in intracranial pressure or by a recent hemorrhage or thrombosis, changes also appear in the E.E.G. The same occurs in epileptic dementia, in the course of an extensive *Alzheimer's* disease, or multiple sclerosis in which the cortex everywhere is riddled with pathological lesions. If, however, there is a loss of specific parts of the brain, *e.g.* destruction by a growing and infiltrating tumor or a thrombotic softening of a specific cortical area, then this does not express itself in the E.E.G. recorded from the surface of the skull at all, once the initial acute phenomena, *e.g.* in the case of a softening, have receded. A case of congenital mental deficiency too in which, if I may say so, certain mechanisms[T43] of the brain are missing, but in which never- theless the overall activity[T44] is normal, shows no changes of the E.E.G. A case of general paresis in which certain mechanisms[T43] of the brain have been destroyed, but the progressive process halted by malaria therapy, also shows no change of the E.E.G. as far as I have been able to determine to date. There is in this case no longer any general disturbance of function[T42]. Such a disturbance most probably occurs, at least transiently, when fresh lesions caused by the spirochetes develop and then also reveals itself in the E.E.G.

At present it seems to me that it is possible to demonstrate general disturbances of function of the cerebrum in the E.E.G. Future investigations must show whether it will be possible to further advance the diagnostic possibilities in this respect. *One* fact, however, which I still wish to discuss, seems to me to give a hint with regard to this. In the many double recordings from various areas of the skull of patients, I have indeed repeatedly found that the E.E.G. recorded from a skull defect sometimes exhibits pathologically altered α-w which are missing in the E.E.G. recorded simul- taneously from forehead and occiput.

Figure 28 shows such an observation. It is that of a 48 year old lady in whom a trepanation over the area of the right frontal lobe had been carried out by Mr. *Guleke* 8 years ago, because of rapidly increasing papilloedema, vomiting, unbearable headaches, etc., associated with definite focal signs[1]. At the site of operation there was a depression of the bone caused by forceps pressure at birth and below it there was a circumscribed serous meningitis with depression of the cerebrum in this area. The bone flap was removed and all signs of raised intracranial pressure receded uneventfully. When a record was taken from this area of defect by means of chlorided silver needles placed 4 cm apart, and simultaneously from forehead and occiput, the two E.E.G.s reproduced here were obtained. A correspondence of the two E.E.G.s in certain segments is again evident, but in between the patterns may be

---

[1] See *Berger* and *Guleke*: Über Hirntumoren und ihre operative Behandlung. Dtsch. Z. Chir., **203**, 104 (1927); especially p. 115, case 5.

different, as was mentioned in more detail above. Of importance to us here is that α-w with an average duration of 130 σ appear in the E.E.G. recorded from the area of the defect, while simultaneously the E.E.G. recorded from forehead and occiput at this point exhibits only waves of 115 σ which would be normal for this lady. Thus, as I repeatedly convinced myself, one sometimes finds pathological E.E.G.s

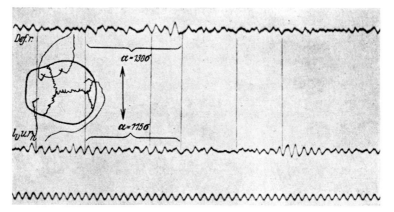

Fig. 28. 48 year old lady. Trepanation on the right[T 45] side in the region of the right planum temporale because of circumscribed serous meningitis. At the top: E.E.G. recorded with needle electrodes located 4 cm apart in the area of the skull defect; below: E.E.G. from the left frontal and the right occipital quadrants of the head recorded with needle electrodes. Time in 1/10ths sec.

with local recordings while such alterations do not appear in E.E.G.s recorded from forehead and occiput. A similar finding I would like to cite is that of a tumor which lay in the depth below a skull defect and caused no general signs of pressure. Over the tumor I found distinct alterations of the E.E.G., whereas the simultaneous recording from forehead and occiput showed an E.E.G. with normal α-w. Just as in this case of a recording from a skull defect, it may in the future be possible by using various locations of electrodes to demonstrate pathological alterations of the E.E.G. when the skull is intact, even *then*, when the E.E.G. recorded from forehead and occiput may at first have shown normal findings; however, this is a matter for future investigations.

After this preliminary survey of the changes of the E.E.G. found up to now in pathological cases, let us briefly consider the nature of the alterations of the records. If, on the basis of what has been reported above, we restrict ourselves for the time being to the changes of the α-w, there exist from a purely theoretical point of view the following possibilities of their alteration: (1) a loss of the α-w, (2) an increase in their length, (3) a decrease in their length, (4) an increase in their amplitude and (5) a decrease in their amplitude. At first and again from a purely theoretical point of view, nine different possible combinations follow from these, of which, however, so far only four have been observed. These are (1) the loss of the α-w, as it occurs transiently with intense attention, or continuously for a longer period of time during narcosis and after administration of scopolamine; (2) the increase in length of the α-w which we see in various disease states, *e.g.* in raised intracranial pressure or also in epileptic dementia, etc.; (3) the increase in the amplitude of the α-w, *e.g.* in the stage of excitation of narcosis or under the effect of cocaine; (4) the decrease in the amplitude of the α-w as *e.g.* in deep sleep. Yet to be added as a 5th alteration would be a disturbance in regularity of the α-w which are at times long,

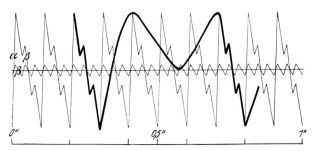

Fig. 29. Diagram of the time course of the α-w and β-w of the normal E.E.G. Heavy line: pathological α-w from Figure 24.

and at times short, as in the cases of dementia paralytica. To date I have not yet observed a definite decrease in the duration of the α-w, just as, for the reasons cited above, it has been as yet impossible to compare the amplitudes of the α-w in different people in view of the different resistances in the electrode circuit. The most frequent pathological alteration was an increase in the length of the α-w, as it clearly appears in the various figures reproduced here. In my second report, with the aid of a diagram, I attempted to represent the mutual relationships of the α-w and the β-w of the E.E.G. and their relationships in time. Either the small β-w appear alone, or there are α-w; in the latter case, however, β-w are always superimposed upon them in the form of notches in a pattern as shown in Figure 29, taken from that paper.

In this diagram I drew with india ink a train of waves from the E.E.G. of Figure 24, which had been obtained in a patient with a severe post-concussion psychosis after skull fracture. One sees that two imperfectly developed pathological α-w correspond to five normal α-w oscillations; one thus recognizes more clearly the alteration which the E.E.G. undergoes under pathological conditions. Even though practical diagnostic results beyond what we already know through other methods of investigations *e.g.* concerning the time course of mental processes in states of somnolence, are unattainable at present, these results nevertheless are of the utmost scientific importance. They allow us to confirm objectively what so far is known to us only from a subjective point of view, by enabling us to record observations in the form of a curve independently of the patients' attitude towards our questions and of their willingness to answer them or not. Moreover, since we are obviously only at the beginning of these investigations, even though I have been involved in them for several years, it is as yet completely impossible to foresee what practical importance they could assume. In any case it already follows from the observations and curves reported here that objective changes in the form of an alteration of the E.E.G. can be demonstrated, when, because of pathological processes, there is impairment of the general functions[T46] of the cerebrum. Precisely these results, however, again argue in favor of a central origin of the E.E.G., as had already been postulated on the basis of numerous other observations. There is no indication and also, according to everything else we know, it is highly unlikely that a difference in the peripheral or central circulation should exist *e.g.* between patients with epileptic dementia and normal individuals. Also, the other assumptions for the origin of the E.E.G. which have been suggested, as its origin from tremor movements of the head or from other muscle movements, cannot be maintained further in the face of this evidence. These movements surely could not produce in an epileptic curves different from those in a healthy individual. It is superfluous to enter once again into further details. I nevertheless considered it necessary to allude explicitly to the importance which these findings have for the determination of the site of origin of the E.E.G.

All the results of the investigations reported here, as well as those contained in my earlier reports on the E.E.G., argue for a *central* origin of this curve. The independence from respiratory oscillations, from transient changes in circulation within and outside the skull, the non-congruence of the pauses which are free of α-w in simultaneous recordings from various sites on the skull and the time differences of the reaction to a stimulus when recording simultaneously from a skull defect and from the skull as a whole, exclude an extracranial cause for the origin of the curves, such as perhaps tremor movements of the entire head. They unequivocally point to a central intracranially located site of origin of the E.E.G. The observations on the influence of stimulating and sleep-inducing[T36] drugs and the reported findings on lesions and diseases of the brain accompanied by disturbances of its functions, argue in the same direction. A unitary explanation of the whole body of observations which I collected in the course of six years with Prof. *Hilpert's* unfailing support, is only possible if one assumes a central origin of the E.E.G. To the question of where the E.E.G. originates, I would answer by stating that it must be most intimately related to the activity of the cerebrum, because only thus can, for instance, the changes during narcosis be explained. The investigators who experimented in animals assumed, as *Fleischl von Marxow*, *Beck* and *Cybulski* and others had done, that the electrical phenomena originate in the cerebral cortex itself and spoke of "cortical currents". *Garten*, as I already emphasized, admonished us to be cautious and stated that the problem is very difficult and that one does not know how much the cortex and how much other parts of the brain are involved in these processes. Nevertheless, on the basis of my experiences reported here in detail, I believe it justifiable to assume that the cerebral cortex is predominantly involved in the genesis of these currents or potential oscillations, the latter being the more correct physical term, even though perhaps other influences may also be involved. As repeatedly emphasized, in my second report I put forward the working hypothesis that the α-w represent concomitant phenomena of those material processes which one terms psychophysical because, circumstances permitting, they may be connected with phenomena of consciousness. The further investigations and my experience concerning the influence of stimulating and paralyzing drugs, as well as the observations in diseases of the brain have thoroughly strengthened my conviction in this respect. As early as 1877 *Danilevsky* alluded to the great importance of such investigations which he performed in animals and stressed: "que l'investigation électromotrice du cerveau nous donne la possibilité d'étudier d'une manière exacte les conditions matérielles, fondamentales, des processus psychophysiologiques"[1,T47]. That *Fleischl von Marxow* expressed himself in a similar vein, I have already emphasized elsewhere. Stimulated by *Mosso's* excellent investigations on cerebral circulation, I had at an earlier date also carried out investigations on the cerebral circulation under the influence of drugs in a patient who was available for such studies. In these investigations, however, I had not obtained *those* results which I had expected and in my study published in 1901 I had come to the conclusion that from the condition of the vascular system of the brain we cannot infer anything concerning the momentary states of the specific elements of the central nervous system. I added: "If we want to obtain information on their momentary states, we have to use other methods". At that time I already entertained the idea of studying the so-called cortical currents, according to the procedure of *Fleischl von Marxow* and of other investigators. I indicated elsewhere how long a path one still had to follow. *Mosso* in his investigations on the temperature of the brain, which he dedicated to *Helmholtz*, stressed[2] that each time we apply exact measuring instruments to the brain, the hope rightly stirs in us that we may learn to recognize the physical bases of consciousness. Even when we do not arrive at a satisfactory result, we could nevertheless be certain, he believed, that we are on the right path to discovery. And thus, I too believe I have followed the right path and have arrived at a proper goal, although today, even in the field of psychophysiology, intuition is more highly regarded in many circles than all the work done in the natural sciences, which I consider to be the only correct approach. I see in the α-w concomitant phenomena of the psychophysical cortical processes. The alteration of the course of the α-w or their loss suggest corresponding changes of these cortical processes. Of the nature of these we can indeed only say that they are physicochemical processes in the cortical grey matter. But I thoroughly maintain the point of view which *von Kries*[3] defended so well against the so frequent erroneous interpretation of *Du Bois'* saying "Ignoramus et ignorabimus", when he considered as not at all hopeless the efforts to identify those material processes which we have to conceive as representing the substrates of mental phenomena, or those with which the latter would have to be associated as regular concomitant phenomena. Certainly we do not know these material processes, but in my opinion we have here in the α-w a concomitant phenomenon of these processes. This may suffice for the time being. For it goes without saying that on this scientific road we can only advance by a slow struggle. In my second report I had explained in detail why I attributed this particular significance to the α-w of the E.E.G. and I stated above what strengthened my belief in this working hypothesis proposed at that time.

The origin of the E.E.G., especially of its α-w, from the cortex itself becomes

---

[1] *Soury, J.*: Système nerveux central, **2**, 1036. Paris, 1899.
[2] *Mosso*: Die Temperatur des Gehirns, **1894**, p. 137.
[3] *Kries, von*: Logik, p. 158. Tübingen, 1916.

a certainty to me by virtue of the following observation: In a 20 year old young man a palliative trepanation had been carried out by Mr. *Guleke* seven weeks earlier, because of a tumor which, according to the clinical manifestations, was thought to be located within the left cerebral hemisphere, but at operation could not be found at the suspected site. The skull defect created by the operation extended from the left lateral frontal to the parietal region. In this patient signs of raised intracranial pressure had recently become again increasingly manifest and a herniation under marked pressure had formed at the site of operation. Because of this it was suspected that the tumor had continued to grow rapidly and might also have invaded the parts of the brain in the region of the skull defect, so that perhaps it could be found and removed in a second operation. By measuring the electrical resistance according to the method indicated by *A. W. Meyer*[1], it was planned to determine whether at this time tumor tissue was present at the site of operation. Instead of the platinum needles I used chlorided silver needles coated with varnish up to their tips. The resistance measurement unequivocally argued against the presence of the tumor in the area of the operative site[2]. It was then possible to combine simultaneously these resistance measurements with the recording of an E.E.G. and, in this manner, with the needles located at different depths, E.E.G.s could be recorded from the cortex and from the hemispheral white matter.

Figure 30 shows the result of such a recording. In this figure two different curves have been put together to afford a clearer view. The upper curve *K1752*

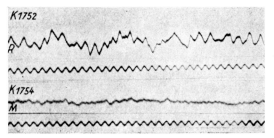

Fig. 30. Young man aged 20 years. Large left-sided palliative trepanation. At the top, *K1752*: E.E.G. recorded from the cortex with silver needles 9 cm apart; at the bottom, *K1754*: E.E.G. recorded with silver needles 7 cm apart, introduced to a depth of 4 cm into the hemispheral white matter.

shows the E.E.G. recorded from the cortex of the herniated part of the brain; the needles are placed 9 cm apart and the resistance in the electrode circuit measures 400 Ohms. The lower curve *K1754* shows the record from the hemispheral white matter taken by means of needles placed 7 cm apart and inserted to a depth of 4 cm, with a resistance in the electrode circuit of 300 Ohms. The considerable difference

[1] *Meyer, A. W.*: Hirn-Rheometrie, eine Methode zum Auffinden von Hirntumoren. Dtsch. med. Wschr., **1928**, 1366 (more precise bibliographic references are also to be found there).
[2] The autopsy of the patient who later died while exhibiting signs of increased intracranial pressure, showed that in fact healthy brain tissue was present at the sites of measurement and that the tumor was located in another, far distant area.

of the two curves is immediately evident; the characteristic E.E.G. is only obtained from the *cortex*, not from the hemispheral white matter! With needles placed in these very locations I also recorded simultaneously from the cortex and the hemispheral white matter to the two galvanometers of the double-coil galvanometer. These records showed the same result. However, because the two galvanometers are not quite equally sensitive, I considered it correct to reproduce in Figure 30 two E.E.G.s recorded one after another, which were both written with the more sensitive system. The E.E.G. thus originates essentially in the *cerebral cortex itself* and this applies especially for the oscillations which I designated as α-w!

The time course of the α-w and also the amplitude of their deflections has been established by a large series of measurements which I have now carried out with three different types of galvanometers — I lately also once had the opportunity to record E.E.G.s with the new *Siemens* oscillograph. Figure 31 shows the course of the potential oscillation which I designated as α-w. All secondarily superimposed waves designated by me as β-w have been omitted from this figure.

The abscissa represents time in epochs of 5 σ, the ordinate deflections in steps of 0.01 mV. *Broca* and *Richet*[1] as early as 1897 published a very interesting study on the refractory time of the cerebral cortex on which subject, as far as I know, more recent investigations do not exist. These two investigators, on the basis of their experiments and a series of findings which they culled from the physiological and psychological literature, came to the conclusion that the "vibration cérébrale" has a duration of 0.1 second. In Figure 6 of their study they give a schematic representation of this "vibration cérébrale" which is completely identical with the schematic

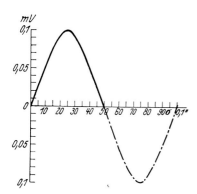

Fig. 31. Diagram. Representation of an α-w of the E.E.G. On the abscissa, time in epochs of 5 σ; on the ordinate, voltage in steps of 0.01 mV.

Figure 31 shown here. They distinguish in the "vibration cérébrale" a positive and a negative phase. The latter would correspond to the part of my diagram indicated by an interrupted line. The negative phase coincides with the refractory time of *Broca* and *Richet*. Today we can cite many more reasons for the limited temporal duration of the "vibration cérébrale" than it was possible to do at the time of those studies. *Alfred Lehmann*[2], the Danish investigator, famous for his excellent research on

---

[1] *Broca* and *Richet*: Période réfractaire dans les centres nerveux. Arch. de Physiol., **1897**, 864.
[2] *Lehmann, Alfred*: Grundzüge der Psychophysiologie, p. 13. Leipzig, 1912.

concomitant phenomena of mental processes, expressed the opinion in his "Psycho-physiology" that 15 images per second are sufficient to create the illusion of a steady movement in a cinematographic performance and that a greater number of images are disturbing. To these statements he adds: "The stream of the ceaselessly changing conscious phenomena is therefore by no means continuous; it rather consists of many mental flashes". He therefore also regards the mental side as being composed of individual component parts which coalesce into a uniform whole. Nevertheless, it was not these general considerations which were decisive for advancing my working hypothesis, but the objective observation of the parallel changes of the α-w and of the mental phenomena in narcosis, etc.[1]. I thus hold to this hypothesis and consider the α-w to be concomitant phenomena of the material processes which we designate as psychophysical. This hypothesis so far also stood the test of practical problems and promises to provide further informations. The material processes which are related to mental phenomena have always particularly absorbed the interest and sagacity of brilliant minds. The great interest which my investigations have aroused in wider circles may in part derive from this. It is most likely also the explanation for many fantastic statements and hopes attached to them which were voiced by non-experts after they had read my reports. Time and again I have emphasized that in the α-w we are dealing only with the concomitant phenomena of the material processes which are connected with the mental ones, but not with these processes themselves! I nevertheless believe that *this* very finding is of the greatest scientific and probably also practical significance.

---

[1] *Note added to proofs*: During the loss of consciousness outlasting a major epileptic seizure, the E.E.G. runs as a straight line, *i.e.* as in deep narcosis. With the gradual return of consciousness after the seizure the E.E.G. step by step regains its known aspects with α-w now reappearing again.

IV

On the Electroencephalogram of Man

Fourth Report

by Hans Berger, Jena

(With 14 figures)

(Received December 16, 1931)

[Published in the *Archiv für Psychiatrie und Nervenkrankheiten*, **1932**, 97: 6–26]

In my investigations reported so far I had worked with the string galvanometer and especially with the *Siemens* double-coil galvanometer. For a few months now an oscillograph system with an amplifier has been available to me[1]. It was especially constructed for my purposes by Siemens and Halske. With it I have since continued my investigations on the electroencephalogram of man. The new galvanometer, as I will call it for brevity's sake, has the advantage of making it possible to measure directly the voltage, not merely the current intensity as had been the case with the coil galvanometer used previously. Furthermore the amplitude of the curve increases in proportion to the increase in voltage. The large resistance within the instrument makes it possible, for practical purposes, to disregard completely the resistance on the skull. With a measuring procedure, designed according to Mr. *Wien*'s suggestions and described elsewhere[2,T48] by Dr. *Dietsch*, the physicist who collaborated with me, it was possible to determine that the ratio of the resistance on the skull to that of the oscillograph was about 1:40. Therefore electroencephalograms of different individuals recorded with the same gain of the oscillograph can be compared from now on. However, in comparison with the coil galvanometer, the new galvanometer[3] has the great disadvantage that its sensitivity decreases fairly rapidly during operation and therefore the calibration curve recorded at the beginning does not remain valid for the whole

---

[1] To the *Carl Zeiss Foundation* I owe the privilege of having been able to obtain this valuable instrument and for this I wish to express here too my most sincere thanks to the gentlemen in charge. Furthermore, I am much obliged to Mr. *Wien* for his interest in my investigations and his expert advice, to Mr. *Esau* for the selection of a suitable young physicist as a collaborator for my investigations and for the many forms of assistance which I received from the Physical-Technical Institute of the University under Mr. *Esau*'s direction. In these, as in all investigations, which have now extended over more than 7 years, Mr. *Hilpert* too helped me by word and deed for which I thank him sincerely.

[2] *Dietsch*: Pflügers Arch., **228**, 644 (1931).

[3] This instrument is capable of reproducing all possible physiological current oscillations, including those of the greatest velocity, such as the most rapid muscle currents.

[133]

recording period. New calibration curves have to be repeatedly interpolated between individual recordings. I hope that with some improvement of the equipment it will become possible to avoid this. Out of prudence I nevertheless till now always had the resistance measured for the individual recordings. The danger of polarization, which in itself is small considering the fairly rapid periods of the alternating current corresponding to the electroencephalogram (E.E.G.), was countered as before by using silver needles coated with silver chloride. The needles were always inserted below the skin and, if possible, introduced below the periosteum of the skull, which of course was only possible by using local anesthesia. Another disadvantage of the new galvanometer, which on the other hand is also its asset, is its high sensitivity. During the recording of the E.E.G. it is of course necessary to turn off X-ray and particularly diathermy instruments, even if they are located in buildings of the clinic which are separate from that containing the examination room. Furthermore all electrical machinery, as is *e.g.* used for the laundry, also has to be switched off. Apart from that it became necessary to provide the lines supplying power for the electrical lights, etc. with extensive shielding devices against interference. During the actual recording the experimental subject and the recording apparatus are located in separate rooms and all electrical signals must be avoided and replaced by purely mechanical devices. A further consequence of the great sensitivity of the galvanometer is a restriction in the selection of suitable patients, because the movements of the patients, when they are connected to the galvanometer, immediately cause the

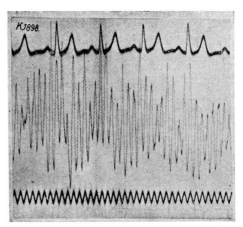

Fig. 1. I.B.[T49], 14 years old. At the top: E.C.G. recorded from both arms (coil galvanometer); below it: E.E.G. recorded with chlorided silver needles from forehead and occiput (oscillograph); at the bottom: time in 1/10ths sec.

light spot to jump off the recording surface. Nevertheless, this oscillograph system represents such a far reaching improvement that I would like to report here on some of the E.E.G.s recorded with it.

Figure 1 shows an E.E.G. obtained in this way. It is that of my 14 year old daughter Ilse and is taken from the left forehead and right occiput; as always it is recorded with chlorided silver needles, as reported in detail earlier. The electrocardio-gram (E.C.G.) written at the top is recorded from both arms by means of lead foil electrodes. I. lies with closed eyes in a slightly darkened room from which noise has been excluded by means of double doors, etc., as much as this is feasible in a clinic. The curve illustrated in the figure is considerably reduced in size in comparison with the original record in which the deflections of the E.E.G. measure on the average 74 mm. The large waves of first order which I designated as alpha waves (α-w) are clearly seen; almost all of them are of precisely equal length with an average of 95 σ in this instance. Superimposed upon them smaller notches can be recognized, some-times merely as thickenings of the rising or falling limbs of the α-w. These notches are the waves of second order which I designated as beta waves (β-w). This curve recorded in I. with the oscillograph system corresponds exactly to the E.E.G.s which I had obtained in her with the double-coil galvanometer; only, of course, the deflec-tions are considerably larger. It would be easy, by selecting a greater sensitivity, to display the E.E.G. with still larger deflections. But of course, under such circumstances with each small disturbance the light spot flies off the recording surface of the appara-tus all the more easily, so that most often one has to be satisfied with a lower sensitivity.

Figure 2 demonstrates that a recording from the surface of the dura yields exactly the same curve. This figure shows the record of a 33 year old man, M.M.,

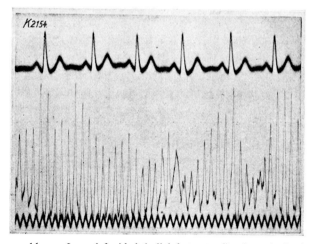

Fig. 2. M.M., 33 year old man. Large left-sided skull defect extending from the forehead to the parietal region. At the top: E.C.G. recorded from both arms; in the middle: E.E.G. recorded with the oscillo-graph by means of chlorided silver needles lying 4.5 cm apart in the epidural space within the bone defect. At the bottom: time in 1/10ths sec.

in whom three months prior to the recording, because of a suspected tumor, a large palliative trepanation had been performed which extended from the forehead to the parietal region. At the time of the recording M. showed no signs of increased intra-cranial pressure and the area of the palliative trepanation had sunk distinctly below the level of the remainder of the skull. Radiotherapy or any other form of treatment had not been carried out. At operation the surface of the cerebral cortex presenting in the area of trepanation had a completely normal appearance. In this examination, records were taken from two points 4.5 cm apart in the midportion of the skull defect. Chlorided silver needles were used which had been inserted through the skin and pushed as far as the dura immediately below it. In the curve reproduced here one sees the large α-w which have an average length of 110 σ and exhibit a potential oscillation of 0.2 mV. The similarity of the curves recorded here from the dura and in Figure 1 from the intact skull can be recognized immediately. If, after all my earlier arguments, proof were still required that the curve recorded from the intact skull is identical with the E.E.G. recorded from the dura or from the cerebral cortex itself (third report, Figure 30), it would be provided by this record.

In my second report I discussed in detail the changes of the E.E.G. under the influence of *sensory stimuli*. Since precisely on this point I have not always been correctly understood, perhaps because I did not express myself clearly enough, I would like to discuss these findings here once more. The E.E.G. changes under the influence of sensory stimuli occur only when the experimental subject has not previously already been distracted and when he actually directs his attention towards the sensory stimulus. Touch stimuli not perceived *e.g.* because of artificial anesthesia of the skin, cause no change of the E.E.G. All events which attract attention elicit an alteration of the E.E.G. Thus, to avoid such disturbances and to keep all sensory stimuli, such as noise, etc. as much as possible away from the experimental subject, one has to use two separate rooms, one for the experimental subject and the other for the recording instruments. It is certainly best, as has been repeatedly mentioned, if the experimental subject lies in a half-darkened room with his eyes closed, leaves free rein to his thoughts and attempts to fall asleep. Pain also causes a change of the E.E.G. exactly like sensory stimuli, probably by continually attracting attention to it. The curves recorded with the oscillograph show the same features as those reported earlier taken with the coil galvanometer; however, the change of the E.E.G. manifests itself even more clearly here in the oscillograph curves.

Figure 3 was obtained from one of my assistants, Dr. C. He lies comfortably on a couch with his eyes closed. At *B* he is touched and stroked along the dorsum of his right hand. At the top is the E.E.G., recorded in the usual fashion with chlorided silver needles from forehead and occiput. Below it, is the E.C.G. recorded from both arms and, at the bottom, time in tenths of a second. The touch at *B* is followed after 0.275 second at *R* by the change of the E.E.G. which I had described earlier in detail. It consists precisely of a disappearance of the α-w, which lasts for a variable period of time, and of their replacement by β-w. The voltage, which as mentioned above, can be recorded directly in such oscillograph curves, thus decreases at *R* to about 1/10th of its pre-existing value.

In my third report I had already emphasized that the changes of the E.E.G. can also be demonstrated in local recordings from the dura within a skull defect. Yet in view of the fundamental importance which just this observation assumes for the explanation of these phenomena, I refer to Figure 4. The record was obtained from the same M.M. from whom another curve had been shown and discussed above in Figure 2. At *S* a pin prick is applied to the index finger of M.'s left hand, while he is lying quietly in a half-darkened room with his eyes closed. After 0.3 second the well known change of the E.E.G. takes place. At this point a drop in potential

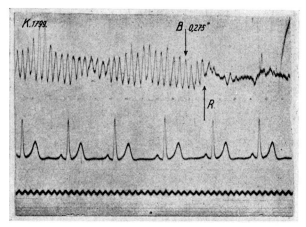

Fig. 3. Dr. C., 30 years old. At the top: E.E.G. recorded with chlorided silver needles from the forehead and occiput (oscillograph); below it: E.E.G. recorded from both arms; at the bottom: time in 1/10ths sec. At *B* touching and stroking the dorsum of the right hand.

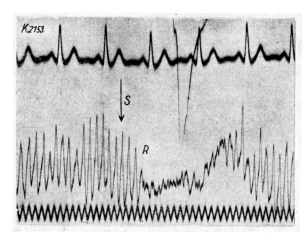

Fig. 4. M.M., 33 year old man. Large left-sided bone defect extending from the forehead to the parietal region. At the top: E.C.G.; below it: E.E.G.; at the bottom: time in 1/10ths sec. The same recording as in Fig. 2. At *S* pin prick applied to the index finger of the left hand; at *R* change of the E.E.G.

to less than 1/10th of the previously existing voltage occurs. Thus we can only be dealing with processes acting directly upon the E.E.G., which originates in the brain, and not with any other intervening phenomena, such as movements, changes in skin resistance, etc. The correspondence is complete between Figure 3, recorded in Dr. C.

from the skull as a whole, and this Figure 4 which shows a recording taken from the dura of a skull defect.

As emphasized earlier in my second report, it would be possible to see a contradiction between these results and the findings in animal experiments. Indeed, in spite of my explanations, some wished to see a contradiction in this, and just for this reason I shall discuss these results again. In the animal experiment, as *Beck*, *Cybulski*, *Fleischl von Marxow* and others found, when one recorded from the cortical sensory centers, a deflection was observed on the galvanometer upon stimulation of the corresponding sense organ. Thus in the monkey *e.g.*, a deflection was observed in the visual area upon exposure of the eye to light. Attempts were also made to determine the limits of the individual sensory centers within the cortex by using this electrical method. Now in man, a diminution in voltage occurs at both recording points under the influence of a sensory stimulus, if the latter absorbs the subject's attention. The recording points are located over the frontal and parietal lobes. We thus record from the skull as a whole and not from a circumscribed sensory center at all. Furthermore, under normal conditions, it is quite impossible to reach the sensory centers in man. Even when one records from the dura of the skull defect in patients with palliative trepanations as in Figure 4, one still does not record from a sensory center. Indeed, in man these centers are situated in areas which are not at all accessible to a recording of this kind. One could assume that it should be possible to record from Cp^{T50}, but the major portion of this sensory center too is located in the depth of the sulcus of Rolando. Thus, in contrast to the animal experiments, the recording of the E.E.G. taken in the manner used to obtain the records of Figure 3 and Figure 4, does not represent a record from a sensory center at all and even less one from the center concerned with touch sensation, but constitutes a recording from other cortical areas. Evidently, what I see are only the distant effects of the touch stimulus on other cortical regions. Probably these have to be explained by assuming that in the area of the involved sensory center, an increased activity takes place, which exerts an inhibitory effect upon the whole remainder of the cortex, as I attempted to make clear in the diagram of Figure 7 of my third report. Thus in Figures 3 and 4 I see an inhibitory effect which emanates from the local center of activity in the cerebral cortex. Such an assumption is in good accord with the physiological concomitants of processes of attention. Already *W. Wundt*[1] designated the inhibitory processes in the central nervous system as the most essential feature for the physiological interpretation of the phenomena of attention. He assumed that inhibitory effects are elicited by excitations conveyed to what he called the center of apperception which he thought to be localized in the frontal lobe. In his hypothetical scheme of the center of apperception inhibitory fibers play a very essential role. Elsewhere *Wundt* speaks of a principle of functional compensation[T51] and amplifies this further by saying that whenever a large part of the central organ, by virtue of inhibitory influences, is in a state of latent function, the excitability of the functioning remainder to stimuli flowing into it is enhanced. As a physiological basis for this law, as *Wundt*

---

[1] *Wundt, W.*: Grundzüge der physiologischen Psychologie, Vol. 1, p. 320 and subsequent pages; 5th edition, 1902.

calls it, one could, according to him, envisage a double mutual interaction, neurodynamic and vasomotor, with the latter appearing after the former. As I emphasized
above, but wish to stress once more, a neurodynamic and more specifically an inhibitory effect, finds its expression in the change of the E.E.G. shown in Figures 3
and 4 which occurs under the influence of a sensory stimulus. As I also emphasized
earlier, the rapidity of onset of this change, which occurs after only 0.275 second, or
even, as I demonstrated elsewhere, as early as 0.09 second following the action of the
stimulus, argues against vasomotor phenomena. According to *Fano* vascular reflexes
take 2–7 seconds to occur. Personally I had previously established that the time between a startling stimulus and the onset of a change in the cerebral vessels measures 2.3
seconds. Apart from this rapid onset, the fact that with sensory stimuli acting for
only a short period of time the change is so evanescent, argues all the more strongly
against vascular processes, which cannot disappear as quickly; 0.5–2 seconds after
the influence of such a stimulus the E.E.G. is again normal. Following the application
of a brief sensory stimulus which holds the attention only very fleetingly, it is sometimes possible to obtain very brief changes of the E.E.G., lasting for only 0.2 second.

Figure 5 shows such an example. Again it is from my daughter Ilse of whom
a record had already been shown in Figure 1. At *R* one can recognize a change in
the E.E.G. which lasted only 0.2 second. It had occurred under the influence of a
brief touch stimulus applied 0.3 second before. Here we are certainly not dealing
with vasomotor processes, but with direct neurodynamic influences upon the E.E.G.
to which later after more prolonged direction of the attention, as *Wundt* also states,

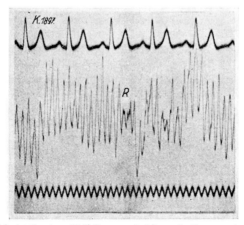

Fig. 5. I.B., 14 years old. At the top: E.C.G. recorded from both arms; below it: E.E.G. recorded
with chlorided silver needles from forehead and occiput (oscillograph); at the bottom: time in 1/10ths
sec. *R*: change of the E.E.G. caused by touching briefly the dorsum of the right hand.

vasomotor processes may become associated. However, we cannot demonstrate
these in the E.E.G. which, as I showed in detail in all my earlier reports, has nothing
to do with vascular processes. *Ebbinghaus* too, according to *Dürr*[1] considers the process

[1] *Dürr, E.*: Lehre von der Aufmerksamkeit, p. 166. Leipzig, 1907.

of attention to be caused by a distribution of excitation in the cerebral cortex. In the state of inattention diffuse excitations which become dispersed are present within the cerebral cortex. By virtue of cortical processes of facilitation and inhibition, these change into concentrated and differentiated excitations when attention is intensified. I believe I see the inhibitory action of the process of attention in the E.E.G. in Figures 3, 4 and 5 and in curves reported earlier, and I am of the opinion that these results agree quite well with those of the animal experiments.

In my earlier reports I had indicated that a more or less distinct change of the E.E.G. also appears when attention is absorbed by a *mental task*, and indeed during its whole duration. I have not yet published any curves relevant to this and would like to do so now.

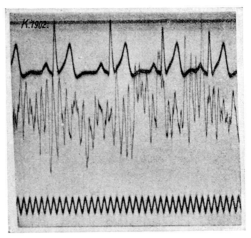

Fig. 6. K.B., 19 years old. At the top: E.C.G. recorded from both arms; below it: E.E.G. recorded with chlorided silver needles from forehead and occiput (oscillograph); at the bottom: time in 1/10ths sec.

Figure 6 shows the E.E.G. of my son Klaus, now 19 years old, taken when he was mentally relaxed. The α-w are fairly large in amplitude and have an average length of 90–110 σ. The resistance measured 6700 Ohms.

Figure 7 shows Klaus' E.E.G. while solving the arithmetic problem "22 × 43". It is clearly evident that the α-w have become much smaller in amplitude and in many places are completely missing. In those segments where β-w alone are present there is a decrease in potential to 1/5th of the previously existing voltage. In a general way one can say, according to my experience, that the potential diminution during mental work does not set in as suddenly as when attention is focussed by an unexpected sensory stimulus, nor does it reach the same degree. But it nevertheless persists more or less distinctly during the entire duration of mental work, while exhibiting certain fluctuations in the amount of voltage diminution. From numerous recordings of this kind taken during mental work, I gained the impression that the degree of mental effort which the performance of the given task demands and which varies according to the experimental subject's practice and education, also finds its expression in the amount of the potential diminution. Very often, especially at the beginning of a mental task, the change does not become too clearly evident, because the mere naming of the expected task already causes focussing of attention.

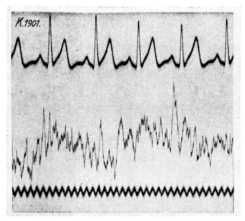

Fig. 7. K.B., 19 years old. At the top: E.C.G. recorded from both arms; below it: E.E.G. recorded with chlorided silver needles from forehead and occiput (oscillograph); at the bottom: time in 1/10ths sec. K.B. solves the problem "23×43"[52].

Figure 8 is taken from a record obtained in my daughter Ilse, of whom other records had been presented above in Figures 1 and 5. In this recording the procedure was somewhat different, insofar as the E.E.G. was written simultaneously with the coil galvanometer and the oscillograph connected in parallel. I believed that it would now be permissible to omit the E.C.G. occasionally after it had been recorded regularly together with the E.E.G. in 2000 curves. The oblique margin of the curve is not attributable to an error, but results from the fact that the light spot of the coil galvanometer and that of the oscillograph were not lined up exactly one above the other. The oblique borderline connects points which coincide in time[1]. At the arrow A an arithmetic problem is given to I. who lies with her eyes closed in a half-darkened room. One sees how very gradually the change of the E.E.G. develops. It consists of a diminution in the amplitude of the α-w, their temporary disappearance, and an increased prominence of the β-w which results from it. The transition from the successfully completed task to a state of rest is much more distinct than the change from what *appears* to be mental rest to activity. In reality mental rest is often non-existent because the experimental subject is internally preoccupied with solving the task as quickly as possible, and is apprehensive lest in the process of doing so he may expose himself to some embarrassment.

Figure 9 which is also taken from a record obtained in my daughter Ilse shows this extremely well. The problem "196:7" given to her is correctly solved. By slightly

---

[1] The same applies for Figure 9.

lifting the right index finger from its support, she indicated to me the moment of completion of the task. Immediately the E.E.G. changes. The voltage which parallels the amplitude of the deflections of the curve shows a tenfold increase. The explanation for the change in the E.E.G. during a mental task, the latter being, of course, associated with an intensification of attention, can only be the same as that given above for the

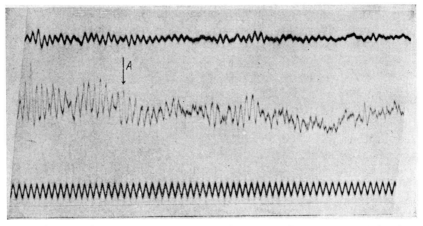

Fig. 8. I.B., 14 years old. At the top: E.E.G. recorded with the coil galvanometer; below it: E.E.G. recorded with the oscillograph. Recording with chlorided silver needles from forehead and occiput. At the bottom: time in 1/10ths sec. At *A* the naming of the problem in mental arithmetic begins.

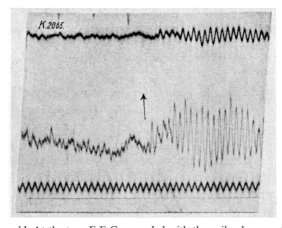

Fig. 9. I.B., 14 years old. At the top: E.E.G. recorded with the coil galvanometer; below it: E.E.G. recorded with the oscillograph. Recording with chlorided silver needles from forehead and occiput. At the bottom: time in 1/10ths sec. — End of mental arithmetic.

phenomena concomitant with the arousal of attention by a sudden sensory stimulus. These are inhibitory effects which are exerted upon the remainder of the cerebral cortex by the center or centers involved in the mental work. After cessation of local work, the entire cortex enters into a state of more or less pronounced activity.

I believe that such an explanation is the most probable one. However, I do not want to leave unmentioned that one could hold completely different views to which I shall refer here particularly for their historical interest. The well known Parisian chemist *Armand Gautier*, who was also greatly preoccupied with biological questions and who was a determined opponent of the concept that mental processes had a material equivalent which was much discussed at the time, expressed his opinion on this question in the following way: "Il faudrait montrer, ou bien que les phénomènes psychiques ne peuvent apparaître qu'en faisant disparaître une quantité proportionelle de l'énergie, cinétique ou potentielle" ... and in the same vein further: "Le cerveau devrait se refroidir, ou son potentiel électrique baisser!"[1, T53]. Now, Figures 7, 8 and 9 indeed show a decrease of the electrical potential during mental work. Yet, I do not believe that this change should be interpreted in this manner. We are dealing here only with a partial phenomenon and in contrast to the decrease in electrical potential, observed at the recording points, there is probably a considerable increase in potential in the centers of activity.

I had explained earlier that in the waking state continuous cortical work is performed to which any incidental mental work only adds a small increment. In view of *Ebbinghaus'* above cited statements on the processes of attention, it even appears to me questionable whether intellectual work does in fact add any significant increment at all and I wonder whether the explanation given by *von Liebermann* is not the more correct one. This explanation to which I had already referred in my second report agrees well with the above demonstrated changes in the E.E.G. during mental work. *Von Liebermann*[2] is of the opinion that cerebral work and the energy expenditure required for it represents an invariable quantity regardless of whether actual intensive (oriented) or extensive (dispersed) mental work is performed. What we call actual mental work, according to him, is distinguished from the other, dispersed, kind only insofar as in the first case attention is concentrated upon a specific object or group of ideas and that the expenditure of energy in the corresponding parts of the cortex is enhanced at the expense of that in other parts. In extensive or dispersed cerebral work many parts of the cortex, even though only fleetingly, are said to become excited whereas in intensive or oriented work specific circumscribed parts of the cortex are involved, but all the more intensely. This would make it possible to explain in the simplest way, why up to the present time, in spite of intensive investigations, it has been impossible to demonstrate that mental work is associated with any considerable increase in the total energy turnover.

In my third report in Figures 25 and 26 I published two *records of epileptics* demonstrating the continuous alteration of the E.E.G. in epileptic dementia occurring on a background of genuine epilepsy. When recording the E.E.G. with the coil galvanometer one finds in this condition, in spite of the variable skull resistance, a surprisingly high amplitude curve with α-w prolonged far beyond normal. Recordings with the oscillograph show the same findings. Also in that third report, I had already pointed out (p. 132, footnote) that during the loss of consciousness outlasting a

---

[1] *Gautier, Armand*: According to *J. Soury*: Système nerveux central, Vol. 2, p. 1265. Paris, 1899.
[2] *Liebermann, von*: Biochem. Z., **173**, 181 (1926).

major epileptic seizure the E.E.G. runs as a straight line, the α-w being completely absent. The E.E.G. in this condition thus corresponds to that obtained in chloroform narcosis. Because hitherto I have not yet published such a curve, I would like to do so now.

In a 55 year old woman suffering from mild arteriosclerosis, occasional epileptic seizures without any focal manifestations occurred since her 53rd year of life. During the preparation for the recording of an E.E.G., one of these attacks occurred, a rare event in this patient. The lead foil electrodes for the recording of the E.C.G. had already been applied to the arms, when suddenly a major epileptic seizure with tonus and subsequent clonus began. Only after the convulsive phenomena had subsided, could the needle electrodes be applied to the skull. A certain amount of time was lost meanwhile because of this and also because the galvanometer had to be ad-

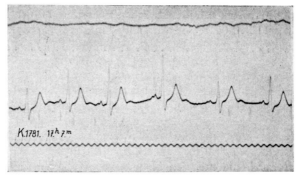

Fig. 10. P.H., 55 year old woman. After a major epileptic seizure. At the top: E.E.G. recorded with chlorided silver needles from forehead and occiput; below it: E.C.G. recorded from both arms (double-coil galvanometer); at the bottom: time in 1/10ths sec.

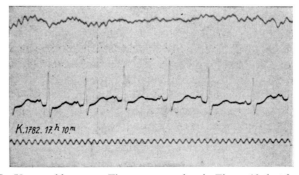

Fig. 11. P.H., 55 year old woman. The same record as in Figure 10, but 3 minutes later.

justed. The seizure occurred at 5:00 P.M. and the first curves, shown in Figure 10, were recorded at 5:07 P.M.

Mrs. H. lies there, breathing stertorously and shows as yet no reaction to any stimuli. No α-w can be seen in the E.E.G. Figure 11 is recorded 3 minutes later, *i.e.* 10 minutes after the onset of the major seizure. Mrs. H. still breathes stertorously,

does not respond when called, but makes some spontaneous arm movements. The
E.E.G. has changed and shows some, albeit still very low voltage α-w and this not
in all parts of the record. Mrs. H. now progressively awakens. At 5:12 P.M. a curve
is recorded of which Figure 12 shows a small segment. Mrs. H. now opens her eyes
and is conscious. The E.E.G., as Figure 12 shows, has undergone a further change;
the α-w have continued to increase in amplitude and are now continuously present

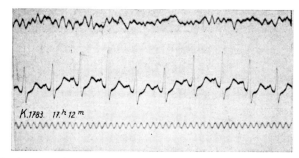

Fig. 12. P.H., 55 year old woman. The same record as in Figure 10, but 5 minutes later.

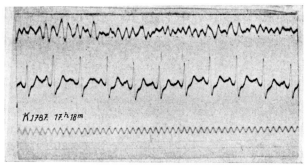

Fig. 13. P.H., 55 year old woman. The same record as in Figure 10, but 11 minutes later.

again. Finally Figure 13 is recorded 18 minutes after the onset of the major seizure.
Mrs. H. is now completely clear in her mind and her thinking is well organized, but
of course she has no recollection of her seizure. It is evident that a steadily increasing
change of the E.E.G. which regains its normal aspect step by step, corresponds to the
gradual awakening from the unconsciousness of the seizure, exactly as is the case
during awakening from narcosis. A detailed review of all E.E.G.s recorded during
this event disclosed furthermore that the α-w do not return suddenly, but during
awakening first appear at regular intervals of 8.5–9.5 seconds; between the α-w, there
are again segments of the curve which are devoid of α-w. These α-w, appearing on the
average every 9 seconds, then remain for increasingly longer periods, so that finally
they are again present continuously. Figure 11 shows at least a suggestion of the
phenomenon which has just been discussed. It appears more clearly only when one
reviews segments of curves which are longer than those that can be reproduced here.
These waves which appear every 9 seconds bear no relationship with respiration

which just during this time had been significantly accelerated. Thus there were 20–21 breaths per minute and a single breath lasted on the average only 3 seconds. There is just as little relationship with circulation. Most likely this is an intrinsic rhythm of the central nervous system to which I repeatedly alluded before, especially in my second report and which also manifests itself in the so-called fluctuations of attention, to the extent to which they are of central origin. This *intrinsic rhythm* of the brain upon awakening from the unconsciousness caused by an epileptic seizure, exhibits in this case a period of 9 seconds as measured from the height of one wave to that of the next; elsewhere, in different individuals, I found in the waking state periods of 1.3–2.65, 2.1–2.5, 1.5–3.9 and 2.3–4.7 seconds. This rhythm is probably a characteristic property of the cerebrum, based on its vital processes, which manifests itself in the mental sphere by various phenomena, which so far are known to us only from their psychic aspect.

It seems to me now first of all necessary to discuss once more the *composition of the normal E.E.G.* As I repeatedly emphasized, the latter exhibits waves of first order which I called α-w, and waves of second order which I called β-w. The α-w normally have a length of 90–120 σ and a maximum amplitude of about 0.2 mV. For the β-w I indicated an average length of 33 σ and a maximum amplitude of 0.1 mV. In my second report I first advanced the working hypothesis that the α-w were concomitant phenomena of those material processes which must be called psychophysical, because they are connected with conscious phenomena. I supported this hypothesis by a series of arguments which I wish to present here once more. Firstly, as stated above, the α-w exhibit a periodic waxing and waning, the period corresponding in time to the phenomena known to experimental psychology as fluctuations of attention. Secondly, any focussing of attention or mental work is associated with a transient arrest or an enduring amplitude diminution of the α-w. As I explained above, one can account for these phenomena most easily in terms of inhibitory effects exerted by a center of activity upon all simultaneous psychophysical processes. Thirdly, the actions of such poisons, as *e.g.* cocaine, which in fact reveal a certain increase in psychical responsiveness, are associated with an increase in the amplitude of the α-w; the same also becomes apparent during the stage of excitation of narcosis. Fourthly, poisons which eliminate mental processes, such as scopolamine and especially chloroform narcosis, on the other hand cause a disappearance of the α-w. Particularly with the latter a parallelism between the depth of narcosis and the disappearance of the α-w becomes evident, which also can be demonstrated particularly during awakening from narcosis. Fifthly, α-w do not disappear during normal sleep, but become smaller in amplitude, which is in complete agreement with our assumption that during sleep the psychophysical processes are by no means extinguished, as is shown unequivocally by dream phenomena. Sixthly, we see an unmistakable alteration of the α-w in pathological states, *e.g.* in a post-concussion psychosis, but perhaps even much more definitely in a severe epileptic dementia with pronounced slowing of all mental processes. Seventhly, at last, the curve reported here too, shows that during the unconsciousness of a major epileptic seizure the α-w likewise disappear and also gradually reappear again, completely in parallel with the gradual recovery of the conscious phenomena. All these observations encourage me to maintain the working hypothesis which I had put forward earlier and which is mentioned above. In my second report I interpreted the β-w as concomitant phenomena of those processes which take place in the living nervous tissue independently of its specific function and I designated them in short as concomitants of the vital processes of the nervous tissue. What prompts me to make this assumption is the fact that the β-w are always present, even when the α-w transiently disappear as *e.g.* when attention is aroused by a sensory stimulus, and the observation that they can be recorded also from a part of the cerebrum which, undoubtedly is no longer capable of functioning, as I then explained. But even during narcosis and during the unconsciousness of the epileptic seizure, β-w are still present while α-w are completely missing. They therefore probably correspond to manifestations of the vital processes of the nervous tissue and represent concomitants of the nutritional processes which are unrelated to the specific[T54] function of the tissue. *Mosso*[1], in his studies on the temperature of the brain, already spoke of organic conflagrations, which in his opinion represent the thermal expression of metabolic phenomena occurring in the organs independently of their special functions. Earlier, and again above, I indicated 33 σ as the average duration of the β-w and 0.1 mV as their maximal amplitude. On the basis of Dr. *Dietsch's* frequency analyses[T55] which he carried out in my clinic, I have to amend these statements somewhat, insofar as according to the records taken with the oscillograph system the β-w comprise waves with a duration of 20–50 σ; also their size generally only amounts to 1/10th of the amplitude of the α-w and thus only to 0.02 mV. As I stressed in my third report, these β-w can be recorded from the cortex as well as from the hemispheral white matter of the human cerebrum. In addition to nerve cells and the nervous elements connected with them, such as neurofibrils, etc., the nervous tissue contains a great number of glia cells, vessels and other components of this kind. It is obviously not possible to determine which particular components through their vital processes cause the appearance of the β-w. They are certainly a *composite quantity*, as has been demonstrated by the results of frequency analyses, which showed that they are composed of waves of very different lengths, ranging from 20 to 50 σ. To summarize, I wish to say that I hold on to the working hypothesis which I had advanced and which postulates that the α-w of the E.E.G. are concomitant phenomena of psychophysical cortical processes and that the electrical phenomena subsumed under the collective term of β-w are concomitant phenomena of those manifestations of vital processes of the nervous tissue which are independent of its specific[T54] function. In pursuing my investigations further there has been to date no cause to substantially modify this working hypothesis or to abandon it, a fate that may sometimes befall a working hypothesis.

I really expected that in persons without brain damage an alteration of the E.E.G. would appear during *fever* with the α-w perhaps becoming shorter and higher in amplitude and the β-w also displaying some changes. To my astonishment, this assumption was not confirmed in two patients treated with malaria and Pyrifer[T56],

---

[1] *Mosso, A.*: Die Temperatur des Gehirns, p. 96. Leipzig, 1894.

who were suffering from tabes and exhibited no mental changes whatsoever. The β-w did not show the slightest changes and in patient R. treated with malaria there occurred an unquestionable lengthening of the α-w from an average length of 100 σ to one of 140 σ during a recording when R. had a temperature of 39.6° after he had already experienced five attacks of malaria during the preceding days. Thus, a lengthening of the α-w took place, as I had found in severe post-concussion psychoses, in increased intracranial pressure, but also in severe epileptic dementia. Perhaps through this unexpected lengthening of the α-w the stupor which not infrequently is present in the highly febrile patient and which also existed in R. at the time of the recording, expresses itself in an easily perceptible manner.

As I repeatedly emphasized, I consider the E.E.G. to represent the electrical concomitant phenomena of the processes involved in the function and the metabolism of the central nervous system. Just as in all active organs of the body more or less distinct changes of the electrical potential occur, so also is this the case in the human brain. These electrical manifestations are an inevitable concomitant of all biological processes. The E.E.G. oscillations are associated with biological cortical processes. As I stated at the end of my third report, both α-w and β-w can be recorded from the human cerebral cortex itself, but from the subjacent white matter of the cerebrum only β-w can be recorded; thus the α-w originate in the cortex. The bioelectric phenomena which find their expression in the E.E.G. are concomitants of excitatory processes, taking place continuously in the central nervous system and especially in the cerebral cortex. According to the available physiological studies, the local excitation of an area of a cell, fiber or tissue leads to a negative electrical charge with reference to the quiescent adjacent region[1]. When recording from two points on the intact surface of a portion of tissue, a diphasic excitatory current arises upon propagation of the excitation from the first to the second point. This wave is the bioelectric end product of the excitatory process (*von Tschermak*). A difference in the concentration of bioelectrically active ions at the excited and at the quiescent point is the cause of the currents which arise. After *Ostwald* had suggested as early as 1890 that bioelectric phenomena could perhaps also be explained in terms of the action of semi-permeable membranes as ion sieves, *Bernstein* in 1902 put forward his membrane theory of bioelectrical phenomena. This theory received excellent support and was further extended by *R. Höber*. The membranes to be considered had to be partially pervious (semipermeable) ones of the kind that have been demonstrated in plant and animal cells. These semi-permeable membranes have gaps through which, purely on account of their size[T57], smaller ions can migrate, while the larger ones are held back. Thus, the positively charged *Faraday* cations pass through the membrane and, through electrical bonds, are held back at the surface of the membrane by the negatively charged anions which because of their size cannot pass through the narrow gaps of the semipermeable membrane. One designates this hypothesis in short as the ion sieve theory.

---

[1] *Bernstein, J.*: Elektrobiologie, p. 87. Braunschweig, 1912. — *Gellhorn, E.*: Neuere Ergebnisse der Physiologie, p. 61, 4. Vorlesung. Leipzig, 1926. — *Höber, R.*: Physikalische Chemie der Zelle und der Gewebe, 6th edition, p. 705 and following pages, 1926. — *Tschermak, A. von*: Allgemeine Physiologie, p. 596 and following pages. Berlin, 1924.

If now a state of excitation occurs within the cell etc., the permeability of the membrane increases, its gaps become larger and the anions, which have been held back purely on account of their size[T57], can now also pass through it and thus the surface of the membrane becomes negatively charged. As *R. Höber* vividly puts it, each cell at the moment of activity behaves as if its plasma membrane had a hole which, upon

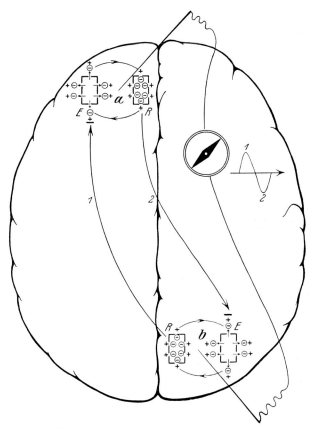

Fig. 14. Diagram. *E*, state of excitation. *R*, state of quiescence. *a* and *b*, the two recording points.

transition to the quiescent state, closes by itself again. In fact it has also now been demonstrated experimentally by *Gildemeister* that the excitation is associated with an increase in cell permeability. On the basis of this conception it is also possible, with the help of schematic representations similar to those sketched by *von Tschermak*, to imagine that the α-w of the E.E.G. are generated in the manner shown in Figure 14. From two points *a* and *b* of the intact surface of the brain, records are taken by means of needle electrodes and a sensitive galvanometer, indicated here by a magnetic needle. If the cortical area at point *a* is in a state of excitation, then an increased permeability of the membrane exists there and the state of negative charge indicated in *E* develops. We assume that there is quiescence, for the time being, at point *b*.

Therefore the deflection of the galvanometer, indicated in the diagram as *1*, occurs. If now at point *a*, after the decay of excitation, quiescence (*R*) occurs, then the negative charge disappears from there. Simultaneously, however, the elements at point *b* may be in a state of excitation and thus a current of opposite direction, indicated as *2*, manifests itself in the galvanometer. Thus *e.g.* on the basis of this so-called ion sieve theory one can form an approximate concept of the diphasic current oscillations which correspond to the α-w of the E.E.G. One therefore must assume that in the waking state tissue elements which are precisely in the opposite phases of excitation or quiescence are always present at both recording points. A state of local quiescence sets in when elsewhere in the brain a center of activity develops which exerts an inhibitory influence upon the local excitation. The α-w then transiently disappear. I wish to emphasize that the ion sieve theory of bioelectric phenomena is not yet established beyond doubt[1] and we do not know yet whether this theory really is the final truth. This is, however, not so important for the interpretation of our results. We know in any case that the bioelectric processes represent concomitant phenomena of the excitatory processes similar to those taking place in every active organ and this, for the time being, is sufficient for us.

Bioelectric phenomena are inevitable concomitant phenomena of vital processes and thus also of the processes of life in the human cerebrum. As *Pflüger*[2] says very aptly, all cells in the living organism are continuously on fire, even though we do not see the glow with our bodily eyes. He also compares the life processes with a singing flame and goes on to say: "This is the way I imagine all living matter to be, but above all the grey matter of the brain. In the waking state its vibrations are the most intense, the singing of the flame the loudest". In the E.E.G. we now indeed, also with our "bodily eye", see before us those vibrations in the form of electrical oscillations. In the light of everything I have demonstrated earlier and in this report, I consider the electrical phenomena which I designated as α-w to be a necessary concomitant of *those* physiological processes of the cerebral cortex to which mental events are correlated in an orderly manner.

---

[1] *Cremer, M.*: Ursache der elektrischen Erscheinungen. *Bethes* Handbuch, Vol. 8, 2, p. 999, 1928.
[2] *Pflüger*: Arch. f. Physiol., **10**, 251 (1875).

V

On the Electroencephalogram of Man

Fifth Report

by Hans Berger, Jena

(With 15 figures)

(Received August 29, 1932)

[Published in *Archiv für Psychiatrie und Nervenkrankheiten*, **1932**, 98: 231–254]

In my last report I gave an account of recordings of the electroencephalogram (E.E.G.) taken with the oscillograph. These recordings[1] have been continued, but very recently, prompted by the report of Mr. *Hess* (Zurich) on the type of insulation he uses for his stimulating electrodes[2] and thanks to his kind help, I changed my technique. Using his procedure, I now provide my silver needles used for recording with a coat of baked varnish. This constitutes a very significant improvement, because with this method the needles hardly increase in thickness and particularly they retain a completely smooth surface, which is not the case with the usual varnish insulation. They can thus be advanced much more easily and without resistance into the sub-cutaneous tissue until they penetrate the periosteum, and one does not have to fear that the insulation might be damaged. In my last report I also referred to the *advantages* of oscillograph recordings of the E.E.G. Since the E.E.G. thus obtained represents a pure potential curve, it is also possible to compare the size of the potentials when recording from the same skull with different distances between the two needle electrodes. With this method it was found that the potential of the E.E.G., measured as the amplitude of its alpha waves (α-w), increases nearly exactly in proportion to the distance between the two needles. With distances between the needle electrodes of *e.g.* 1 cm, 7 cm and 11 cm, with reference to the underlying cortical surface, α-w amplitudes of 4.2, 10.0 and 15.0 mm were found, when these were recorded with the oscillograph and the setting of the sensitivity remained unchanged. In the same individual, with different distances between the needle electrodes, the length of the α-w, however, remains the same. In the case just discussed, the α-w always had a length of 100 σ, whether they were recorded over a distance of 1 cm, 7 cm or 11 cm.

---

[1] Mr. *Hilpert*, as he has done in all my investigations for the past 8 years, has helped me by word and deed. For this I would like to thank him again at this time.

[2] *Hess, W. R.*: Die Methodik der lokalisatorischen Reizung und Ausschaltung subcorticaler Hirnabschnitte, p. 44. Leipzig, 1932.

The statement which I made several times, that the amplitude of the α-w of the human E.E.G. measures 0.2 mV, refers to measurements of the α-w taken in recordings from the skull as a whole, with the needles placed on the forehead and on the occiput and with a distance of about 22–24 cm between them, when measured along the scalp surface.

K. *Wachholder*[1], in an excellent paper on the general physiological principles of neurology, also reported on my investigations on the E.E.G. He took this opportunity to raise some objections against the technique of my investigations. The criticism that my report lacks proof that the instruments are capable of following higher oscillation frequencies than those which I have found, should such frequencies have been present, becomes, one may assume, untenable when one points to the use of the oscillograph, which allows the recording of all frequencies. In 1931, in my third report on the E.E.G., on page 131, I had already reported on this matter, and this probably escaped Mr. *Wachholder's* notice, probably because at that time I had not published curves relevant to this problem, like those that are now available in my fourth report[2]. *Wachholder's* other criticism, that between the two recording sites there lie an almost infinite number of cells which certainly do not all subserve the same function, I readily admit is well taken. It is, however, impossible to proceed in man as in an animal experiment. In spite of this, one is able to make very important observations. This I believe to have proved by the investigations I have made to date. I have pointed out time and again, and as recently as in the detailed arguments presented in my fourth report, that my observations on the E.E.G. of man recorded under conditions involving sensory attention merely represent distant effects of the localized, but to us completely inaccessible excitatory processes. I conceived of these changes of the E.E.G. as inhibitory phenomena which are elicited from the active center itself. I often racked my brains about these changes in the E.E.G. of man which, as I already stressed in 1930 in my second report, I had not expected at all, and I have taken into consideration the most diverse explanations for these changes. In view of the unequivocal results in the animal experiments, however, my explanation seemed to me to be the most probable one. A concept which would lead to the assumption that completely *different* laws apply, whenever in man mental processes are involved, as of course is the case in a conscious sensation, appears to me to be a mystical explanation, founded on no evidence, which one would have to discard as a matter of principle. One could, however, consider whether the sudden flattening of the E.E.G. under the influence of a sensory stimulus to which attention is directed, as shown *e.g.* in Figures 3 and 4 of my 4th report, could be attributed to the fact that a continuous excitation is taking place at that time at the two recording points *a* and *b* of the diagram, reproduced in that paper as Figure 14, so that no current could flow to the galvanometer from either point. However, among the arguments against this assumption is, firstly, the fact that in recordings taken from various areas

---

[1] *Wachholder, Kurt*: Die allgemeinen physiologischen Grundlagen der Neurologie. Fortschr. Neur., **4**, No. 2, 90 (1932).

[2] Moreover I had also recorded E.E.G.s for several years with the large *Edelmann* string galvanometer, before I changed to the coil galvanometer.

of the skull, or even from skull defects situated in completely different regions, one always obtains a flattening of the human E.E.G. in response to a sensory stimulus. One would therefore have to assume that with each sensation which arouses attention, thus *e.g.* with a fleeting touch of the hand, the entire cerebral cortex goes into a state of continuous excitation, an assumption which decidedly contradicts other views, which we hold. Secondly, it is extremely likely that a continuous excitation is also composed of individual waves which correspond in their length to the α-w of the E.E.G. and probably differ from the usual α-w only by their larger amplitude. One would therefore have to assume that whenever in a recording from points "a" and "b", a lack of current occurs, the continuous excitation composed of individual waves coincides precisely in time at the two points, so that at any given time excitation or quiescence exists with exact simultaneity and in periodic alternation at points "a" and "b", an assumption which is also very improbable.

The beautiful animal experiments[1] recently reported by *Kornmüller* and *Fischer* confirm the results of earlier investigators. Their studies also present for the first time excellent curves which make it possible to check the measurements precisely. They also showed for the first time in a really incontrovertible manner that, *e.g.*, the area in which cortical currents can be recorded in rabbits and cats when the eye is exposed to light, coincides with the anatomically defined region of the striate or visual area. Their results, it is true, could be criticized because they have not recorded from two areas of the cerebral cortex, as earlier investigators had done, but from the eye on the one hand and from the cortex on the other, a criticism which in the present case is of no great importance. The curves reported by *Kornmüller* and *Fischer* also show, as I had assumed it to be the case for man, that the excitatory states associated with the activity in the involved sensory center, consist of individual oscillations, which correspond to the α-w of the human E.E.G. They also demonstrate that a large number of individual oscillations correspond to longer lasting excitations. Thus, these animal experiments confirm that it is indeed legitimate to assume that a continuous excitation of the human cerebral cortex also consists of individual oscillations, *i.e.* of α-w. For this reason, it seems to me that the flattening of the E.E.G. under the influence of a sensory stimulus which focusses the attention cannot possibly be explained by postulating a continuous excitation at the two recording sites[T58]. I therefore reverted time and again to the explanation of this process given earlier, which postulates an inhibitory effect emanating from the center of activity. In humans with intact skull, and even in those with trepanations, it is, however, not possible to take a record with the galvanometer from a sensory center itself, because of the hidden location of the sensory centers. In 1930 in my second report, I expressed the opinion that the conditions in the animal experiment must be similar. One may assume that there, too, when a cortical current is elicited in a sensory center by the

---

[1] *Kornmüller* und *Tönnies*: Registrierung der spezifischen Aktionsströme eines architektonischen Feldes der Grosshirnrinde vom uneröffneten Schädel. Psychiatr.-Neur. Wschr., **1932**, Nr. 10. — *Kornmüller*, *A. E.*: Architektonische Lokalization bioelektrischer Erscheinungen auf der Grosshirnrinde, J. de Neur., **44**, 447 (1932). — *Fischer*, *M. H.*: Elektrobiologische Erscheinungen an der Hirnrinde. Pflügers Arch., **230**, 161 (1932).

appropriate sensory stimulus, the continuous action currents are inhibited simultaneously everywhere in the cortex, except in the involved sensory area. Therefore a decrease of the electrical potential should occur. I wrote at the time that the reason why such changes had not been observed in animal experiments may be that for recordings outside the stimulated sensory center, the sensitivity of the galvanometers used was not sufficient to permit the detection of these small and fleeting changes of the electrical activity. Curves on which I could have checked such measurements were then not available in the literature. I have not carried out any further animal experiments on the influence of sensory stimuli upon cortical currents since 1910, after I had convinced myself that in order to perform such experiments correctly the animals should not receive any sedative drugs and under no circumstances should be anesthetized. Now *Kornmüller's* and *Fischer's* animal experiments are available which are documented with good curves. I am inclined to believe that Figure 4c in *Fischer's* paper provides confirmation of the assumption made above. There, in the cat, during illumination a record was taken from a region outside the striate area. If one considers *Fischer's* statement, "that the marking of the stimulus (illumination) was carried out manually and therefore is sometimes grossly imprecise", it is evident that the onset of illumination as well as its cessation is associated with a clear decrease of the spontaneous electrical oscillations in this cortical area. This decrease each time lasts for 0.3 second and measures about 0.1–0.2 mV. However, precisely in this curve 4c, such a decrease occurs once before apparently without any external cause. However, we do not know to what extent this may represent the distant effect of a sensory stimulus which affected the animal. The deflections of the coil galvanometer, which I used for recording the E.E.G. of man, are about 20 times larger than those of *Fischer's* string galvanometer at the setting used by him, and the deflections of my oscillograph are many times larger still than those of my coil galvanometer. Moreover, I also indicated that the maximal amplitude of the α-w of the human E.E.G. was only 0.2 mV and not 1.0 mV. The observation of electrical processes occurring in the animal experiment in regions outside the stimulated sensory center, are in my opinion of the utmost importance for explaining the findings which I obtained in man and which concern the alterations of the E.E.G. under the influence of sensory stimuli, etc.

In my last report I already referred to the *disadvantages* of the oscillograph which result from its excessive sensitivity to currents of all kinds. Of course this excessive sensitivity manifests itself not only with regard to currents coming from outside, but also with regard to all those which are caused by events in the body of the experimental subject himself. Because of this excessive sensitivity I committed a serious error which I would like to correct now, especially because on this *particular* point I made inaccurate statements at the 32nd Meeting of Middle German Psychiatrists and Neurologists in Chemnitz on October 25, 1931[1] and at the meeting of the Medical Society in Jena on November 11, 1931. I committed the error of confusing in epileptics muscle currents with the beta waves (β-w) of the E.E.G. An epileptic who, as a consequence of frequent attacks, had developed mental deterioration,

---

[1] Report on the 32nd Meeting of Middle German Psychiatrists and Neurologists in Chemnitz. Arch. f. Psychiatr., **96**, 746 (1932).

exhibits the striking E.E.G. shown in Figure 1. One immediately recognizes that the
α-w are of large amplitude and that they are prolonged on the average up to 180 σ,
in contrast to the α-w of healthy indiduals, which have a length of 90–120 σ. When
this epileptic patient has a brief absence which lasts for about 3 seconds and is not
associated with any visible excitatory motor phenomena, one obtains with the same

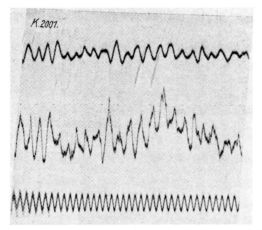

Fig. 1. S. S., 14 years old, with epileptic dementia. At the top: E.E.G. recorded with the coil galvanometer; below it: E.E.G. recorded with the oscillograph. At the bottom: time in 1/10ths sec.

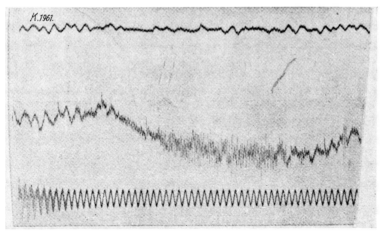

Fig. 2. S. S., 14 years old, with epileptic dementia, during an absence lasting for about 3 sec. At the
top: E.E.G. recorded with the coil galvanometer; below it: E.E.G. recorded with the oscillograph.
At the bottom: time in 1/10ths sec.

kind of recording an E.E.G. as shown in Figure 2. During the absence the α-w
disappear, just as they do during the unconsciousness associated with a major epileptic
seizure (compare Figures 10–13 in my fourth report!). Simultaneously, however, it
seems that a significant change in the β-w also sets in; they increase considerably
in amplitude. I was repeatedly struck by this change of the presumed β-w in epileptics,

but only in those whose curves were recorded with the oscillograph. I became convinced that this sudden amplitude increase of the β-w had to be considered as a state indicative of an impending seizure, and that in the major epileptic seizure too, a

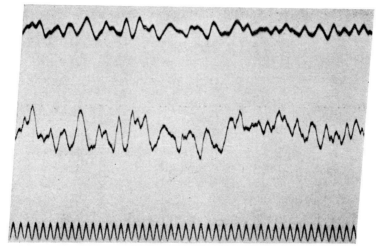

Fig. 3. R. B., 9 years old, with epileptic dementia. At the top: E.E.G. recorded with the coil galvanometer; below it: E.E.G. recorded with the oscillograph. At the bottom: time in 1/10ths sec.

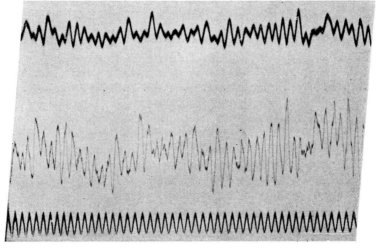

Fig. 4. G. F., 9 years old, suffering from epileptic seizures, but without impairment of mental function. At the top: E.E.G. recorded with the coil galvanometer; below it: E.E.G. recorded with the oscillograph. At the bottom: time in 1/10ths sec.

considerable amplitude increase of the β-w should occur simultaneously with the disappearance of the α-w. I assumed the same to be true for an absence and earlier I had made a statement to this effect. Additional investigations and experiments carried out repeatedly, however, proved to me that the presumed high amplitude β-w which occur in Figure 2 are not β-w at all, and are not part of the E.E.G. as such, but are incompletely reproduced muscle action currents of the temporalis muscle. Even an absence in an epileptic, which is not associated with any externally recognizable motor manifestations, is probably, according to my recent experience, always associated with excitatory motor phenomena. These need not at all become manifest in an obvious manner and may be missed even in the most careful observation. This applies *e.g.* to a slight trismus which immediately becomes associated with muscle action currents of the temporalis muscle and is recorded by the sensitive oscillograph. I therefore amend my earlier verbal reports and those contained in the proceedings of the above mentioned meeting, to the extent that during an epileptic seizure and also during an absence definite changes in the β-w *cannot* be demonstrated. In my third report I pointed out that the alterations of the α-w are by no means found in all epileptics, but only in those who have developed mental deterioration. Figure 3 shows the E.E.G. of a 9 year old severely demented epileptic boy which I shall compare with Figure 4. This record is that of a 9 year old boy, who is thus exactly the same age. He is also epileptic, but in spite of fairly frequent seizures, he has not yet developed mental deterioration. The differences in the length of the α-w are striking. The length of the α-w, in Figure 3 measures on the average 230 σ, in Figure 4 on the average 105 σ.

I had already recorded earlier E.E.G.s of *children*, but only in a few, isolated instances when the opportunity by chance presented itself. However, I had not recorded any in children below the age of 5. Through Mr. *Henkel's* and Mr. *Ibrahim's* courtesy, it became possible for me to extend these investigations to younger children. I was able to record E.E.G.s in 17 children ranging in age from 8 days to 5 years. In these recordings the needle electrodes, which I otherwise employed, could not be used because at this age local anesthesia seemed to me not to be without risk. I made these recordings with silver foil electrodes, because I had already repeatedly convinced myself that with these electrodes it is also possible to obtain perfect E.E.G.s[1]. A silver foil was placed on the forehead and another on the occiput of the child, each about as large as the palm of the hand. Under each of these a slightly larger piece of flannel soaked in warm physiologic saline was placed and each foil was covered by a second equally moistened flannel pad. By winding a thin rubber bandage around the child's skull, these electrodes were fastened and protected against drying. For moistening the flannel pad physiologic saline was used instead of the 20% sodium chloride solution at body temperature, which I otherwise employed in such cases, because the possibility existed that some of the solution could get into the eyes of the children. This naturally increased the resistance considerably. Many of the small children and smallest infants quietly tolerated the application of the electrodes, especially when they had been nursed immediately before. A few children, however, screamed incessantly and became so restless that it was impossible to obtain the kind of continuous records necessary for interpretation. For recording, the coil galvanometer with a highly sensitive insert[T6] was used exclusively, because it was clear from the start that oscillograph recordings would only very seldom be successful in the children who were often very restless. From the successful records, however, it becomes

---

[1] Arch. f. Psychiatr., **87**, 527 (1929), especially p. 548 [this book p. 54] and following pages, and **94**, 16 (1931), especially p. 35 [this book p. 111].

clearly apparent that in six children aged 8–13 days, an E.E.G. could *not* yet be demonstrated. Figure 5 shows the record of a 10 day old healthy boy who lay completely still during the recording. As has been said, the record is taken with the coil galvanometer. One observes slight fluctuations in the galvanometer curve which are caused by the child's cerebral pulsations (the fontanelles are still widely open),

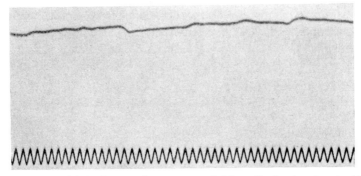

Fig. 5. Boy G., 10 days old. At the top: the curve recorded from forehead and occiput by means of silver foil electrodes and with the coil galvanometer. At the bottom: time in 1/10ths sec.

respiratory and other movements. However, one sees no trace of the characteristic α-w of the E.E.G. I succeeded, however, in demonstrating an E.E.G. in a 35 day old healthy and very strong boy. This is the youngest child in whom I was able to record an E.E.G. During the recording he lay completely still and began to fall asleep, so that it could be performed without any difficulties. Figure 6 shows the E.E.G. of this boy recorded with the coil galvanometer. Again one sees very distinctly the cerebral pulsations which have been attributed to the open fontanelles. However, already the α-w of the E.E.G. unmistakably are superimposed upon these cerebral pulsations. The α-w in this instance have a length of 160σ and thus exhibit a much slower course than is usually the case in adults and somewhat older children. In all records of healthy and strong children who were examined by me and were older than 2 months, the E.E.G. could be demonstrated. The α-w clearly increased in amplitude with increasing age of the children, whereas simultaneously the cerebral pulsations became less distinct. Figure 7 originates from a strong boy aged 6 months and 5 days who was initially very restless during the recording, but then quietened down a little, so that nevertheless, to some extent, this recording was successful. One sees very distinctly the α-w of the E.E.G. which have increased in amplitude in comparison to Figure 6, even though the resistance of the electrodes, which was always measured, is about the same. The α-w in this case have an average length of 175σ. All children of older age who were examined showed the E.E.G. clearly, but in a 4 year old child the length of the α-w still measured on the average $135–160 \sigma$, and thus was increased in comparison with that of the adult. In my investigations I found values of the α-w of $110–120 \sigma$ only from the 5th year of life onward. These values thus corresponded to those which in numerous examinations I had found in adults and also in children beyond the 5th year of life. If one enters on graph paper the average length of the α-w of children from the beginning of the 2nd month of life up to the age of 5 years, one finds a steadily declining curve. However, this curve is not a straight line, but fluctuates. It declines in an oscillating fashion to a value of 110 σ.

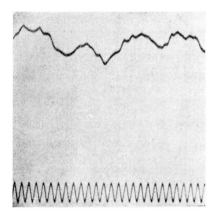

Fig. 6. Boy R. T., 35 days old. At the top: the curve recorded from forehead and occiput by means of silver foil electrodes and with the coil galvanometer; in it the α-w of the E.E.G. can be recognized. At the bottom: time in 1/10ths sec.

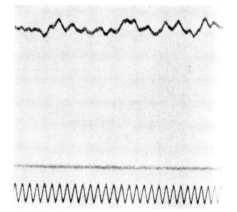

Fig. 7. Child E., 6 months and 5 days old. At the top: the E.E.G. recorded from forehead and occiput by means of silver foil electrodes and with the coil galvanometer. At the bottom: time in 1/10ths sec.

    I am inclined to explain the absence of the E.E.G. in the first weeks of life by the fact that the cerebral cortex from which, evidently, according to my observations (third report, Figure 30), the E.E.G. is derived, has not yet assumed its function. This is in good agreement with the physiological observations in the newborn and especially also with *Flechsig's* anatomical studies on the development of myelin in the human cerebrum. The human infant is born with an immature cerebrum. It is true that at birth a number of cortical areas, *Flechsig's* so-called primordial regions, are already predominantly myelinated, yet large regions of the cerebral cortex are still without myelin. In *Flechsig's* so-called intermediary regions, myelination starts only within the first month after birth and is completed within the first 6 weeks of life. In the terminal regions this process starts only after the 2nd month of life. According to *Flechsig*, the completion of myelination in the tracts made up of coarser fibers takes place in about the 4th month of life, if the child was born at term[1]. I believe that the absence of the E.E.G. in newborn infants and until the beginning of the 2nd month of life can be attributed to this lack of development of the cerebral cortex. *Peiper*[2], in an excellent study, pointed out that the brain of young infants is also immature in a physiological sense and that the phylogenetically youngest parts of the brain are not yet capable of functioning. According to him, the ability to form conditioned reflexes develops only in the second trimester of life and signs of the awakening intelligence, and thus of the most important activity of the cerebrum, appear only in the third or fourth trimester of life. Also very convincing is *Peiper's* sagacious allusion that, in the course of dying, the path is retraced in exactly the opposite direction to that followed during the gradual awakening of the cerebral activity of the newborn. The ability of the brain to function is first extinguished in the youngest and last in the oldest parts of the brain. Till now I have always declined to follow the suggestions made to me from various sides subsequent to reports on my investigations, that I should study the gradual extinction of the E.E.G. in a *dying* person, for I hold such investigations to be inadmissible on moral grounds. However, already years ago I had observed the gradual extinction of the E.E.G. in the animal experiment and had found that the α-w coalesce more and more, become longer and flatter, similar to what I have been able to observe in pathological cases. These findings too can very well be compared, in the sense proposed by *Peiper*, with the gradual development of the E.E.G., which we have just now been able to identify in the developing child. I believe that these E.E.G. changes observed in the animal experiment are of fundamental significance with regard to the pathological alterations of the E.E.G., which I had already described earlier. For this reason and because of findings to be reported below, I wish to discuss in a few words these earlier, as yet unpublished observations.

Figure 8 shows a recording obtained from a 4 year old female dog of which I had already published Figures 1, 2 and 3 in my first report in 1929. About 5 hours prior to the recording of the E.E.G., she had received 1.5 gram of Veronal by mouth and, one hour prior to the beginning of the preparatory operation, 0.03 gram of morphine subcutaneously. The E.C.G., in accordance with a proposal by *Einthoven*, was recorded with freshly amalgamated zinc rods which had been inserted under the skin of the chest. For the recording of the E.E.G., small, freshly amalgamated, tiny zinc plates were used, which were inserted into the subdural space through a slit and lay over the right and left cerebral hemispheres. The skull and skin wounds were closed again over the operative site in order to avoid drying and other effects of this kind. It is evident that the E.E.G. of the dog brain is somewhat distorted by cerebral movements which in their turn, as I had already explained earlier, cause the tiny plate electrodes to rest with varying firmness on the cerebral surface. The oscillations of the E.E.G. are, however, not caused by the motion of the blood in the brain[T59]; but they are probably greatly modified by it because not only the degree of filling

---

[1] *Flechsig, Paul*: Gehirn und Seele. Leipzig, 1896. — Anatomie des menschlichen Gehirns und Rücken-
    marks. Vol. 1, p. 11 and following pages. Leipzig, 1920.
[2] *Peiper, Albrecht*: Das Erwachen der Hirntätigkeit des Säuglings. Z. Neur., **139**, 781 (1932).

of the arteries, but also that of the cerebral veins, which is related to the respiratory movements, causes the pressure between the electrode and the brain surface to vary. Thus, in many places, individual oscillations of the E.E.G. are considerably increased and in others again attenuated. As a consequence of this, the E.E.G. of the dog, which in this case was also under the influence of Veronal and morphine, actually appears

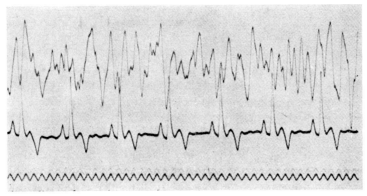

Fig. 8. 4 year old female dog. At the top: E.E.G. recorded with amalgamated tiny zinc plate electrodes placed in the subdural space; below it: E.C.G. recorded with amalgamated zinc rods inserted under the skin. At the bottom: time in 1/10ths sec.

with greater clarity only after cessation of respiration when the heart beats have become less frequent, as is the case in Figure 9 to which I shall return below. The individual oscillations of the E.E.G. of the dog have an amplitude of 0.2 mV and are thus five times smaller than the "spontaneous oscillations" on which *Fischer* reports in his study. His "spontaneous oscillations" reproduced in Figures 1 and 2 are in fact much larger and in any case do not represent what I consider to be an E.E.G. They could be spontaneous oscillations which are markedly distorted by other electrical processes and one would have to consider what kind of interference could be involved. It is possible, however, that they could be caused by simple experimental errors which, as I emphasized above, can creep in even if one has been engaged in such investigations for many years, as I have been. It is quite conceivable that under certain circumstances when one records from the eye and the brain, currents having nothing at all to do with the processes that are being investigated could enter into the record. As I explained in my first report in 1929, I had many difficulties because of the intrusion into the E.E.G. of electrical oscillations originating from the heart, whenever I recorded not from the skull alone, but from the skull and any other part of the body. Indeed I have repeatedly observed that even when one recorded from two points on the skull which were not placed completely symmetrically with regard to the heart, individual waves of the E.C.G. appeared in the E.E.G. of many people, especially Einthoven's R-, but also the T-wave, so that already then I wrote of the ubiquity of the E.C.G. This was the reason which for many years prompted me to write the E.C.G. simultaneously with all recordings of the E.E.G. The "spontaneous oscillations" shown by *Fischer* are reminiscent of such distortions. Furthermore, it could be possible that these oscillations represent, after all, the effect of sensory stimuli which escaped the experimenter's notice and which, if they were to originate from the interior of the animal's body, he would also be totally unable to observe. The use of curare with the ensuing inability to move voluntarily any part of the body, and the induction of artificial respiration, puts the animal into completely different physiological conditions, as *E. Weber*[1] justly emphasized. It is completely impossible to appraise what states of irritation originating in the body may act on the cerebral cortex of the fully awake animals. Such irritations could be elicited by drying of the trachea, overinflation of the lungs, furthermore by pain originating from the wounds, thirst, uncomfortable positioning, etc. *Fischer* himself, in correct appreciation of this situation, pointed out that even with the greatest precautions one can probably never eliminate all the stimuli. All this, it seems to me, has to be taken into account when judging the oscillations shown in Figures 1 and 2 of *Fischer's* study. According to my experience, these do not represent spontaneous oscillations corresponding to the E.E.G. This experience, it is true, is based on only a few investigations in the dog, and not on any carried out in the species of animals used by *Fischer* and *Kornmüller*, namely rabbits and cats, but it nevertheless extends over a great number of investigations in man carried out over several years. Some waves in Figure 4b of *Fischer's* study and some in Figure 2 of *Kornmüller's* study, according to their length and their order of magnitude, would most likely seem to correspond to the true "spontaneous oscillations" of the dog brain and to the α-w of the human E.E.G. These are the three waves in Figure 4b of *Fischer's* study which occur in the cat before illumination and on the average have a length of 133 σ with an amplitude of 0.1 mV. And in Figure 2 of *Kornmüller's* study of the rabbit, these are the waves which occur after illumination, between the initial and terminal deflection, which have a length of about 160 σ and likewise show an amplitude of about 0.1 mV. During the action of the sensory stimulus which one intends to test, one really never knows which impressions affect the animal, either simultaneously during stimulation or during the so-called resting pauses. This makes the interpretations of the results extremely difficult and even sometimes impossible. These circumstances and the fact to which I alluded above, that the experiments in higher animals have to be carried out without the use of any sedative drugs and without general anesthesia, made me lose interest in the continuation of these investigations as early as 20 years ago. This was precisely what prompted me to explore time and again whether it would be possible to carry out similar investigations in man, in which the subject would not sustain any damage nor experience any pain, until at last in 1924 I succeeded in discovering the E.E.G. of man. In needle recordings of the E.E.G. from the human skull or from skull defects in patients with trepanations, just as with needle recordings of the E.C.G., distortions of the E.E.G. cannot be produced because of the smallness of the needle tip which picks up the current and because the surrounding tissue is pressed more or less firmly against the recording surface. Such distortions inevitably occur when

---

[1] *Weber, E.*: Der Einfluss psychischer Vorgänge auf den Körper. 1910. p. 146.

applying larger electrodes of various sizes to the pulsating surface of the brain or to other tissues, *all* of which in fact do exhibit pulsations. However, let us return to our illustrations.

The distortions of the E.E.G. of the dog brain present in Figure 8 are actually without importance for our subsequent consideration. The curve of Figure 9 was

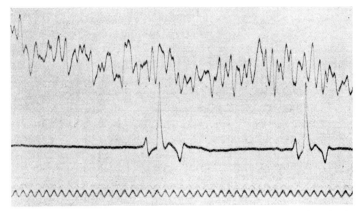

Fig. 9. The same female dog as in Figure 8 with the same recording arrangement. Respiration stopped^{T60} cardiac beats somewhat slower. Time in 1/10ths sec.

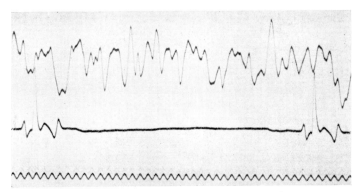

Fig. 10. The same female dog as in Figures 8 and 9 with the same recording arrangement. Respiration stopped and marked slowing of the heart beats. Time in 1/10ths sec.

recorded soon after respiration had been eliminated by careful cervical cord transection, carried out without great blood loss and after the animal had received 0.05 gram of muscarine intravenously, which induced slowing of the heart beat. After elimination of respiration and slowing of circulation, the spontaneous electrical oscillations of the cerebral cortex of the dog appear much more distinctly in this figure because they are undistorted, as was mentioned above. It will therefore be best if we choose the E.E.G. of this illustration as the starting point of our further considerations. Figure 10, which was recorded only a few minutes later, shows that the heart beats have become still slower. Whereas between the single heart beats shown in Figure 9, about two beats had failed to occur, now about 5 beats have dropped out while respiration is completely absent. By this time, the E.E.G. too has undergone a distinct change which at first concerns only the duration of the individual oscillations. A fusion of the single oscillations corresponding to the α-w of the human E.E.G. has taken place. There is at first no evidence for an amplitude diminution of the α-w; however, such

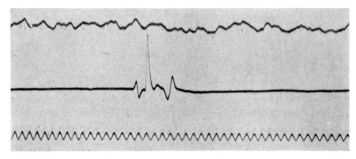

Fig. 11. The same female dog as in Figures 8, 9 and 10 with the same recording arrangement. Respiration stopped, still further slowing of the heart beats. Time in 1/10ths sec.

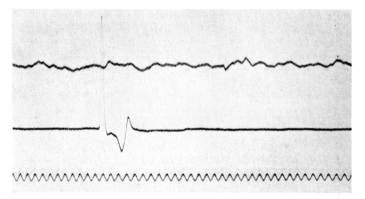

Fig. 12. The same female dog as in Figures 8, 9, 10 and 11 with the same recording arrangement. Respiration stopped; only sporadic heart beats. Time in 1/10ths sec.

a diminution appears very rapidly with longer duration of the apnea and a further decrease in the number of heart beats, as is shown in Figure 11 in are cording taken a few minutes later. The amplitude of the individual oscillations has now decreased very considerably, whereas simultaneously, through further fusion of several oscillations into a single one, their length has increased still more. These processes now very rapidly progress further, as shown in Figure 12. Now there are only very sporadic heart beats which occur after long intervals and then exhibit considerably larger E.C.G. deflections[T61] than under normal conditions. The animal no longer reacts to any stimuli. The E.E.G. progressively approaches a straight line on which the very much slowed single oscillations are only recognizable as very feeble deflections. One may assume that in the dying human the E.E.G. behaves in the same way as is shown in the dying dog. There too, during the gradual extinction of life, the α-w will probably become progressively slower and of smaller amplitude, until the galvanometer records only a straight line as an indication that the cerebrum has irrevocably ceased its activity.

I have also further pursued the recording of the E.E.G.s in pathological states. In four patients, I had the opportunity of investigating the effect upon the E.E.G. of *illuminating gas poisoning* of varying severity. In the least severe of these cases of poisoning, that of a 23 year old girl who had been only transiently unconscious, lengthening of a few α-w of the E.E.G. was found on the day following the intoxication. This change had completely disappeared in a second recording taken in the same girl 14 days later. In a 41 year old woman, the intoxication had been considerably more severe. She had been unconscious for 12 hours and had also suffered a severe epileptic seizure after the poisoning. Twelve days later, a lengthening of the α-w of the E.E.G. to an average duration of 130–150 σ was still found in this patient, who was then completely clear in her mind and not confused. Still more severe alterations of the E.E.G. were found in a 55 year old woman who, after the intoxication, had been unconscious for 18 hours and who had suffered a severe epileptic seizure. These changes were present in a record taken on the 5th and again still in another taken on the 20th day after the poisoning. At the time of the second recording this patient still exhibited extremely severe disturbances of recent memory and a state of confusion. In a fourth patient, a 50 year old man who, together with his wife, had poisoned

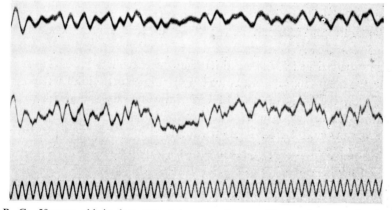

Fig. 13. R. G., 50 years old, in deep stupor, because of severe illuminating gas poisoning. At the top: E.E.G. recorded with the coil galvanometer; below it: E.E.G. recorded with the oscillograph. At the bottom: time in 1/10ths sec.

himself with illuminating gas, I had the opportunity, thanks to Mr. *Veil's* obliging kindness, to record an E.E.G. while the severe stupor caused by the illuminating gas poisoning still persisted. Figure 13 shows this record. Through appropriate measures taken in the Medical Clinic, it had been possible to obviate any immediate threat to life posed by the intoxication. At the time of recording G. was still deeply stuporous, so that *e.g.* a local anesthesia was unnecessary when the needle was inserted. The recording took place in the afternoon of the day on which earlier in the morning the patient had been found unconscious in his apartment. After the recording of the E.E.G., severe stupor persisted for an additional 4 days. The E.E.G. shown in Figure 13 is somewhat low in voltage and shows extreme lengthening of the α-w to an average of 195–300 σ. Lengthening of the α-w of the E.E.G. still persisted in two further recordings taken in the same patient and performed on the 17th and on the 20th days after the intoxication, at which time he exhibited most severe disturbances of recent memory, even though his thinking appeared well organized. This lengthening was not as marked as in the first record; it measured on the average 130–165 σ. There is no doubt that intoxications which are associated with such severe cerebral signs, as is the case in illuminating gas poisoning, cause distinct changes of the E.E.G. These alterations, just as the mental defects, considerably outlast the acute period of intoxication.

Earlier already I had repeatedly examined people with severe *heart diseases* in order to determine whether irregularities of the E.C.G., which might occur, could affect the E.E.G. However, I made no observations in these studies which could be interpreted in this way. Thus no influence of the very irregular heart beats on the pattern[20] of the E.E.G. was found in a 54 year old patient who since the age of 10 years, after an acute cardiac condition, continued to suffer from heart disease and in whom, at the time of my investigations, a mitral stenosis, pulmonary congestion and a continuous arrhythmia had been diagnosed by the internist. The E.E.G., as always, had been recorded with needles from the forehead and occiput. However, a persistent alteration of the E.E.G. existed in this patient who, for many months, had shown mental changes, and upon more precise testing exhibited considerable disturbances of recent memory. There was a consistent lengthening of the α-w to an average of 130–150 σ. Therefore some impairment of the activity of the cerebrum must have occurred which expressed itself in the E.E.G. and which perhaps in this case indicated the presence of extensive lesions in the cortex itself, of the kind which *Bodechtel*[1], on the basis of his histological investigations performed on cardiac patients, was able to demonstrate in his beautiful study.

I have now collected E.E.G.s of 29 patients with *general paresis*, after having slowly but steadily continued these investigations. In untreated cases of general paresis alterations of the E.E.G. were always found during the progressive course of the disease. They appear frequently in the form of a surprisingly low voltage of the E.E.G., which becomes evident in the oscillograph curves. This low voltage even exists when there is no reason to suspect that attention has been diverted by sensory stimuli, fear, pain and other factors. Especially on days after a paralytic attack, the voltage of the E.E.G. is particularly low. Furthermore, as I stressed in my third report, the alteration of the E.E.G. in general paresis in comparison to that of a healthy individual consists of a strikingly unequal length of the α-w which follow immediately upon each other in a segment of the curve. In such cases I sometimes had the impression that occasionally in general paresis, shortening of the α-w could also occur. However,

---

[1] *Bodechtel, G.*: Gehirnveränderungen bei Herzkrankheiten. Z. Neur., **140**, 657 (1932).

I do not dare to decide on this question at present, in spite of the large material which has been studied, because according to the frequency analyses[T55] carried out by Dr. *Dietsch*, the β-w exhibit a much greater range of variation in length than I originally assumed and thus could sometimes be mistaken for very low voltage and shortened α-w. In general paresis one also finds at times more or less prominent and consistent increases in the length of all the α-w of the E.E.G. In general paresis too, the E.E.G. only gives information on the momentary physiological state at the recording sites of the cerebral cortex and probably also on that existing in the areas of the cerebrum lying between them. However, it can give no information on the further course of the general paresis. Also there is no characteristic E.E.G. of general paresis, as I had emphasized in that earlier report. As I explained there too, it is sometimes no longer possible to demonstrate any definite pathological changes of the E.E.G. in patients with general paresis in whom the progress of the disease has been arrested after malaria therapy, even though it may have left a considerable mental defect. As I stated earlier, there evidently has been a loss of specific cerebral mechanisms[T43] in these cases, but no longer are there any general disturbances of function[T42] of the kind that manifest themselves in the E.E.G.

In two cases of severe *Korsakoff's psychosis* with extreme disturbances of recent memory and confabulation, I was also able to establish the presence of distinct alterations of the E.E.G. In a 43 year old woman, the wife of a liqueur manufacturer, who for 13 years had been drinking a great deal, an average increase in length of the α-w of the E.E.G. to 130–165 σ was found. In a 62 year old beer distributor's wife who had been drinking beer and brandy for many years, the average increase in length of the α-w of the E.E.G. amounted to 140–190 σ. There can be no doubt that these are pathological E.E.G. changes.

Marked changes of the E.E.G. were also found in severe cases of *senile dementia*. These again consisted of distinct lengthening of the α-w of the E.E.G., whereas in mentally healthy old people, even beyond the 60th year of life, I have not to date observed any lengthening of the α-w of the E.E.G. For instance in a 64 year old woman who exhibited the nocturnal states of restlessness of senile dementia and moderate disturbance of recent memory, an increased length of the α-w of the E.E.G. to 135–150 σ was found. In a 76 year old civil servant who showed a most severe disturbance of recent memory, to a degree where one could actually speak of complete abolition of recent memory, an E.E.G. recorded in the usual fashion with needles from the forehead and occiput exhibited the changes shown in Figure 14. It was found that the rather high voltage α-w of the E.E.G. were on the average lengthened to about 145–220 σ, the values being most often close to the upper limit of this range. Thus, just as in pronounced instances of *Korsakoff's* psychosis, one finds in severe cases of senile dementia distinct changes in the E.E.G. which exhibits a considerable lengthening of the α-w, and this the more markedly so, the more severe the clinical deficit in the mental sphere.

In my third paper, I also reported on investigations of the E.E.G. in patients with *oligophrenia* — patients with mental debility and imbeciles. At that time I had been unable to establish any deviation of the E.E.G. in imbeciles from that of mentally normal subjects, when only the *length* of the α-w was compared. I pointed out, however, that if one uses coil galvanometer records it is impossible to make accurate comparisons of the amplitudes of the α-w, because of the variable resistance of the skull in different subjects. Thanks to Dr. *Dietsch's* investigations, I have now performed a much more precise measurement of the resistance and with the oscillograph,

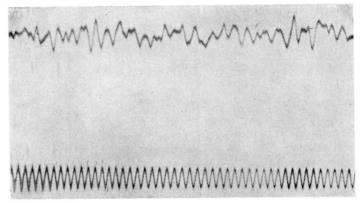

Fig. 14. J. S., 76 year old, with severe senile dementia. Above: E.E.G. recorded with the coil galvanometer; below: time in 1/10ths sec.

as I mentioned in my fourth report, I am no longer dependent upon the local resistance on the skull, so that it is now possible to compare the amplitude of the α-w of the E.E.G. in different persons. If I now compare E.E.G.s recorded with the oscillograph in three imbeciles with those of mentally normal subjects, I find the former surprisingly low in voltage, with α-w of normal length. Such E.E.G.s could, however, very well also have originated from normal subjects whose attention had been diverted by an event in their environment, by pain, or by similar factors. Because obviously one can never fathom what is going on in another person's mind and since imbeciles especially are incapable of giving sufficient information concerning their possible fears, etc. in the course of the recording of the E.E.G., prudence is always indicated when interpreting the amplitude of the potentials of the recorded E.E.G. To be sure, the records in the three patients were taken repeatedly to eliminate as much as possible the element of novelty and unexpectedness in the recording of an E.E.G. In these repeated recordings, the same low voltage was found. Because in spite of all efforts I could not arrive at a sufficiently convincing result, I recorded in addition E.E.G.s in four idiots who had not learned to speak. Recording these E.E.G.s was associated with very great difficulties because of the restlessness and the recalcitrance of these patients. Sedatives could not be given, because they were certainly apt to influence the E.E.G. which one expected to record. I finally adopted the procedure of having the patients bathed in warm water for several hours at a time, so that they developed considerable fatigue. The E.E.G. could then be obtained without great difficulties. In a 6 year old idiot boy, in addition to the low voltage of the E.E.G., distinct lengthening of the α-w on the average to about 133–250 σ was found. Repeated records from another

6 year old idiot boy showed an average length of the α-w of 140–200 σ. A 26 year old idiot who, like the others, has never learned to speak, is always incontinent and has to be fed, showed an E.E.G. as shown in Figure 15. I owe to Mr. *Boening* the opportunity of investigating this patient. The curve shown here immediately strikes one by its low voltage. The E.E.G. in Figure 15 reminds one of the curve of the electrical

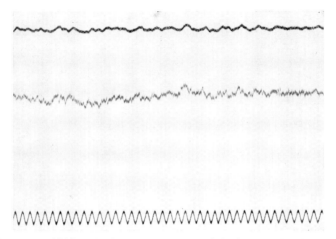

Fig. 15. W. H., 26 year old idiot. At the top: E.E.G. recorded with the coil galvanometer; below it: E.E.G. recorded with the oscillograph. At the bottom: time in 1/10ths sec.

oscillations of the dying dog reproduced in Figure 12. Of course in this case one could think of the possibility that the low voltage of the curve had been caused by diversion of the attention by fear, pain and other factors of this kind. But when the recording was repeated, the E.E.G. was equally low in voltage with a skull resistance that was relatively low. Furthermore the eyes of the patient had been covered with a light bandage and cotton wool had been inserted into the external auditory canals, precautionary measures which obviously do not prove that diversion of attention did not occur in spite of them. However, in view of the behavior otherwise exhibited by this extremely retarded idiot, I hold it to be impossible that his mind had been distracted. Furthermore the very flat α-w of the E.E.G. also show a distinct lengthening to 160–230 σ. In many places between them, it is true, normal α-w of 100 σ duration are also interspersed. In a 43 year old female idiot a similar E.E.G. was recorded. Thus in the most severe forms of mental retardation such as in idiots, one certainly finds obvious alterations of the E.E.G., in comparison to that of a mentally normal individual. Therefore, I now no longer hesitate to reject possible distraction of attention as the explanation of the strikingly low voltage of the E.E.G. observed in imbeciles, for such distraction would have had to continue with the same intensity during the entire duration of the record, and with each renewed recording in the same patient it would have to recur constantly in the same manner. Instead I consider this low voltage to be a characteristic property of the physiological processes in the cerebrum, even when the α-w are not significantly altered in their time course.

In my third report on the E.E.G. I already stressed that among all the possible pathological alterations of the E.E.G., when recording with the coil galvanometer, one finds only the following: an increase in the amplitude of the α-w, their flattening, or their temporary or more prolonged loss, furthermore lengthening and finally irregularity of the α-w. At that time a shortening of the α-w could not be demonstrated unequivocally and the situation today is still exactly the same. As emphasized above, one sometimes has the impression that there may be a shortening of the α-w in the E.E.G.s obtained in patients suffering from general paresis. However, in view of the larger range of variation of the β-w of the E.E.G., this question can still not be settled. In the meantime I investigated a series of other diseases, but these observations added nothing fundamentally new to the earlier ones. The use of an oscillograph which reproduces the E.E.G. as a pure potential curve and, as was emphasized elsewhere, with respect to the height of its deflections is independent of the local resistance of the skull, makes it possible to compare the amplitudes of the α-w of the E.E.G. of different individuals. I continued to carry out resistance measurements on the skull according to the procedure devised by Dr. *Dietsch* even though this was not at all necessary in these cases. It became apparent from these studies that the α-w of the E.E.G. are strikingly low in voltage after a paralytic attack and in idiocy, which suggests that the biological processes in the cerebral cortex which are associated with these electrical phenomena are less intense. However, here again I wish to point out particularly that, when making use of the amplitude of the α-w in comparing the E.E.G.s of different human subjects, extreme caution is indicated even if one bases such comparisons on oscillograph curves. Mental processes markedly influence the voltage of the E.E.G., as I demonstrated again in my fourth report. Especially in patients who give only fragmentary or no information at all about their subjective experience, it is often impossible to exclude this source of error. I pointed out earlier that directing the attention to a sensory stimulus can cause a decrease in voltage of the E.E.G. to 1/10th of its original value and that the same voltage decrease also occurs during a continuous mental task. Physical pain, fear, excitation, etc., act in the same way. In patients it is at times not possible to eliminate these factors, even if one repeats the records on different days. I often followed this procedure in order to demonstrate to the patients that nothing happens to them which was likely to cause them fear or pain. In an entirely normal and intelligent human subject, for example, I was able to obtain an E.E.G. with the same low voltage as that shown in Figure 15 which was taken in a markedly defective idiot, but only when the normal subject was preoccupied with a task which absorbed his whole attention *continuously* and to the highest degree. A normal person may be given the task of holding a thin wire within the slit of a steel spring attached vertically to a frame at a comfortable height, with the added stipulation that the wire should not touch the rim of the slit anywhere. To perform this task the subject must direct his whole attention upon the image of the slit, the position of the wire in relation to its rim and upon the position of his fingers, his hand, the arm and the whole body, so that he is fully preoccupied if he wants to perform this task conscientiously. When I performed this experiment in one of my assistants, a completely healthy and very intelligent young man, I was indeed able to obtain an E.E.G. which for the whole period of recording exhibited the same low voltage as the E.E.G. shown in Figure 15. But in spite of this there exists a fundamental difference between the E.E.G. of the healthy subject, totally absorbed in this extremely demanding task, and Figure 15. It is true that in the healthy individual, the α-w are also remarkably low in voltage and are even completely absent at times, but when they are present they have a normal length of 100 σ, whereas in Figure 15, in addition to the low voltage, they exhibit distinct lengthening. Furthermore I am of the opinion that such a profoundly defective idiot, as the one from whom the E.E.G. of Figure 15 had been recorded, would be completely incapable of maintaining such marked concentration of attention for the whole duration of the recording. Indeed here in Figure 15, I see in the low voltage of the oscillograph curve a sign that in this case[T62] the biological processes of the cerebral cortex, whose electrical concomitants the E.E.G. represents, continuously take place with a very low energy expenditure. In spite of the use of the oscillograph, however, the surest way to demonstrate pathological changes in the E.E.G. is still the measurement of the length of the α-w. When making such measurements, the normal range of variation has to be taken into consideration and it is very important not to interpret as pathological occasional α-w with a length greater than 120 σ, but only the *average* lengthening in a longer series of consecutive α-w.

VI

On the Electroencephalogram of Man

Sixth Report

by Hans Berger, Jena

(With 7 figures)

(Received February 1, 1933)

[Published in *Archiv für Psychiatrie und Nervenkrankheiten*, **1933**, 99: 555–574]

In my publications I repeatedly emphasized that, when using several, very sensitive galvanometers, one always obtains at different times the same electroencephalogram in one and the same individual, if he is mentally and physically relaxed. Its principal or alpha waves (α-w) exhibit a definite length. I have now performed many investigations[1] on the alteration of the electroencephalogram (E.E.G.) under the influence of startling stimuli. Naturally, under these conditions, distortions of the E.E.G. by unintentional movements occur very easily. But in *those* cases in which these are sufficiently unobtrusive, so as not to disturb the recording, one finds that startle, as any other stimulus which absorbs the attention, leads to a decrease in voltage and to a loss of the principal waves of the E.E.G. After a brief period of time the principal waves return again. However, they repeatedly disappear and return again until the E.E.G. reassumes the form it had before the influence of the startling stimulus. In a 25 year old physician who had been vigorously startled by the unexpected firing of a cap pistol, the drop in voltage persisted initially for 19 seconds; then for 5 seconds there was an increase in voltage and subsequently a renewed decrease set in which persisted for 17 seconds. In other experimental subjects, the time course of this waxing and waning of the after-effects of the startling stimulus was different. The duration of the first decrease in voltage, its repeated recurrence and finally the duration of the decrease recurring at any given time, depend upon the intensity of the emotional effect. Precise measurements of the length of the α-w at the time of their return following a startling stimulus repeatedly showed that they can be considerably shortened to as much as half of their previous length. These findings now give the key for the interpretation of E.E.G.s of many healthy persons in whom a considerable shortening of the α-w was found. These were invariably people who, in spite of their assurance to the contrary, awaited the recording of the

---

[1] As in all these investigations, Mr. *Hilpert* has again helped me faithfully, for which here too I thank him cordially.

E.E.G. with a certain apprehension. An example of such an E.E.G. is shown in Figure 1 which was obtained from a healthy lady who had approached me with the offer of being a subject for the recording of an E.E.G. It is evident that the α-w are considerably shortened in comparison with those found in a state of rest. They exhibit a length of only 55 σ, whereas I had repeatedly indicated a value of 90–120 σ

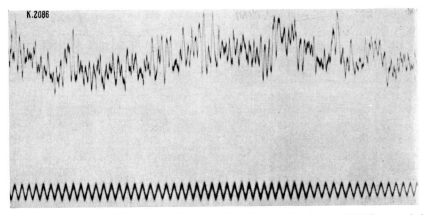

Fig. 1. Mrs. K., 29 years old, in a state of emotional excitement. At the top: E.E.G. recorded with the oscillograph; below: time in 1/10ths sec.

as their normal average length. From other curves in which the electrocardiogram had been recorded simultaneously, one could demonstrate that during the recording the pulse was considerably accelerated. This is proof that a state of mental relaxation certainly could not have been present. On the basis of such records in which a certain acceleration of the pulse was always noted, I became convinced that in healthy individuals a decrease in the duration of the α-w can occur under the influence of anxious excitement. In very pronounced instances it appears, moreover, that the principal waves not only become shortened to half their normal length, but that a decrease in their voltage also occurs. The α-w become smaller in amplitude. When comparing the E.E.G.s of different individuals, the influence of emotional excitement caused by the recording itself, as well as distracting stimuli must therefore, among other things, also be taken into consideration. Particularly when recording the E.E.G.s of patients with diseases of the cerebrum, one will have to take into account the influence of possible emotional excitement. This is one more factor which can render comparisons difficult. However, in pronounced pathological states, I found without exception an *increased duration* of the principal waves of the E.E.G. beyond 120 σ. Nevertheless, in future investigations, the possibility of a shortening of the α-w by emotional factors must also be taken into consideration.

The α-w, as I stressed in my fifth report, have the *same* length in one and the same human individual, even in different types of recordings. I would like to add they also have the same form, even when the recording electrodes are placed on very different parts of the skull. With different recording distances, the voltage of the E.E.G.

increases with the distance between the two recording sites. However, the α-w maintain their form and length, though the recording electrodes certainly lie over cortical areas with completely different structure. Even when one records from the dura within a bone defect and compares the E.E.G. obtained in this manner with an E.E.G. recorded simultaneously from the whole skull, one obtains the same form and length of the α-w. I would like to stress this expressly with regard to the E.E.G. of *man*. This observation is also in accord with the animal experiments reported by *Travis* and *Dorsey*[1] in which simultaneous multiple recordings were carried out, as far as one can gather from the report in the "Zentralblatt". In this report it is particularly emphasized that the same action current was always obtained when records were taken from areas of the animal cerebral cortex which differ completely in their structure. A certain contradiction exists between these findings in the animal and *Kornmüller's*[2] investigations which were also carried out in animals. *Kornmüller* was able to confirm the old observation that when sensory stimuli are presented, currents occur in the related cortical center. On the basis of his findings, he also believes that the action currents differ in their form and course, depending upon the anatomical structure of the cortical areas from which they are recorded. The statement made by *Fischer*[3] is also to be understood in this sense, when he says that the spontaneous electrical oscillations in the animal display different patterns[T120] in different cortical areas. Thus there is no agreement concerning the results obtained in *animals*. In *man*, in any case, the situation is as follows: The E.E.G. recorded from various areas of the cortex, either from the skull as a whole or from skull defects in different locations, always exhibits the same form of the principal waves in one and the same individual. This is the case even if the cortical areas over which the needle electrodes are placed have a completely different structure and therefore also subserve completely different functions. Double recordings especially, several of which I already published in Figures 4, 5, 6, and 28 of my third report, show this perfectly well. Double recordings from various areas of the intact skull also demonstrate this. I shall reproduce here some E.E.G.s recorded one after the other with the oscillograph from the same individual, a 24 year old physician. The recording method used in these studies becomes evident from the small drawings inserted in Figure 2. The principal waves are everywhere the same; only small variations in their length occur, ranging from 85 σ to 92 σ. These variations are similar to those also found with the same recording arrangement[T63] in the course of a longer segment of a curve. From such records, and even more convincingly from double recordings which I published earlier, one cannot fail to gain the impression that when one records from the various areas of the cerebrum with these different recording arrangements, one studies one and the same process, which finds its expression in the E.E.G. This process is independent of the structure and the function of the cerebral cortical area lying below

---

[1] *Travis* and *Dorsey*: Action current studies of simultaneously active disparate fields of the central nervous system of the rat. Abstract Zbl. Neur., **65**, 635 (1932).

[2] *Kornmüller, A. E.*: Architektonische Lokalisation bioelektrischer Erscheinungen auf der Grosshirnrinde. J. Psychol. u. Neur., **44**, 447 (1932).

[3] *Fischer, M. H.*: Elektrobiologische Erscheinungen an der Hirnrinde. Pflügers Arch., **230**, 161 (1932).

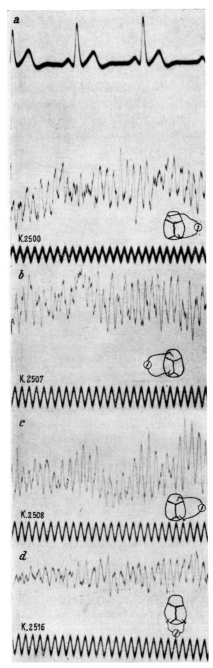

Fig. 2. Dr. W., 24 years old. Four different recordings of the E.E.G. taken with the *oscillograph*. In curve *a*, at the top, E.C.G. recorded from both arms with the coil galvanometer. Time in 1/10ths sec. In each sample the site of recording is indicated in the small drawing of the skull.

the recording site. In particular, however, I would like to emphasize that in pathological cases the alterations of the α-w of the E.E.G. can be demonstrated in the most diverse recording arrangements. Thus *e.g.* the considerable lengthening of the principal waves of the E.E.G. present in a case of epileptic dementia is just as clearly apparent in a recording taken from forehead and occiput, as in one in which the needles are placed over the right and left parietal eminences. This uniformity of the process which is represented by the E.E.G. revealed itself also by the fact that the latter always responds in the same way to the most diverse stimuli to which the attention is directed, and this with the most diverse recording arrangements. Thus the truly amazing sensitivity of the E.E.G. towards interfering sensory stimuli becomes apparent time and again, so that *e.g.* an accidental creaking of the experimenter's chair is capable of absorbing the experimental subject's attention to such an extent that further[T64] investigations become impossible. Therefore one has to assume according to the results of my studies that in all areas of the cerebral cortex outside the sensory center affected by the stimulus, a decrease in the voltage of the E.E.G. and a transient disappearance of the α-w take place, as shown particularly in Figures 3 and 4 in the fourth report. The animal experiments, however, — and here we can now rely upon *Kornmüller's* and *Fischer's* beautiful curves — prove that in response to the appropriate stimulus an action current originates in the corresponding sensory center. This current takes the form of individual oscillations. We can assume that the same is true for *man*, as I already emphasized in 1930. We therefore arrive at a concept which is represented in Figure 3 in the form of a sketch.

A is meant to demonstrate that in a state of mental and physical rest one obtains the same α-w in all recordings from *a* to *b*, *b* to *c*, *c* to *d*, *d* to *e*, *e* to *f*, and of course also when recording from *a* to *f* etc. In the latter case, according to earlier explanations, the amplitude of the α-w increases. *B* represents the recordings taken simultaneously from the same areas when the contralateral hand has been touched. Subsequent to this a decrease in the voltage of the E.E.G. and an absence of the α-w develop at points *a*, *b*, *c*, *e*, and *f*. Only at point *d*, which corresponds to the excited sensory center, a considerable increase of the α-w takes place. The purpose of the schematized record labelled *a*[T65] is to demonstrate once more a continuous recording of the E.E.G. at point *a*. The point in the record designated by *1''*[T66] (1 sec) indicates that the contralateral hand has been touched. A decrease in voltage and a loss of the α-w occurs which in the drawing here extends from the line indicating *1''* (1 sec) to that indicating *2''* (2 sec). The purpose of the schematized record labelled *d*[T67] is to display a continuous recording of the human E.E.G. from an active sensory center, the pattern of the E.E.G. being inferred from animal experiments. Again the touch stimulus was applied shortly before *1''*[T66] (1 sec); the α-w of the E.E.G. increase in amplitude and exceed a certain limit which is designated in the diagram as *I–S*[T68], the internal threshold as defined by *Fechner*[1]. In the schematic representation this increase in amplitude lasts from *1''* to *2''*[T66] and is subsequently replaced again by the usual pattern[T20] of the E.E.G. However, I wish to lay particular stress on the fact that in *man* nobody

---

[1] *Fechner*: Elemente der Psychophysik. Second part, p. 377.

till now has seen this pattern of the E.E.G. in the area of an active sensory center of the cerebral cortex. This pattern is merely inferred from animal experiments, such as those performed by *Caton*, *Beck*, *Fleischl* and many others, and more recently by *Kornmüller* and *Fischer*. That the voltage decreases and the α-w disappear out-

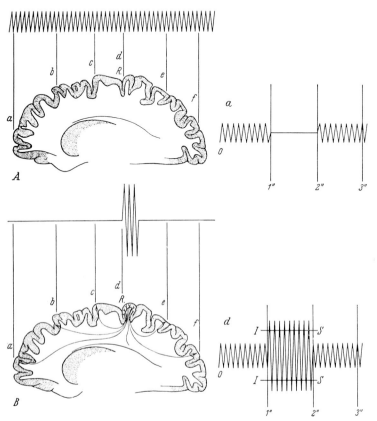

Fig. 3. Sketch. Explanation in text.

side of the active center, I was able to demonstrate in numerous investigations. This inhibition of the E.E.G. activity[T69] in all cortical areas not directly affected by the stimulus can surely only serve the purpose of increasing the efficiency of the active center itself, or that of creating the conditions which are required for the occurrence of a conscious sensation. *Fechner* assumed that the psychophysical motion, which he imagined to occur in the form of oscillations, has to attain a certain magnitude in order to be associated with conscious phenomena. *Jodl*[1] indicated that from the point of view of the natural sciences, no fundamental objections can be raised against such a concept because, according to him, the observation of nature everywhere shows

---

[6] *Jodl*: Lehrbuch der Psychologie. Vol. 1, p. 44. Stuttgart, 1903.

us that increases which apparently are merely quantitative, beyond a certain level also imply qualitative changes. Thus, he points out, steady increase in pressure at low temperature leads to liquefaction of a gas; the fluid has properties which are not inherent in the gas, even in a rudimentary form. Against such a view, *Linné's* dictum "natura non facit saltus" has been repeatedly quoted, which however has lost much of its power of conviction in the light of modern quantum theory and other newer concepts in science. In any case the interpretation of the events as given above is the most likely one, particularly if one considers the fact that we will most probably never be able to unveil their true nature.

In mental work too, even in its most *diverse* forms, when one records from *different* regions of the intact or the trephined skull, there always appear the *same* changes in the E.E.G., in the form of diminution in voltage and a transient loss or diminution in amplitude of the α-w. Under these circumstances, something else can be seen which becomes evident in Figure 4.

This is a small segment of a very long curve which was recorded in a 24 year old physician while he solved a problem of applied mental arithmetic which obviously required much effort. This figure contains two simultaneous recordings of the E.E.G. with two galvanometers which were not connected to each other. From the right side of the skull a record was taken with a coil galvanometer, from the left side another was obtained with an oscillograph. Because the light spots are not in precise vertical alignment, simultaneous points of the curves are connected by lines drawn with india ink. One sees how the E.E.G. at *a*, *b*, *c* and *d* repeatedly assumes the *particular* form which it generally does during mental work or when a sensory stimulus holds the attention. This change is most distinct at the beginning of *b*, the least pronounced at the beginning of *d* and it always appears more clearly in the lower curve obtained with the oscillograph. Following *a*, *b* and *c* large α-w appear, as they are found in a state of rest. Thus very distinctly one recognizes an intermittently recurring[T70] change in the E.E.G. which usually lasts only for fractions of a second, though in one instance (at *b*) it did last for 2 seconds. These intermittently recurring alterations correspond to the momentary periods of work. It is known from psychology that even when solving a difficult arithmetic problem we are not engaged in work continuously, but the work is composed of individual parts, a fact that we can see graphically reproduced in the E.E.G. Furthermore we recognize that the periods of work are often very short and interrupted by pauses of equal and in many cases even longer duration. Here also during the periods of work we are dealing, according to our concept, with the effect of inhibitory processes. These inhibitory effects are exerted by the momentarily active center which is inaccessible to us and which affects the remainder of the cortex from which we record. As *Pflüger* already stressed[1] we have to distinguish between two processes in the cerebral cortex: (1) excitatory processes which are correlated with mental phenomena and (2) conduction processes which occur without such mental concomitants. It is therefore also conceivable that only the excitatory processes in the cerebral cortex act in an inhibitory manner upon

---

[1] *Pflüger, E.*: Über den elementaren Bau des Nervensystems. Pflügers Arch., **112**, 1 (1906).

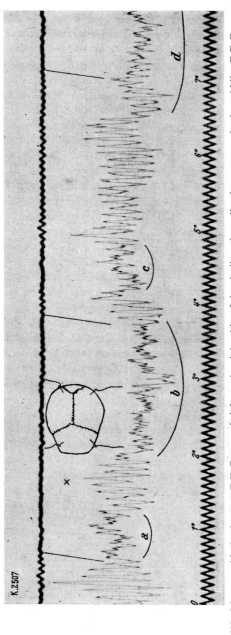

Fig. 4. Dr. W., 24 years old. At the top: E.E.G. recorded from the right side of the skull to the coil galvanometer; in the middle: E.E.G. recorded from the left side of the skull to the oscillograph; at the bottom: time in 1/10ths sec. — Record taken while solving a difficult problem of applied arithmetic which requires considerable time. Simultaneous points of the two E.E.G.s are connected with india ink lines.

the other parts and that the constantly intercalated conduction processes which, of course, require a certain amount of time, remain without such a distant inhibitory effect exerted upon the entire cortex. If we were to make such an assumption, we would expect to obtain this same composite picture in the E.E.G. during any mental work of fairly long duration. The results of cortical stimulation experiments on which *Bechterev*[1] reports on the basis of *Wedensky's* investigations are also in favor of the concept that the decrease in voltage of the E.E.G. which is caused by the influence of a sensory stimulus or which appears during mental work, does in fact represent an inhibitory effect. In animal experiments *Wedensky* was able to show that when a cortical motor area of one hemisphere was stimulated, the excitability of the corresponding cortical area of the other hemisphere was diminished and the excitability of the antagonistic cortical center enhanced. *Braunstein's* and *Weiler's*[2] beautiful investigations suggested that the pupillary dilatation occurring in man under the influence of psychic stimuli, the so-called psychoreaction of the pupil, is very likely dependent upon an inhibition of the sphincter tone which originates in the cerebral cortex. *Bumke*[3] agreed with this concept and stressed that the inhibition of the sphincter tone may originate almost anywhere in the cerebral cortex. The investigations on the latency of this psychoreaction of the pupil agree well with the results of my measurements concerning the time which elapses until the inhibitory effect manifests itself in the E.E.G. Indeed the change in the E.E.G. takes place much earlier. *Weiler* indicates a latent period of 0.44 second as the shortest time for *sensory* stimuli, when involvement of the dilator of the pupil probably occurs in addition to inhibition of the sphincter tone. In contrast I found a change in the E.E.G. following a sensory stimulus as early as 0.23 second after the stimulus. This figure leads to an important consideration. *Ziehen*[4] states that the sensory reaction time for cutaneous stimuli applied to a finger is 200 σ. This sensory reaction time includes centripetal conduction, the central process and centrifugal conduction with all the various latent periods. For centripetal conduction and the central process one can thus allow half of this value, $= 100 \, \sigma$, and this estimate certainly seems to be a little too high. Upon touching the finger of an experimental subject, a decrease in voltage occurred after 0.23 second, *i.e.* 230 σ in the E.E.G. recorded from forehead and occiput. If now one assumes that, from the time of its application to the skin, it took this stimulus 100 σ to influence the sensory center in the postcentral gyrus, then $230 - 100 = 130 \, \sigma$ would be the remaining time for the central conduction of the inhibitory process from the postcentral gyrus to the recording sites and for the latent periods. This is more than the conduction time from the finger to the cortex including all latent periods. In any event one conclusion which follows from this is that the central conduction seems to be considerably slower than the peripheral one. I already indicated elsewhere[5] that the conduction in the fibers of the human brain-stem and spinal cord, *e.g.* in the pyramidal fibers,

[1] *Bechterew*: Die Funktionen der Nervenzentra. H3, p. 1388. Jena, 1911.

[2] *Weiler*: Untersuchungen der Pupille und Irisbewegungen beim Menschen. Z. Neur., **2**, 101 (1910).

[3] *Bumke, O.*: Die Pupillenstörungen bei Geistes- und Nervenkrankheiten. 2nd edition. Jena, 1911.

[4] *Ziehen*: Physiologische Psychologie. 12th edition, p. 541. Jena, 1924.

[5] *Berger, H.*: Zur Physiologie der motorischen Region des Menschen usw. Arch. f. Psychiatr., **77**, 321 (1926).

must be considerably slower than in peripheral nerves, as had been suggested earlier by animal experiments. We now have to assume that in the cerebrum itself there is a considerable further decrease in conduction velocity as compared to that in the spinal cord and brain-stem, for this is what the considerations which have just been presented suggest. The increasing slowness of conduction in fiber systems as they approach the center corresponds to a similar process in the grey matter, whose excitatory states likewise have an increasingly slower time course the closer they are to the center. Finally, in the cortex itself, there are only 8–11 principal waves of the E.E.G. in 1 second.

As I explained in detail earlier, the α-w of the E.E.G. originates in the human cerebral cortex itself. The E.E.G. probably represents the electrical phenomena which are concomitant to the various states of rest and excitation of the cortical cells. This assumption received further support through the experimental studies in animals carried out by *Bishop* and *Bartley*[1]. They concluded that the electrical concomitant phenomena which can be recorded from the cerebral cortex of animals reflect potentials of ganglion cells and not of nerve fibers. As *Wachholder*[2] rightly emphasized, one can assume that between my two recording points a myriad of nerve cells of completely different function and different structure are interposed, a fact to which I specifically referred above. The sum of the manifestations of excitation of all these interposed nerve cells results in the relatively simply patterned E.E.G., with its principal waves which exhibit a periodic waxing and waning. If the "all-or-nothing law" also applies to the cerebral cortex, as is affirmed by some but denied by others[3], one would have to assume that the number of nerve cells active at any time varies. If this is the case the rhythmic waxing and waning of the voltage of the E.E.G. is caused by the fact that a number of the interposed nerve cells enter into a state of complete quiescence, only to completely resume their full activity again after a brief pause. *Herring*[4] emphasized that all organs of the body are not simultaneously active in all their parts, but that in these parts periods of quiescence and activity constantly alternate, some cells being active while others are resting. He called this the law of fluctuation. In the waxing and waning of the E.E.G. we are probably confronted with this fluctuation.

In my further investigations it became necessary to follow the course of the E.E.G. still more precisely by means of multiple *simultaneous* recordings. I had already reported earlier on simultaneous recording of the E.E.G. from various regions of the skull, or from trephine openings and from the skull as a whole. I then came to the conclusion that simultaneously recorded E.E.G.s do indeed exhibit a certain degree of correspondence; however, there is certainly no identity of the simultaneous curves. The various parts of the curves between concordant segments can exhibit

---

[1] *Bishop* and *Bartley*: Electrical activity of the cerebral cortex as compared to the action potential of excised nerve. Abstract in Zbl. Neur., **65**, 634 (1932).

[2] *Wachholder, K.*: Die allgemeinen physiologischen Grundlagen der Neurologie. Fortschr. Neur., **4**, No. 2, 90 (1932).

[3] *Brücke, Th.*: *Bethes* Handbuch der normalen und pathologischen Physiologie. Vol. 9, p. 34, 1929.

[4] *Herring*: The "law of fluctuation" or of alternating periods of activity and rest in living tissues. Brain, **49**, 209 (1923).

an entirely different pattern. By means of simultaneously recorded coil galvanometer and oscillograph curves, I followed up these questions further. In such records it could be established that when one records from the right forehead and the right occiput, and simultaneously from the left forehead and left occiput, using different galvanometers, E.E.G.s result such as that of Figure 5.

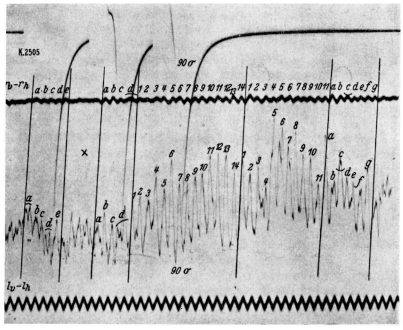

Fig. 5. Dr. W., 24 years old. At the top: E.E.G. recorded with the coil galvanometer from the right side of the skull; in the middle: E.E.G. recorded with the oscillograph from the left side of the skull. At the bottom: time in 1/10ths sec. Simultaneous points of both E.E.G.s are connected by india ink lines.

The light spots are not in exact vertical alignment, therefore simultaneous points of the curves are connected by lines drawn with india ink. One sees the marked correspondence of the E.E.G.s recorded from the right and left sides of the skull of a healthy 24 year old physician. In the segment of the curve on the right side of the first india ink line, one looks at the first α-w matched to each other by the letters a, b, c, d and e. One sees that the individual α-w of the right and left side are congruent not only in their time course, but also in their form, as far as this can be assessed by a comparison of curves recorded with galvanometers of different design. The same can be seen on the right side of the third india ink line. I also wish to draw attention particularly to the correspondence of the principal waves designated with d in the upper and lower curves. The same applies for the other specifically identified parts of the two curves and among these I draw attention in particular to the principal waves c in the last segment of this illustration outlined by two india ink lines. That this correspondence does not always exist, however, becomes apparent from the second outlined segment of the curve which is marked by a cross. One obtains exactly the same correspondence and circumscribed discrepancies of multiple recorded curves when one records simultaneously from the right side anteriorly to the left side posteriorly, and from the left side anteriorly to the right side posteriorly, as well as in recordings over short distances, oriented longitudinally on the right or the left side. If in these recordings by chance one fails to take care that correspondingly located electrodes are connected to corresponding poles of the galvanometer, one obtains mirror image curves which can immediately be transformed into identical curves by reversing the polarity of one of the galvanometers. Immediately the impression forces itself upon the unprejudiced investigator that the process being recorded here from the right and from the left half of the skull is one and the same and that it only transiently exhibits local deviations. The precise correspondence of the time relationships and the configuration of the individual principal waves in the two recordings confirm this. This may lead to a complete identity of their form insofar as this can be expected with different galvanometers. The deviations which from time to time encompass longer or shorter intervals of the two simultaneously recorded E.E.G.s remain considerably less obvious. *Travis* and *Dorsey*, in multiple recordings in the animal, were able to observe a "synchonism" of the course of the action currents of homologous cortical areas of the right and of the left hemisphere. This observation agrees with what is reported here, *i.e.* the congruence of the *E.E.G.s* recorded from the right and left half of the skull of *man*. I would like to stress in particular once again that this congruence in time applies not only for E.E.G.s recorded from the two entire halves of the skull, but also for the recording from limited segments on the right and left side, provided these are oriented in the same anteroposterior longitudinal direction. The *E.E.G.s* reproduced above which were recorded simultaneously from the right and left side of the skull of *man*, however, show much more than this mere *simultaneity* of the course, they even show an *identity*, which reveals itself unmistakably in single principal waves. Thus one comes to the conclusion that in man it is *one and the same* process which is recorded from both cerebral hemispheres and which occasionally, and only transiently, is masked or altered by local events.

Juxtaposition of other simultaneous recordings leads even further. For if one records from an anterior and posterior location, *i.e.* from forehead and occiput, and simultaneously at a right angle to this arrangement from both parietal eminences, the *E.E.G.s* in this case too frequently seem to be congruent, but only because the principal waves have the same length. These principal waves, however, by no means conform to each other in their details; they are not identical in the two recordings. Under such conditions one can, however, also obtain E.E.G.s in which a pervading difference between the two records exists with regard to their time course. In such a case, coincidence in time of single segments of the two curves is out of the question. Figure 6 shows this clearly.

This is a record taken in the same gentleman as Figure 5, however, the upper coil galvanometer curve records from the left side anteriorly to the right side posteriorly, and the lower oscillograph curve records from the right and left parietal eminences. Because the light spots of the two curves are again not in precise vertical alignment, simultaneous points on the curves are connected by india ink lines. If we look at the first segment on the right side of the first india ink line, the very distinct α-w in the antero-posterior recording are designated with the numbers *1–7*. These by no means coincide with the α-w labelled *a, b, c, d, e, f, g* and *h* of the recording between the right and left side. One also sees the same in the further course of the two E.E.G.s. Measurements in this case also demonstrate that the principal waves in the two recordings are not of equal length. In the coil galvanometer curve, in

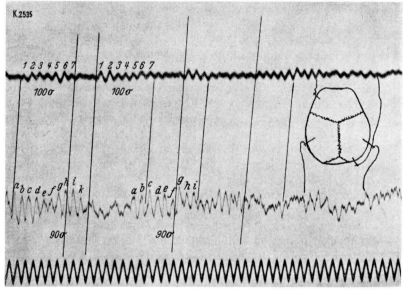

Fig. 6. Dr. W., 24 years old. At the top: E.E.G. recorded with the coil galvanometer from the left frontal and the right occipital quadrants of the head; in the middle: E.E.G. recorded with the oscillograph from the region of the right and left parietal eminences. At the bottom: time in 1/10ths sec. Simultaneous points of the two E.E.G.s are connected by india ink lines.

the first outlined segment, the α-w have a length of 100 σ, in the oscillograph curve one of 90 σ. In other subjects when using the same arrangement, these time differences are not always as evident. However, there too one finds a difference in the time course[T71] of the two E.E.G.s which is not just transient. The E.E.G.s are consistently different and congruent segments are lacking. This finding as well as the observation reported above reinforce my view that in the E.E.G. a process becomes manifest which spreads over the cerebral cortex in a very definite *direction*, a progressing wave of activity moving from front to back (or if one wishes, from back to front, because the two directions cannot be separated on the basis of the galvanometer curves). We thus come to the conclusion that this is a uniform process involving both cerebral hemispheres and moving in a fixed direction, which finds its visible expression in the E.E.G.

Till now I have believed that the corpus callosum insures this coordination of the two cerebral hemispheres into a single unity, especially since I attributed the diminution of the excitability of the homologous motor center on the contralateral side in *Wedensky's* experiments to an effect mediated by callosal fibers. The report of the above mentioned American investigators, who proved that the "synchronism" of homologous cortical areas of the right and left side in the rat persists even *after* cutting the corpus callosum, calls for a cautious approach. One could of course say that in man conditions are different. Yet one cannot simply disregard these findings and at least one will have to consider whether the coordination of the two cerebral hemispheres into common activity could not also be brought about by deeper structures. The animal experiments of the Americans point to more deeply lying centers from which the course of the cortical processes with regard to their simultaneity (synchronism) could be regulated. Likewise the directed and synchronized course of the E.E.G.s of the right and the left hemisphere of man could also be regulated from a center lying outside the cortex. Quite naturally one thus arrives at the ideas of *Berze, Reichardt* and others. For instance, *Berze*[1] considers the thalamus to be a center from which the tonus of the organ of consciousness is regulated and from which the psychocerebral apparatus, *i.e.* the cerebral cortex, can be turned on and off. It is entirely possible that this also applies to the course[T72] of the E.E.G. Undoubtedly, however, this question still has to be left open. In many pathological cases, thus *e.g.* in a young man with a tumor in the depths of the left cerebral hemisphere, I found the coordination of the two cerebral hemispheres to be disturbed in the E.E.G.s, recorded simultaneously from the two sides. However, I do not yet wish to take up these observations in more detail. One would also have to consider whether the *inhibition*, which, upon the influence of a sensory stimulus manifests itself in the E.E.G. everywhere in the cerebral cortex, may also originate in a center localized outside the cortex and thus may arise in the thalamus. This seems to be a likely interpretation for the changes taking place in response to a startle, for this surely is a defense reaction of the organism. From the biological standpoint we can interpret in a similar manner the processes taking place when attention is aroused by an unexpected sensory stimulus. However, these processes, compared with a startle, may be attenuated[T73] in proportion to the lesser degree of arousal[T74]. One can therefore not immediately discard the possibility that with a startling stimulus the facilitation and inhibition in the cortex originate from a center located outside it. Yet on the other hand unequivocal experimental observations indicate that facilitatory and inhibitory processes can originate in the cerebral cortex itself. In this regard I would like to refer once again to *Wedensky's* investigations. As far as the progression of mental work or of any thought process is concerned, it is certainly easier to assume that the facilitatory and inhibitory events originate from the cortical center of activity involved at any given time. I would like to assume the same in the case of simple sensory stimuli.

When interpreting mental processes including those of man, rightly their biological significance is increasingly taken into account and their gradual phylo-

---

[1] *Berze, Josef*: Bewusstseinstonus. Wien. med. Wschr., **1911**. — Psychischer Antrieb und Hirnstamm. Wien. med. Wschr., **1932**, No. 11.

genetic evolution is considered, as was first done by *Herbert Spencer*[1]. Attempts have been made to reduce the three types of mental processes, defined according to the customary classification as sensation, emotion and goal seeking[T75], to *one* of these as the only basis for all. Such attempts, which have been made by *Spencer, Horwicz*[2], *Höffding, Münsterberg* and many others, did not receive universal recognition. However, there is agreement that mental processes too have evolved from the simplest beginnings and according to their biological importance have become increasingly perfected. One is inclined to favor the view that all three above named types are already contained in the simplest psychical processes. *Jodl* expressed this view most forcefully and stated that sensation, emotion and goal seeking are three different ways in which the general process of the primary psychical reaction manifests itself. This is also *Müller-Freienfels'*[3] opinion, who speaks of all mental phenomena as being only differentiations of a mental "primordial phenomenon" in which the active character of all mental processes already becomes apparent in the reaction and the attitude towards external influences. *Berze*[4] who like *Wundt* sees in goal seeking the fundamental element of all mental processes, developed his view with great clarity and advocated a unitary concept of psychophysical function. According to his view, there corresponds to this unitary psychophysical function a unitary *physiological* process distributed over the entire extent of the cerebral cortex. He distinguishes in the cerebral cortex, or in the "psychocerebral apparatus", as he also calls it, two regions which he designates as spheres and he localizes them in certain layers of the cerebral cortex, referring to anatomical views first expressed by *von Monakow*. In accordance with his psychological conception of the importance of actions for mental life in general, *Berze* calls the layers in which material processes associated with psychical events occur the intentional sphere. In this sphere, according to his view, no localization exists at all. He claims for it the three upper cortical layers, *i.e.* according to the customary nomenclature cortical layers 1 to 3. The other sphere, the impressional, comprises the 4th to the 6th cortical layers; in it, in contrast to the intentional sphere, there exists a sharp localization; it is here that one has to look for the sensory centers, the fields of engrams, central regions for other cortical functions and purely motor areas. Even though the anatomical basis for this concept does not correspond to facts, (especially should one assume that the upper three cortical layers exhibit a uniform structure over the entire cerebral cortex), I nevertheless believe that this objection is not sufficiently serious to invalidate such a view. It is quite probable that such a sharp anatomical separation of these two spheres cannot be made at all. This, however, by no means argues against the, in my opinion, very felicitous distinction between these two regions which, of course,

[1] *Spencer, Herbert*: Prinzipien der Psychologie. Translated by *Vetter*, Vol. 1. 1903.

[2] *Horwicz*: Psychologische Analysen. Halle, 1872.

[3] *Müller-Freienfels*: Das Denken und die Phantasie. Leipzig, 1916.

[4] *Berze, Josef*: Die primäre Insuffizienz der psychischen Aktivität und ihr Wesen usw. Leipzig and Vienna, 1914. — Zur Lokalisation der Vorstellungen. Z. Neur., **44**, 213 (1919). — Schizophrenie und psychologische Auffassungen. Allg. Z. Psychiatr., **77**, 58 (1921). — Zur Frage der Lokalisation psychischer Vorgänge. Arch. f. Psychiatr., **71**, 546 (1924). — Störungen des psychischen Antriebs. Z. Neur., **142**, 720 (1932).

collaborate most closely with each other. Many anatomical facts argue in favor of the particular importance of the upper cortical layers for mental processes[1]. *Kaes*[2] demonstrated that a continuing physiological development of the external zone of the cortex takes place until the 45th year of life. Such an observation clearly points to the particular significance of the upper cortical layers, just as do many pathological findings. Of these I only wish to emphasize those in *Pick's* cortical atrophy. As I stressed above, an intimate collaboration of *Berze's* two spheres would indeed have to be postulated, with the implication that the inherited structures existing in the impressional sphere become modified under the influence of the intentional sphere and that new mechanisms[T43] are constructed or assembled out of available parts, also always under the influence of the intentional sphere. Through such structural alterations, which can no longer be reversed, the individual brain experiences its historical evolution[3]. In addition to the greater endowment with inherited mechanisms, the acquired mechanisms naturally determine the profound differences between the brains of different human individuals and between the animal and the human brain. *K. Goldstein*[4] propounded views similar to those of *Berze*, even though he speaks of fundamental functions and not of a unitary psychophysical function as *Berze* does. To these fundamental functions corresponds, according to his view, the cortical performance in general. He then continues by saying that the individual functions, such as perceiving, imagining, thinking, feeling etc., are only special ways in which these fundamental functions are elaborated from different materials supplied by the activity of the senses or the motor mechanisms. It appears to me therefore that the difference between his and *Berze's* view is not at all significant; in their fundamental concepts both are in agreement. *Berze* thus assumes a unitary *physiological* process as the concomitant phenomenon of psychophysical processes, which take place everywhere in the cortex, perhaps in certain cortical layers, *i.e.* in his intentional sphere. Now, in the E.E.G. we are confronted with the electrical concomitants of a uniform process distributed over the entire cortex; in its genesis the nerve cells of the cortex are involved. This process is uniform and is independent of local structural differences of the cortical areas. It proceeds in a very definite direction over the entire cerebral cortex which in this manner appears to be integrated into an undivided whole. The principal waves of the E.E.G., as I demonstrated in many instances, are intimately connected with conscious phenomena. They disappear in the unconsciousness of chloroform narcosis, return gradually with the reawakening of consciousness, undergo profound alterations when mental processes are severely disturbed, *e.g.* in epileptic dementia, and so forth. All this led me earlier to propose the working hypothesis that the principal waves of the E.E.G. are concomitant phenomena of those material cortical processes which one terms psychophysical because, circumstances permitting, they can be associated with phenomena of consciousness. According to the findings

---

[1] *Von Economo* and *Koskinas*: Cytoarchitektonik der Hirnrinde des erwachsenen Menschen. Text volume. Berlin, 1925, p. 116, 179 and 183.

[2] *Kaes*: Die Grosshirnrinde des Menschen. Jena, 1907. Text p. 45.

[3] *Lieder, Franz*: Die psychische Energie und ihr Umsatz. Berlin, 1910, p. 369 and following pages.

[4] *Goldstein, Kurd*: Zur Funktion des Nervensystems. Arch. f. Psychiatr., **74**, 370 (1925).

reported above, I therefore conceive of the E.E.G. as representing the electrical concomitants of a wave of activity proceeding in a definite direction over the human
cerebral cortex, which integrates the two hemispheres into an undivided whole reacting
in unison. This activity is automatic, but it is altered by external influences and shows
a periodic waxing and waning. I am inclined to believe that we are here indeed confronted with the continuous activity of *Berze's* intentional sphere.

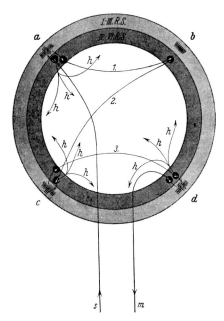

Fig. 7. Sketch. Explanation in text.

If we choose to make this assumption, we arrive at a concept as represented in
the sketch shown in Figure 7.

The cortex, *Berze's* psychocerebral apparatus, is represented as an undivided
whole in the form of a closed circular ring. A boundary between *Berze's* intentional and
impressional spheres within this circular ring is suggested, the all too sharp separation
of the two being perhaps permissible in such a sketch. A sensory stimulus arrives
through fibers S at the corresponding sensory center within the impressional
sphere. It causes, at point a, an excitatory process which, after having attained a
certain magnitude, affects the intentional sphere, which lies above it and is intimately
connected with the impressional sphere. In the intentional sphere, psychophysical
processes take place *continuously* which manifest themselves in the form of the E.E.G.
Immediately there is an inhibition of the automatic activity of the entire intentional
sphere[1] and thus the internal threshold is exceeded at point a^{T76}. This event in
the intentional sphere again elicits processes in the impressional sphere and a further

---

[1] In Figure 7 the pathways through which these inhibitory phenomena pass, are indicated by h.

conduction of the excitation through pathway *1* to point *b* takes place. There the process may merely occur in the impressional sphere and the continuous psycho-physical process in the intentional sphere which manifests itself in the E.E.G. may not become involved. Yet a further conduction through pathway *2* to point *c* may occur where the same process takes place again as at point *a*. From here too con-duction may proceed still further through pathway *3* to point *d* and hence further still through fiber *m* to deeper parts of the brain. This is how, on the basis of my investigations and with reference to *Berze's* views, I imagine the psychophysical cortical processes to occur. According to this view the E.E.G. would represent the continuous automatic activity of *Berze's* intentional sphere which from time to time at certain points exceeds the internal threshold and then becomes associated with conscious phenomena.

Naturally this is only an image born of the general human need to arrive at a unified concept. Yet, with regard to these processes, we shall hardly ever arrive at anything other than such images, which are adapted as closely as possible to the physiological and psychological facts available at any given time and therefore are being improved time and again.

VII

On the Electroencephalogram of Man

Seventh Report

by Hans Berger, Jena

(With 14 figures)

(Received April 28, 1933)

[Published in *Archiv für Psychiatrie und Nervenkrankheiten*, **1933**, *100*: 301–320]

There is hardly any need for me at this point to dwell on the close dependence of the cerebral activity upon the blood circulation. In my third report I discussed in detail the relationships between cerebral circulation and the electroencephalogram (E.E.G.) and I demonstrated in illustrations that the occasional dropping out of single cerebral pulsations, caused by extrasystoles, has no influence upon the course of the E.E.G. Accelerated cardiac activity, as found in fever, exerts no corresponding influence upon the course of the E.E.G. Quite unexpectedly, on the other hand, in high and prolonged fever, a distinct lengthening of the principal waves of the E.E.G. occurs in comparison to the normal record found in the same individual, as I emphasized in my fourth report. This lengthening of the alpha waves (α-w) considerably exceeds the average length of the principal waves found in healthy persons and indicates that in fever there is some impairment of cerebral cortical processes which may be completely reversible. These deleterious effects are reminiscent of the lengthening of the α-w of the E.E.G. occurring *e.g.* in carbon monoxide poisoning; I presented such E.E.G.s in my fifth report. Bacterial toxins, if they affect the cerebral cortex, also cause a distinct alteration of the E.E.G., even when they do not lead to major elevations of temperature. Figure 1 shows the E.C.G. (electrocardiogram) and the E.E.G. of a 44 year old man who became ill with severe purulent basal meningitis following actinomycosis.

Because of neck stiffness which led to considerable posterior retraction of the occiput, he could only lie on his side and there was therefore some difficulty in recording the E.C.G. from both arms. He was fully conscious, although at times he showed transient periods of confusion and was unable to distinguish between real and imaginary events. At the time of the recording, however, he was able to give a correct account of things. The axillary temperature was 37.6°; the pulse was markedly accelerated with 132 beats per minute. The principal waves of the E.E.G. are high and distinctly formed; on the average they show considerable lengthening to 140 σ.

[191]

Thus one finds in this instance also slowing of the principal waves of the E.E.G. in spite of the significant acceleration of cardiac activity. On the day following this recording, the man succumbed to his illness after respiratory paralysis of sudden onset. The autopsy (Prof. *Berblinger*) confirmed the purulent meningitis limited to

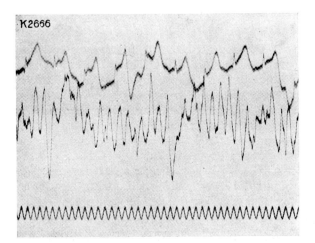

Fig. 1. H.E., 44 year old, with basal purulent meningitis. At the top: E.C.G. recorded from both arms to the coil galvanometer. Below it: E.E.G. recorded with needles from forehead and occiput to the oscillograph. At the bottom: time in 1/10ths sec.

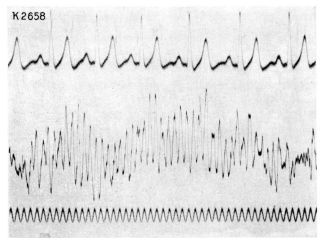

Fig. 2. I.B.[T49], 16 years old. At the top: E.C.G. recorded from both arms to the coil galvanometer. In the middle: E.E.G. recorded with needles from forehead and occiput to the oscillograph. At the bottom: time in 1/10ths sec.

the base of the brain which had been suspected during his life. For comparison I again show in Figure 2 the E.C.G. and E.E.G. of my daughter Ilse who is now 16 years old.

In the fourth report I had already published E.E.G.s of I. which were taken in her 14th year of life. The principal waves of the E.E.G. have maintained the same form and the same average duration of 95 σ; no change has occurred in the course of the years.

In my sixth communication I explained in detail why I came to the conclusion that the E.E.G. is the manifestation of a directed wave of activity which integrates the cerebral cortex of both cerebral hemispheres into a unified whole. There I also reproduced several simultaneously recorded E.E.G.s. Figure 3 again shows such an observation in a 24 year old healthy physician in whom records were taken from the right and left sides of the skull.

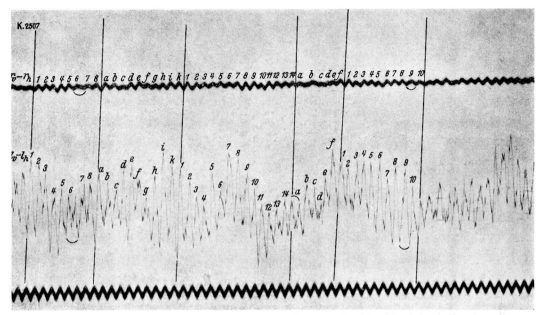

Fig. 3. Dr. W., 24 years old. At the top: E.E.G. recorded from the right side of the skull to the coil galvanometer; in the middle: E.E.G. recorded from the left side of the skull to the oscillograph. At the bottom: time in 1/10ths sec. Simultaneous points of both E.E.G.s are connected with india ink lines.

A correspondence of the principal waves of both E.E.G.s labelled with the same numbers or letters is found which includes all details. I already reported in the earlier paper (p. 186) that in pathological cases I sometimes found this correspondence of the E.E.G.s recorded from the two sides of the skull to be disturbed. In a 21 year old man with a tumor in the depth of the left cerebral hemisphere I found a distinct discrepancy of the two curves, when I recorded the E.E.G.s simultaneously from the right and left sides of the skull 4 weeks after a palliative trepanation. This applied to the time relationships as well as to the form and amplitude of the principal waves of the E.E.G. In a 48 year old man who also had a tumor in the depth of the left hemisphere, I made the same observation 5 weeks after palliative trepanation when I recorded simultaneous E.E.G.s from both sides of the skull. In this older man the findings were verified at autopsy. Both patients at the time of the E.E.G.

recordings were very easily fatigued, the older man somewhat stuporous, the younger one euphoric. In spite of this the latter subsequently fully recovered while the tumor became calcified. In a 31 year old lady, who also had a deep frontal tumor involving the midline, the E.E.G.s from the right and left sides of the skull, simultaneously recorded 4 weeks after a large left sided palliative trepanation[1], showed the findings illustrated in Figure 4. According to the results of the encephalogram[T40], the tumor had widely separated the two frontal horns of the lateral ventricles.

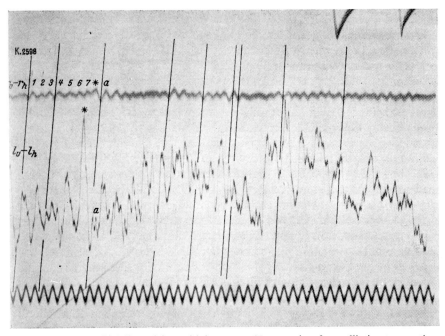

Fig. 4. F.B., 31 years old. Bilateral frontal lobe tumor. Four weeks after palliative trepanation. At the top: E.E.G. recorded from the right side of the skull to the coil galvanometer; in the middle: E.E.G. recorded from the left side of the skull to the oscillograph. At the bottom: time in 1/10ths sec. Simultaneous points of both E.E.G.s are connected with india ink lines.

The upper coil galvanometer curve shows the E.E.G. recorded from the right frontal and the right occipital quadrants of the head. The line in the middle records the E.E.G. obtained with the oscillograph from the left side of the skull. The anterior needle electrode is placed on the dura in the area of the trephine opening, the posterior one on or below the cranial periosteum at the occiput. Simultaneous points of the curves are connected with india ink lines. It is immediately evident that this time, in contrast to Figure 3, the two E.E.G.s do not correspond. For instance, opposite the three principal waves in the upper E.E.G. on the right side of the first india ink line there are only two principal waves in the E.E.G. from the left side. Also the form and amplitude of the two principal waves show no correspondence whatsoever

---

[1] All the operations mentioned here were performed by Mr. *Guleke* in our Surgical Clinic.

in the two recordings. There is a disturbance in the coordination of the activities of the right and left sided cortical areas. At that time the patient was clear in her mind and her thinking was well organized; her marked euphoria had to be attributed to the severe frontal lobe damage caused by the tumor growing into both hemispheres.

In a 32 year old man with a deep right posterior frontal tumor, as suggested by the encephalographic[T40] findings and the clinical manifestations, simultaneous E.E.G. recordings taken on the right and left side of the head demonstrated a congruence of the two curves, exactly as shown in Figure 3 for a healthy subject.

In my sixth report I already discussed the question of the site from which the coordination of the activity of the cortical areas of both hemispheres, their marching in step if I may use this expression, is being regulated. I pointed out that I had considered the corpus callosum to be the organ which mediates this coordination, but that, in view of *Travis'* and *Dorsey's* investigations, I wavered and began to consider whether perhaps this integration could be effected from the thalamus. I tried to pursue this question further. Simultaneous recordings of E.E.G.s in a 26 year old man with a severe metencephalitis[T77] with long lasting oculogyric crises and all other known manifestations of damage to the basal ganglia, failed to disclose any disturbances of coordination of the activity of the two cerebral hemispheres. In this context I also wish to mention that simultaneous recordings in a 33 year old patient with a pronounced mental defect, who had suffered from dementia praecox for two years, also failed to demonstrate a disturbance in the coordination of the activity of the two cerebral hemispheres. Because in the cases of cerebral tumors mentioned above it is impossible to determine which neurological[T78] deficits are to be interpreted as focal signs and which as distant effects, the question as to the site from which the coordination of activity of the two cerebral hemispheres is regulated must still remain unsettled. One thing is *certain*, however, that the coordination of activity of the two sides can be impaired also by local processes in the cerebral cortex itself, as I already showed in Figure 28 of my third report. The recording from the site of trepanation reproduced there shows principal waves different in form and time course from those in the simultaneous recording from the skull as a whole. In this case damage to the cortex was found at the site of operation. Likewise in a 70 year old lady who had recovered from a mild stroke involving the left cerebral hemisphere, I still found several days later a correspondence in the time relationships of the E.E.G.s recorded from the right and from the left side of the skull, but there was a marked difference between the principal waves of the right and left side with regard to their form and especially their amplitude. I made the same observation in women suffering from dementia paralytica in whom severe mental deterioration had developed in spite of malaria therapy. In other cases of dementia paralytica a precise correspondence of the E.E.G.s recorded from the two cerebral hemispheres was found, just as in healthy individuals; but on the other hand the α-w were lengthened or showed in both recordings striking irregularities which were simultaneous, a fact to which I had again alluded in my fifth report. Figure 5 shows these features in a 35 year old woman who has been suffering from paralytic attacks for half a year and who underwent malaria treatment.

One sees E.E.G.s recorded simultaneously from the right and the left sides of the skull, in which once more simultaneous points are connected with india ink lines. Mutually corresponding principal waves in the two E.E.G.s are again indicated by identical letters, numbers or signs. The synchronization of the activity of the two cerebral hemispheres is preserved and the forms of the principal waves are approxi-

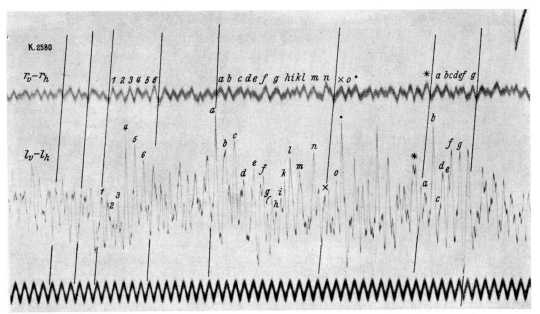

Fig. 5. M.R., 35 years old. Suffering from dementia paralytica. At the top: E.E.G. recorded from the right side of the skull to the coil galvanometer; in the middle: E.E.G. recorded from the left side of the skull to the oscillograph. At the bottom: time in 1/10ths sec. Simultaneous points of the two E.E.G.s are connected with india ink lines.

mately congruous; however, there often is no correspondence of the amplitudes of the deflections occurring on the right and on the left side[T79]. Thus e.g. the amplitudes of the deflections of the α-w labelled 1–6 shown on the right of the third india ink line are different over the two hemispheres. The same again is true for the α-w a, b and c on the right side of the fifth, or for the principal waves labelled with a cross, circle and dot on the right of the sixth india ink line. That the form too is often markedly different can be observed especially in the α-w labelled with a cross and also in the waves labelled a on the right side of the seventh india ink line. As mentioned such observations can also be made in other patients suffering from general paresis. As in the case of an arteriosclerotic cortical lesion described above, the cortical lesions of general paresis disturb the coordination of the activity of the two cerebral hemispheres insofar as the two halves of the brain, though still responding at the same time to a simultaneous stimulus, no longer do so with the same intensity.

In another patient, also suffering from general paresis, more profound differences were found when the E.E.G. was recorded simultaneously from the right and left sides of the skull. This was a 45 year old woman who had shown personality changes for years and in whom a severe epileptiform paralytic attack with residual motor aphasia and paralysis of the right arm had occurred, which led to her admission to the clinic. In the clinic the paralytic attack with clonic jerks of the right side recurred. On the following day simultaneous and bilateral E.E.G. recordings from the right and the left side were obtained as illustrated in Figure 6.

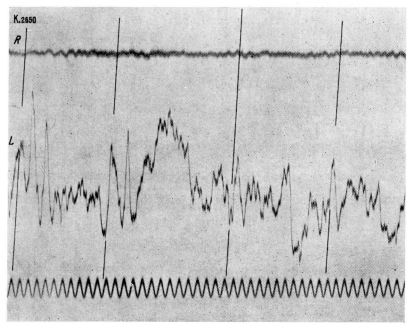

Fig. 6. Mrs. K.N., a day after an epileptiform paralytic attack accompanied by right sided convulsive phenomena. At the top (R): E.E.G. recorded from the right side of the skull to the coil galvanometer; in the middle (L): E.E.G. recorded from the left side of the skull to the oscillograph. At the bottom: time in 1/10ths sec. Simultaneous points of the two E.E.G.s are connected with india ink lines.

Records were taken from the right forehead and the right occiput to the coil galvanometer and from the left forehead and left occiput to the oscillograph. Simultaneous points are again connected with india ink lines. It is immediately evident that the two E.E.G.s differ markedly. This could also be demonstrated repeatedly in many other recordings on the same day and also when the two galvanometers were exchanged. On the right side strikingly brief α-w with an average duration of 55–70 σ predominated, whereas on the left the α-w had a length of 140–200 σ. Synchronization of the two sides cannot be demonstrated. The principal waves of the right and left side differ in their time course, in their form and in their amplitude. Therefore here too one has to assume that the local damage, which according to the clinical manifestations affected primarily the left cerebral hemisphere, interfered with the coordination of the activity of the two cerebral hemispheres which exists in healthy subjects and that because of this, it disturbed the regular course of the directed wave of activity of the entire cortex. Precisely this pathological case, however, provided the opportunity for further important observations. Clonic jerks of the right arm, the right hand and the fingers were observed in this patient, who also continued to exhibit motor aphasia. Consciousness was preserved while these jerks occurred. They recurred after intervening pauses of several minutes, but sometimes also at shorter intervals and then again stopped for a longer period of time. These clonic jerks were present when the recording of the E.E.G. from both sides of the skull was repeated four days after the recording reproduced in Figure 6. Figure 7 shows such a tracing. The profound differences between the records from the right

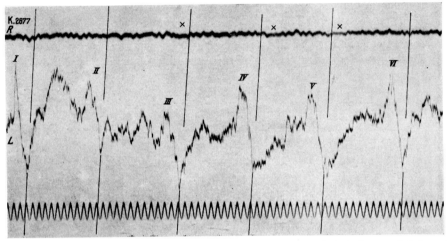

Fig. 7. Mrs. K.N., recorded 4 days later than Figure 6. At the top (*R*): E.E.G. recorded from the right side of the skull to the coil galvanometer; in the middle (*L*): E.E.G. recorded from the left side of the skull to the oscillograph. At the bottom: time in 1/10ths sec. Simultaneous points of the two E.E.G.s are connected with india ink lines.

and from the left side of the skull are again immediately evident. Especially striking is the fact that the tracing from the left side displays the sudden drops in potential marked with *I–VI*, which are not matched by any corresponding changes in the record from the right side. Another recording was made a few minutes later during the same session, after the galvanometers had been exchanged. Records were now taken from the left side of the skull to the coil galvanometer and from the right side to the oscillograph; these yielded the picture shown in Figure 8. The galvanometer, connected to the electrodes placed over the left forehead and left occiput, records no real oscillations at all; the E.E.G. curve is lacking. On the right side there are α-w with an average length of 100 σ. The suspicion arose that the rises and falls in potential marked in Figure 7 with *I–VI* could be related to the isolated clonic jerks of the fingers of the right hand which were also repeatedly observed during the recording. In order to verify this, records were taken in the following manner[T80]: an E.E.G. was recorded from the right side of the skull with the coil galvanometer. Furthermore two silver needles, which served as the recording electrodes for the oscillograph, were inserted on the right and left side and advanced until they penetrated under the periosteum. Each was placed in *that* region of the skull which by means of *Kocher's*

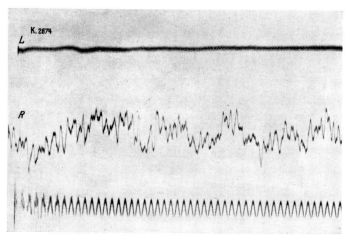

Fig. 8. Mrs. K.N., recorded on the same day as Figure 7. At the top (*L*): E.E.G. recorded from the left side of the skull to the coil galvanometer; in the middle (*R*): E.E.G. recorded from the right side of the skull to the oscillograph. At the bottom: time in 1/10ths sec.

cyrtometer[T81] had been identified as being located over the area of the hand and arm centers of the precentral convolution. The record yields the picture shown in Figure 9.

The record taken with the oscillograph from the region of the hand and arm centers of the left and right precentral convolutions displays once more the rises and falls in potential designated by *I–IV*, which again are not matched by corresponding changes in the recording from the right side. It was therefore extremely likely that these rises and falls in potentials had, after all, a causal relationship to the clonic jerks which repeatedly occurred in the fingers of the right hand, and that perhaps

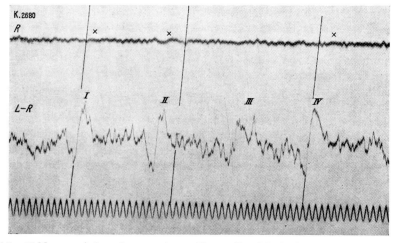

Fig. 9. Mrs. K.N., recorded on the same day as Figures 7 and 8. At the top (*R*): E.E.G. recorded from the right side of the skull to the coil galvanometer; in the middle (*L–R*): E.E.G. recorded to the oscillograph from the areas lying over the left and right precentral convolutions. At the bottom: time in 1/10ths sec. Simultaneous points of the two E.E.G.s are connected with india ink lines.

these represented periodic discharges of the cortical centers to which these clonic twitches were related?[T82] One would therefore have to interpret the absence of the E.E.G. on the left side in Figure 8 as a state of exhaustion consequent to a series of discharges of the left sided motor centers. Because of the patient's general condition, however, these investigations had to be discontinued for some time. After the patient's condition had improved, it was possible to resume the investigations three days later. The woman had made a good recovery and enjoyed the visit of her relatives; the paresis of the right arm had clearly subsided, but she was not yet able to talk. Clonic jerks in the right arm, in the right hand and especially in the right fingers still occurred from time to time. At some hours of the day these jerks were very brisk. A record was taken with the coil galvanometer from the right frontal and the right occipital quadrants of the head. On the left side another record was taken with the oscillograph from two points, one of which was located 2 cm in front, the other 2 cm behind the middle of the precentral convolution. Furthermore, as to their vertical position, they were situated at mid distance between the superior and middle frontal sulci. During the recording the clonic jerks were closely observed and the moment at which they occurred was recorded by me on the photographic paper of the galvanometer in each instance. This was achieved by means of pneumatic transmission, electrical signals being out of the question as I already explained in earlier reports, because of their disturbing influence upon the oscillograph. Many such recordings were made, for during this session very numerous clonic jerks occurred. Figure 10 shows such a tracing.

The E.E.G. recorded from the right side of the skull with the coil galvanometer is written at the top. It was recorded as a matter of precaution in order to demonstrate that gross movements or other experimental artefacts[T10] had not by chance occurred and distorted the oscillograph curve which was the one of crucial importance. The middle curve displays the record from the region of the left motor area. Oscillations

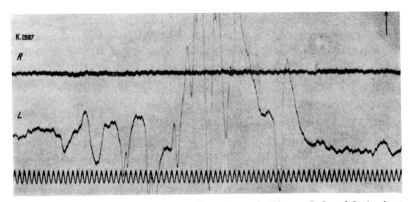

Fig. 10. Mrs. K.N., three days later than recordings shown in Figures 7, 8 and 9. At the top (R): E.E.G. recorded from the right side of the skull to the coil galvanometer; in the middle (L): oscillograph curve recorded from the skull over the area of the middle of the left central convolutions. At the bottom: time in 1/10ths sec. The arrow indicates the time of occurrence of an observed clonic jerk of the right arm.

began which progressively increased in amplitude until they could no longer be recorded in their whole extent on the photographic paper. The upward pointing arrow indicates the moment at which a clonic jerk of the right arm was observed and marked on the photographic paper by me. One can see that this clonic jerk is preceded by very considerable oscillations. The time relationships can of course not be evaluated more precisely because considerable errors in the time measurement are introduced by the act of observing, the transfer of the information to the signalling hand etc. As mentioned above, observations similar to the one shown here were made repeatedly during this session. Mr. *Hilpert*, who, as he had always done, helped me in these recordings and with another physician operated the galvanometer in the recording room separate from the one in which the patient lay, was able to observe the light signals given by me, which each time indicated a clonic jerk. From changes in the oscillograph curve, *i.e.* from the occurrence of larger potential oscillations he was always able to tell his colleague beforehand, as he assured me later, that a light signal would soon be given by me to indicate an observed clonic jerk. Figure 11 shows a similar observation from the same session. In it only the oscillograph curve from the region of the left motor area is recorded.

The movement was one of sudden flexion of the fingers of the right hand which led to closure of the hand. The arrow again indicates the moment when the observed clonic jerk occurred which I recorded by means of pneumatic transmission. One sees here that the larger oscillation is preceded by smaller deflections recorded on the oscillograph; then a steep drop in potential occurs followed by a new rise and a second drop which is somewhat slower. Then the potential curve proceeds relatively evenly. In this instance too the time between the appearance of the potential oscillations and the observed clonic jerk seems to be relatively long.

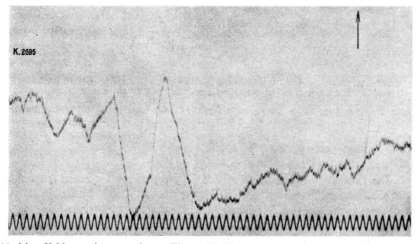

Fig. 11. Mrs. K.N., on the same day as Figure 10. The curve reproduces the oscillations recorded with the oscillograph from the skull in the area of the middle of the left central convolutions. At the bottom: time in 1/10ths sec. The arrow indicates the time of occurrence of an observed clonic jerk (flexion) of the fingers of the right hand.

During the same session I made a few experiments with the aim of having the moment of the clonic jerk recorded by the patient herself. I achieved this by connecting the coil galvanometer with the *Edelmann* pulse telephone which records the finest movements instantaneously. I put the pulse telephone into the patient's half-closed right hand and the clonic jerks, which at that particular time induced predominantly flexion movements of the fingers, were then recorded automatically on the photographic paper. Figure 12 was obtained in this way.

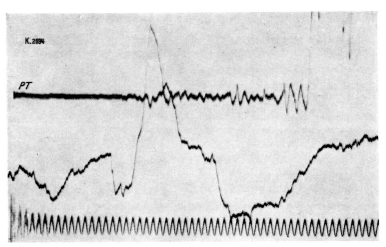

Fig. 12. Mrs. K.N., on the same day as in Figures 10 and 11. The upper line (*PT*) represents the movements of the right hand written by the coil galvanometer and recorded with the *Edelmann* pulse telephone. The middle line reproduces the oscillations recorded with the oscillograph from the skull in the area of the middle of the left central convolutions. At the bottom: time in 1/10ths sec.

PT reproduces the record of the pulse telephone placed in the palm of the right hand. At first it records a straight line; then slight tremulous movements of the hand occur and finally a clonic jerk which can be recognized by the sudden large deflection. The oscillograph curve from the left motor region, recorded below, shows first a slight decrease in potential, then a considerable rise, which is followed by a steep drop which takes place in two or three steps. Here too, the potential oscillation *precedes* the clonic jerk by a considerable interval. The time relationships agree well with the time values in the preceding curve obtained by the manual recording method, if one takes into consideration the sources of error inherent in the latter. These observations, however, (and I would like to stress this particularly) *cannot* be used for time measurements[T83], because we are dealing here with a severely affected patient, in whom probably all processes within the cerebrum, at least those within the predominantly damaged left cerebral hemisphere, are pathologically altered and probably also slowed down. These observations, however, confirm the conjecture made above when discussing the second recording of this patient, that the sudden rises and falls of the electrical curve are related to local discharges within the motor region and to the observed clonic jerks. For years already I had waited for the opportunity to make such an observation, in which the clonic jerks would be restricted to the arm or leg and would not be apt to lead to faulty recordings on account of the involvement of the face or other muscles. Epileptics[T84] are not suitable for such observations. These slight clonic jerks which persist for several days and occur without any large movements capable of disturbing the recordings, are actually observed only after epileptiform paralytic attacks which, according to my experience, are much rarer now than in earlier years. A similar observation made earlier, in which clonic jerks of the right leg appeared during the recording, was unsatisfactory because the strong clonic jerks of the thigh induced displacements of the whole body which were also transmitted to the head, so as to make it impossible to exclude artefacts[T14]. After further progressive improvement of her condition, the patient, from whom the curves reproduced above had been obtained, died 18 days after the last recording as a consequence of bronchopneumonia caused by aspiration. The autopsy confirmed the diagnosis of general paresis. Intense chronic leptomeningitis increasing in severity towards the frontal lobe was found with prominent external hydrocephalus over the anterior regions of the cerebrum, more pronounced on the left than on the right side. On the left side in the region of the foot of F3[T85] and at the same level, behind the postcentral convolution, two large fluid filled cysts were found on the depressed surface of the cerebrum. The convolutions in Broca's region and in the neighboring gyri as well were narrowed in a crest-like fashion. On the right side the changes were much less pronounced. There was moderate internal hydrocephalus. The microscopic investigation confirmed the presence of severe alterations of the cortex characteristic of general paresis. These were more marked in the left frontal lobe than in the right; furthermore, in myelin stained preparations circumscribed focal defects were found on the left side.

The large potential oscillations appearing in Figures 10, 11 and 12 therefore represent local discharges having a causal relationship with the subsequent clonic jerks. According to our present anatomical and physiological knowledge, we have to localize the site of origin of these discharges in the very region from which the records were taken. The potential oscillations originating locally are so large that they reveal themselves also in the antero-posterior recording shown in Figure 7. Of course, they also appear in a recording such as that shown in Figure 9 in which one needle electrode is located immediately above the involved area. Evidently, in the antero-posterior recording, between the two recording sites, large areas of cortex with innumerable ganglion cells are interposed which, however, also include those of the motor area. The latter are in a pathologically altered state and exhibit recurrent discharges which also find their expression in the E.E.G. Of course, the potential oscillations are most distinct when, without the interposition of other nerve cells, one records from their site of origin itself, just as is shown in Figures 10, 11 and 12. The pathological process responsible for the paralytic attack which, including its sequelae, extended over several days, also affected the contralateral cerebral hemisphere, as shown in Figure 6. First of all, considerable shortening of the α-w can be demonstrated on that side. The processes of repeated discharges, when occurring in rapid succession, lead to a state of exhaustion, so that transiently the α-w of the E.E.G. on this side disappear completely, as is shown in Figure 8, to which I already referred above. However, on closer inspection it becomes evident from Figure 7 and likewise from Figure 9, that transient alterations of the coil galvanometer curves on the right side, each indicated by a cross, often correspond to the rises and falls in potential of the oscillograph curve, which are labelled with Roman numerals. There is transient disappearance of the α-w which already are of very low voltage and short. Every time it occurs, the discharge on the left side apparently also exerts an inhibitory action upon the remainder of the cortex. It is true that this change is not always very pronounced; it can, however, also be recognized in Figure 10. At any given time the clonic jerks in the hand and arm are *preceded* by considerable potential oscillations in the region of the corresponding cortical motor centers of the precentral convolution. According to their anatomical location these centers very likely extend to the cortical surface which lies immediately below the dura and therefore are much more advantageously located for our recordings than all sensory centers of man.

Naturally the idea suggested itself that similar processes also take place in epileptic seizures and that there as well, in the so-called clonic stage of the major attack, large discharges occur within the motor region, which one should be able to demonstrate in the oscillograph curve. But the hope that such an observation might be made in any fully developed epileptic seizure of man appears futile from the start. The movements associated with the attack, the numerous muscle currents which appear during the seizure, the displacements of the electrodes, etc. make it impossible to obtain a satisfactory record, especially in view of the enormous sensitivity of the oscillograph to all kinds of interference. In my fifth report I had pointed out that in short losses of consciousness, which occur as absences in many forms of epilepsy, a transient disappearance of the α-w can be demonstrated in the E.E.G. recorded from forehead and occiput. I had to amend my additional statement made verbally on an earlier occasion, that the accessory waves[T86] simultaneously increase in amplitude. I indicated that these were not in fact accessory waves, but muscle action currents. They originate from the temporalis muscle and correspond to a slight trismus which in the patients investigated occurred each time during the brief absences and which at first had escaped my notice. Furthermore, in my fourth report, i documented with illustrations that during the loss of consciousness which outlasts the major epileptic seizure the α-w of the E.E.G. are missing and that they reappear only very gradually, keeping pace with the reawakening consciousness. I had hoped that by studying patients with cortical seizures which are quite commonly observed, I would come closer to understanding the events taking place in the cortical motor centers during the occurrence of clonic jerks. However, all attempts directed to this end failed time and again. It is evident that only those individuals could be selected in whom the occurrence of facial twitches or the participation of the eye muscles in the convulsions could be excluded, because in convulsions associated with these movements muscle currents could reach the recording electrodes and thus distort the pattern of the curves. Thus there remained only cortical seizures confined to the arm or leg which are not very frequent and the patients, after the insertion of the needles, never obliged me by having a seizure with the hoped-for clonic jerks during the recording session, even when hyperventilation was carried out. They occasionally developed a seizure; but precisely during these recordings the facial musculature was also involved in the attack, so that the curves obtained were unsatisfactory. As mentioned above, I had searched for years for a patient with isolated clonic jerks outlasting a paralytic attack for several days, such as the one which finally became available to me.

In view of this observation[87] and on the basis of *Fischer's*[1] beautiful investigations on the electrobiological effects of convulsive poisons in animal experiments, I believe that I am now in a position to correctly interpret an observation which I had already made in 1930, but which I did not publish, because time and again I suspected the presence of artefacts[14] which might have escaped my notice. I once recorded a long curve in an 18 year old girl, who since her 13th year of life had suffered from sporadic major epileptic seizures with tongue biting and urinary incontinence, but who in addition also had had numerous minor seizures and absences. Figure 13 reproduces a small segment of this record.

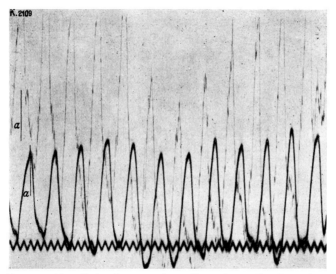

Fig. 13. G.G., 18 years old, suffering from genuine epilepsy. Recording from the right side of the forehead and the left side of the occiput to an oscillograph and coil galvanometer connected to the same electrodes[88]. At the top: the oscillograph curve; below it: the coil galvanometer curve. At the bottom: time in 1/10ths sec. *a* and *a* indicate simultaneous points of the two curves.

The needle electrodes were placed over the forehead and occiput and the two galvanometers, namely the coil galvanometer and oscillograph, were both connected to these electrodes[88]. During the recording the girl was lying with her eyes closed, exactly as in preceding examinations. The respiration suddenly changed a little and the house physician who observed the patient with me remarked that she suddenly tapped her thigh rapidly with her left hand. No other movements could be observed.

---

[1] *Fischer, M. H.*: Elektrobiologische Auswirkung von Krampfgiften am Zentralnervensystem. Med. Klin., **1933**, No. 1.

At the end of the recording, the patient spontaneously said that she had just had a minor seizure. The galvanometer curves showed steeply rising and falling potential oscillations of sudden onset, each with a duration of 0.34 to 0.36 second, which occurred in regular succession and disappeared just as suddenly after 26 seconds. I had thought at the time that I and the physician who had observed the patient with me, had perhaps missed some head movements or clonic twitches of the face, which might have rhythmically displaced the needle electrodes, and for this reason I shelved this observation for the time being. From the experience I gained through my own observations reported above and in the light of what I learned from *Fischer's* investigations, particularly his Figure 5, it seems certain that these recurring potential fluctuations in Figure 13 must have had a causal relationship to the clonic twitches. In this case the twitches appeared as flexion movements of the fingers of the left hand, and the potential fluctuations probably preceded them.

Therefore intense local processes, of the kind which in this instance occurred in the motor region[T89], can also be demonstrated in an E.E.G. recorded from forehead and occiput, especially when by this very process all other simultaneous cortical processes are inhibited and eliminated. However, the events occurring under the influence of a sensory stimulus in sensory centers of the cortex which in man are inaccessible to direct recording, are relatively insignificant and too restricted to a circumscribed area to become apparent in the form of an increase in potential, even at recording points lying in close proximity to the involved area[1]. In this instance one finds just as in mental work, merely a decrease in potential, which represents an inhibitory effect. This inhibitory effect, however, is usually very distinct and can also easily be demonstrated at very remote recording points. This general decrease in potential in my opinion is at least of equal importance for the psychic aspect of these processes, perhaps even more important than the local increase.

If one reviews many E.E.G.s obtained in epileptics it is not rare at all to find in these records segments of curves such as that shown in Figure 14. It was obtained

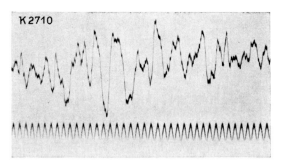

Fig. 14. W.G., 23 years old, suffering from genuine epilepsy. Recording with needle electrodes from the right frontal and the left occipital quadrants of the head to the oscillograph. At the bottom: time in 1/10ths sec.

---

[1] See the beautiful results of the animal experiments made by *Kornmüller*: J. f. Psychol., **44**, 447 (1932); **45**, 172 (1933) and by *Fischer*: Pflügers Arch., **230**, 161 (1932) which confirm the occurrence of action currents following sensory stimuli in the related sensory centers of the cortex and their close confinement to a specific structurally characterized cortical area.

in a 23 year old epileptic who has suffered from many seizures and twilight states since his 12th year of life and who shows incipient epileptic dementia.

One sees that in the middle of the segment of the curve shown here suddenly a steep drop in potential followed by a rise occurs, which vividly recalls the discharges in the records shown above (*e.g.* Figure 11). This strongly suggests that after frequently repeated discharges a tendency to produce high potentials with a steep voltage drop persists. Thus these large potential oscillations are perhaps a characteristic peculiarity of the E.E.G. of epileptics who are prone to have many seizures. It is a fact that in such epileptic patients one finds E.E.G.s of this type in the most diverse recordings. Perhaps in this manner the E.E.G. expresses graphically the presence of the existing predisposition to seizures of the cerebrum.

VIII

On the Electroencephalogram of Man

Eighth Report

by Hans Berger, Jena

(With 6 figures)

(Received September 20, 1933)

[Published in *Archiv für Psychiatrie und Nervenkrankheiten*, **1934**, *101*: 452–469]

In 1930, in my second report, I advanced the working hypothesis that the alpha waves (α-w) of the electroencephalogram (E.E.G.) are concomitant manifestations of those material cortical processes which one calls psychophysical, because under certain circumstances they are associated with phenomena of consciousness. I have found it possible to adhere to this working hypothesis until now. In diseases of the cerebrum which are associated with altered mental processes I also found changes in the E.E.G. consisting of loss, lengthening, increase or decrease in amplitude or irregularity of the α-w. One must conclude that the vital processes which are the basis of these bioelectric phenomena have also undergone corresponding changes. Thus the fundamental process in the cortex must either have ceased to function, or become enhanced or diminished or become altered in its time course. In the earlier papers, I reported on the influence of *drugs* upon the pattern[T20] of the E.E.G. I described that in deep scopolamine–morphine sleep the α-w of the E.E.G. disappear, that the same occurs in chloroform narcosis and that with gradual awakening from anesthesia the α-w return and again disappear upon renewed deepening of narcosis. The α-w are also lacking during the unconsciousness which outlasts a major epileptic seizure and reappear again with the gradual return of consciousness. At the time I also indicated that in an alcoholic during the excitation stage of narcosis the α-w increase in amplitude and I published records which demonstrated these changes. I also reported that under the influence of cocaine the same changes may occur.

Over the years I have had further opportunities to investigate the influence upon the E.E.G. of potent drugs which must occasionally be administered to agitated mental patients[1]. I found that scopolamine without added morphine in doses of 0.001 gram, given by injection, often did not exert any definite sleep inducing effect.

---

[1] In the performance of these investigations Mr. *Hilpert* has always helped me with word and deed, for which here too I would like to express to him my cordial thanks, as I also thank Messrs. *Witzleb*, *Lemke* and *Stefan* for their help.

Correspondingly it also caused only a general diminution in the amplitude of the deflections of the E.E.G. without any fundamental alteration of the α-w, as I reported earlier. Scopolamine given together with 0.01–0.02 gram of morphine in accordance with its more pronounced sedative and sleep inducing action also had a much more distinct influence upon the E.E.G.: the α-w were markedly flattened or absent, which confirms findings reported earlier. There were great individual differences in the effects on the E.E.G. of doses of 0.02 gram of morphine alone when given in severe anxiety attacks. These effects were entirely related to the variable degree of sedative action. If a distinct morphine effect with complete sedation and somnolence occurred, the duration of the α-w was increased beyond their normal length and they tended to fuse with each other. Sodium Luminal too, which is used in severe states of agitation, when given by injection at a dose of 0.4 gram[T90], caused no discernible alteration of the α-w of the E.E.G. if, in spite of a pronounced sedative effect, the patient had not gone to sleep. A dose of 0.3 gram of Luminal in aqueous solution given intramuscularly in extremely agitated patients, in keeping with the more pronounced sedative and sleep inducing effect it exerts upon the patients, had a distinct influence upon the E.E.G.; the α-w showed an increased length, on the average up to 135–150 σ, they became strikingly low in voltage and the tendency of the α-w to fuse, already mentioned when discussing the effect of morphine, also occurred. In any case when using these drugs it became apparent that there was mutual correspondence between the changes of the α-w of the E.E.G. and the effects upon mental processes; whenever a significant action of the drug upon the latter failed to occur, visible alterations of the α-w of the E.E.G. were also lacking.

The action of *anesthetics* upon the E.E.G. of course merits very special consideration and reference was already made to the earlier observations on the effects of chloroform narcosis. However, a whole series of drugs for induction of anesthesia exist and in operating a large clinic their use in agitated mental patients often becomes necessary, *e.g.* when performing a lumbar puncture, fluoroscopy, gynecological examinations, small surgical interventions and finally also for control of the most severe and long-lasting states of agitation. I made all the observations on the changes of the E.E.G. under the influence of such anesthetics only in extremely agitated mental patients. However, I believe that in comparison to their action upon the E.E.G. of the healthy human subject, the action of these drugs on agitated psychotics is different only in degree, but not fundamentally. Thus when giving Avertine[1,T91] by the most commonly used rectal route of administration, a sufficiently deep narcosis was obtained to permit small surgical interventions. Figure 1 shows an E.E.G. recorded during such an Avertine narcosis. The 26 year old patient who had suffered from dementia praecox for many years received, after the usual preparations, 4.4 grams of Avertine in the appropriate solution by enema and thereupon fell into deep sleep with stertorous respiration. Painful stimuli still elicited a slight defensive movement, but no longer provoked any expression of pain. Forty-five minutes after the administration of Avertine the E.E.G. and E.C.G. were recorded simultaneously

---

[1] *Blume*: Über Avertin in der Psychiatrie. Dtsch. med. Wschr., **1927**, Nr. 31, 1307. *Sioli* and *Neustadt*: Avertin in der Psychiatrie. Klin. Wschr., **1927**, 1851.

in the usual manner. The E.C.G. deviates somewhat from normal, because the patient has a well compensated mitral valve lesion. The E.E.G. recorded with the oscillograph set at a high sensitivity exhibits very distinct α-w which, in comparison with the α-w of the waking state, have considerably decreased in amplitude and also show a slight decrease in duration to an average of 72 σ. Twice more I had the opportunity

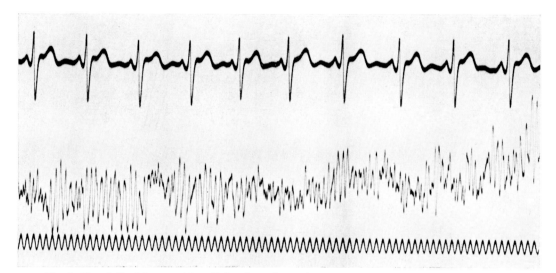

Fig. 1. Mrs. L.E., 26 years old, suffering from dementia praecox; 45 min after rectal administration of 4.4 grams of Avertine. At the top: E.C.G. (mitral valve lesion). In the middle: E.E.G. At the bottom: time in 1/10ths sec.

to record E.E.G.s of two other patients during Avertine sleep induced by rectal administration of the drug. Strikingly low amplitude α-w were always found, but there was no complete disappearance of the α-w as occurs during a pronounced chloroform effect. Furthermore, in all three cases defensive movements in response to painful stimuli were not completely abolished. It can therefore be assumed that Avertine, when administered by rectum at the usual dose, does not lead to as complete an elimination of the cerebral cortical processes as does chloroform in deep narcosis.

Very frequently in my clinic Pernocton[1,T92] is used intravenously for small surgical procedures and often also to perform an encephalogram[T40]. I therefore had the opportunity to record E.E.G.s in patients while under the influence of Pernocton. These records immediately caused me a great surprise. The findings in the E.E.G. did not at all conform to my expectations; indeed they appeared to be contrary to these in every respect. Figure 2 shows the E.E.G. recording of 30 year old Miss E.G. who came from a well educated family and who for many years had suffered from dementia praecox accompanied by very severe states of agitation. Fifteen minutes prior to this recording she had received 5 ml of the usual Pernocton solution

---

[1] *Reck* and *Haack*: "Pernocton", ein neues injizierbares Schlaf- und Beruhigungsmittel, seine Anwendung bei erregten Geisteskranken. Allg. Z. Psychiatr., **91**, 417 (1929).

intravenously and had fallen into a deep sleep during its slow infusion into the vein. Painful stimuli no longer elicited any reaction whatsoever. The E.E.G. strikes one immediately by its surprisingly high voltage α-w which are clustered into peculiar groups. One of these has been specifically marked at *c*. As a glance at the figure shows, these groups bear no relationship with the heartbeat, *i.e.* with the movement

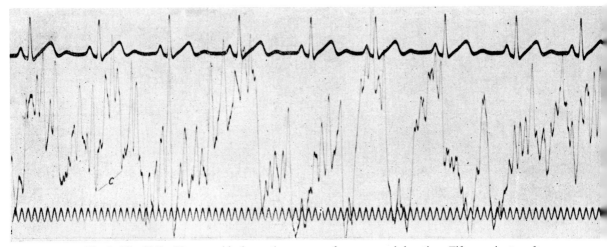

Fig. 2. Miss E.G., 30 years old; dementia praecox of many years' duration. Fifteen minutes after intravenous administration of 5.0 ml[T93] of Pernocton. At the top: E.C.G.; in the middle: E.E.G.; at the bottom: time in 1/10ths sec.

of the blood, nor is there any relationship with the much slower respiration which is not specifically shown on the curve. These groups extended over a period of 0.4–0.65 second, as has been shown by measurements in a longer curve of which only a small segment is reproduced in Figure 2. That these changes do not represent an individual characteristic peculiar to Miss E.G. was shown by two further recordings of E.E.G.s during Pernocton sleep which were obtained in two other patients. It was always found that the α-w were strikingly large in amplitude and time and again clustered in a peculiar way into groups with a duration ranging between the two extremes of 0.35 and 0.7 seconds. This peculiar group formation reminded me of the illustration shown in my fifth report which demonstrates the E.E.G. of a dog slowly dying because of cardiac arrest. However, there the amplitude of the α-w soon decreased and they showed a distinct increase in length. Here on the other hand, we find an amplitude increase of the α-w, besides their grouping, with a normal average duration of each clearly developed α-w. In all three cases studied, consciousness was completely abolished as far as we were able to determine. This was a finding which appears to be completely at variance with the views I held to date concerning the significance of the α-w and which I expressed in the working hypothesis reiterated above.

Evipan[T94] also, when given intravenously, produces a brief narcosis and causes exactly the same change in the E.E.G. It has been used in my clinic in many cases, as briefly reported by Mr. *Stefan*[1]. The effect on the E.E.G. is shown in Figure 3. The 24 year old patient, M.B., suffering from schizophrenia, received 9.0 ml^{T93} of Evipan solution intravenously. During the slow intravenous infusion, the anesthetic effect became clearly apparent; 27 minutes later a curve was recorded of which a small segment is shown in Figure 3. In this instance too, no flattening, let alone disappearance of the α-w as occurs under the influence of chloroform, can be seen. On the contrary one sees strikingly large amplitude α-w of normal duration and the same marked tendency to group formation as had been shown in Figure 2 under the influence of Pernocton. That this was in fact not a chance result, but a reflection of a predictable

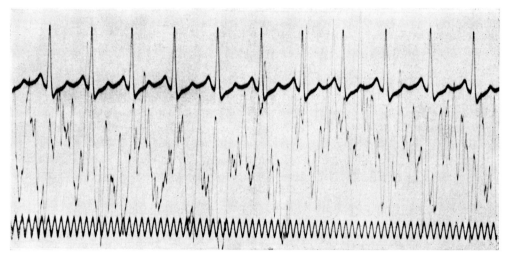

Fig. 3. Miss M.B., 24 years old, has been suffering for many years from schizophrenia superimposed upon mental retardation^{T95}. Twenty-seven minutes after intravenous administration of 9.0 ml^{T93} of Evipan. At the top: E.C.G.; in the middle: E.E.G.; at the bottom: time in 1/10ths sec.

influence of Evipan upon the E.E.G., became apparent from two additional E.E.G. recordings which I made under short Evipan narcosis. The same picture has repeatedly been found and the records appear so similar to the E.E.G.s obtained in Pernocton sleep, that they could be easily mistaken for one another, even though they were obtained from different patients. That in fact the α-w have increased in amplitude considerably in comparison with those seen in an awake and fully conscious individual, is shown by Figure 4, which was recorded from the same patient as Figure 3. This recording was obtained 9 minutes later. The patient is fully awake, responds to commands, but is already quite restless and makes all kinds of movements with her arms; because of this the E.C.G. is distorted. The α-w of the E.E.G. recorded with the same sensitivity of the oscillograph are, however, considerably smaller in amplitude than in Figure 3; furthermore, the peculiar group formation, which occurs in Pernocton as well as in Evipan sleep, has completely disappeared. Again the E.E.G.

---

[1] *Stefan, H.*: Klinische Erfahrungen mit Evipannatrium. Münch. med. Wschr., **1933**, 808.

shows an occasional decrease in amplitude, (indicated in this figure by a cross), as is always the case during wakefulness. The contrast to the action of chloroform is also very clearly evident in Figure 4. Upon awakening from chloroform narcosis the α-w return and gradually increase in amplitude. However, precisely the opposite occurs here. The α-w decrease in amplitude, often by more than half, upon awakening

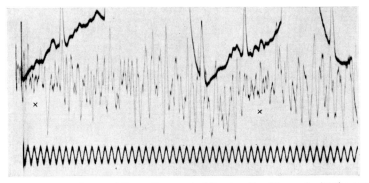

Fig. 4. From the same patient as Figure 3, recorded 9 min after Figure 3. At the top: E.C.G. distorted by movements; in the middle: E.E.G.; at the bottom: time in 1/10ths sec.

from narcosis, and the group formation of Pernocton and Evipan sleep which is present during anesthesia, disappears. I also wish to call attention to the differences between these curves and that reproduced in Figure 1 which shows the Avertine effect. These findings in the E.E.G. under the influence of Pernocton and Evipan appear to me to be so significant as to require more detailed discussion.

First of all it is necessary to obtain some information about the mode of action of the drugs discussed here. In this matter I follow the expert leadership of Messrs. *Molitor* and *Pick*[1]. It should first be emphasized that compounds with a completely different chemical structure may exert an identical anesthetic effect and that hypnotic drugs which belong to the same group may exert quite different biological actions. Furthermore one must not lose sight of the fact that, although a primary site of action of these drugs within the nervous system does exist, their action when given in higher doses is by no means confined to this site, but may affect any other part of the nervous system. Finally, the most important investigations were evidently carried out in animals and one has to exert a certain degree of caution in carrying over the results of these to the conditions in man. *Molitor* and *Pick* distinguish between cortical and brain-stem hypnotics. The primary site of action of the cortical hypnotics is in the cerebral cortex; its activity is reduced or abolished by their action. To the cortical hypnotics belong ether, chloroform, alcohol, morphine and the bromides. Avertine, being a tribromoethyl alcohol, must probably also be included among this group of drugs. My earlier reported findings that in chloroform narcosis the α-w disappear and gradually return in parallel with the reappearance of the phenomena of consciousness, agree well with a primary cortical site of action of chloroform.

---

[1] *Molitor* and *Pick*: Pharmakologie der Schlafmittel. In *Sarason*: "Der Schlaf", p. 76. Munich, 1929.

The amplitude reduction of the α-w in Avertine sleep would also fit with this inter-pretation. Scopolamine, which eliminates the activity of the cortical motor regions when given together with morphine, also causes disappearance of the α-w of the E.E.G. when the effect of the two drugs is fully developed. The simultaneous adminis-tration of the two drugs must therefore be considered as tantamount to the applica-tion of cortical hypnotics. Brain-stem hypnotics, which are also called subcortical or thalamic hypnotics, have their first site of action outside the cortex, in the brain-stem, probably in the sleep regulating center or its vicinity. To *von Economo*, the excellent investigator who unfortunately died so early, we owe the more precise localization of this center to which he gave its name. He distinguishes between brain sleep and body sleep[1]. Here we are only concerned with brain sleep. According to *von Economo* its characteristics consist of partial blocking of the pathways mediating afferent and efferent excitations and of abolition of consciousness. He emphasizes particularly that one can only form a hypothetical concept of the mode of action of the sleep regulating center, but that in all likelihood brain sleep should be regarded as an inhibition which originates in this center and that the effect of this inhibition is exerted upon the cerebrum and diencephalon. The primary site of action of the brain-stem hypnotics is therefore not in the cortex, but precisely in the sleep regulating center of the brain-stem in the region of the thalamus. Luminal and Pernocton belong to these brain-stem hypnotics, besides many others which do not concern us here. Among these we should certainly also include Evipan in view of its chemical composi-tion and more particularly because of its biological mode of action. The three drugs just mentioned are barbiturates which exert a pronounced hypnotic action. Luminal in general is not given in sufficiently high doses to induce a marked anesthetic effect. I was therefore not in a position to report observations concerning its action. Per-nocton and Evipan however, as mentioned, are very frequently given intravenously to induce a brief narcosis. *J. Keeser*[2] established in animal experiments that, after intravenous injection of hypnotic doses of Pernocton in the rabbit, the presence of the drug can be demonstrated by the microsublimation technique in the diencephalon and in other parts of the central nervous system, but not in the cerebrum. According to a communication I received from the I.G. Farben Company, no analogous animal experiments have been carried out with Evipan; however, one may assume the situation to be the same as for Pernocton. The animal experiment has thus proven that Pernocton does in fact act first precisely where, according to the clinical manifestations, one would expect it to exert its effect. These unequivocal results of the animal experiment, which are in excellent agreement with the clinical manifestations in man, may there-fore unhesitatingly be applied to man. The primary site of action of Pernocton and Evipan is not in the cortex, but subcortical in the region of the thalamus, and this is in complete agreement with our observations on the E.E.G. In contrast to chloro-

---

[1] *von Economo*: Der Schlaf als Lokalisationsproblem. In *Sarason*: "Der Schlaf", p. 38. Munich, 1929.

[2] *Keeser*, *J.*: Beitrag zur pharmakologischen Wirkung der Barbitursäurederivate, Pernocton und Somnifen. Schmerz, Narkose und Anästhesie, **1929**, fasc. 7: 260. Nach *Pernocton*[T96], 2nd edition, p. 16. Berlin: Riedel A.G.

form narcosis we found that the α-w of the E.E.G. were not abolished; they persisted, even increased in amplitude and underwent the peculiar change which I designated in brief as group formation. The activity of the cerebral cortex which finds its expression in the E.E.G. is therefore not abolished in this instance, but undergoes a change which we must consider in greater detail insofar as it manifests itself in the E.E.G.

We do not wish to start this discussion by considering the marked increase in amplitude of the α-w which becomes apparent when comparing Figures 3 and 4 taken from the same patient, but prefer to deal first with the group formation. In earlier papers I repeatedly indicated that a certain rhythmicity in the sequence of the α-w is apparent in the E.E.G.[T97]. In healthy individuals this rhythm has a period of 1.3–4.7 seconds. Upon awakening from the unconsciousness of an epileptic seizure this period was prolonged to 8.5–9.5 seconds. In Pernocton and Evipan sleep we find a pronounced rhythmic organization of the E.E.G. curve. When Pernocton is given the period measures 0.35–0.7 second and with Evipan 0.3–0.9 second. In comparison with the values found in healthy individuals the process which I earlier called the intrinsic rhythm of the brain is therefore considerably shortened. However, the peculiar group formation is not completely explained by this. Another condition must still be fulfilled. This can be most easily explained by referring to Figure 5. In *a* the α-w of the E.E.G. were drawn on ruled paper in their proper sequence.

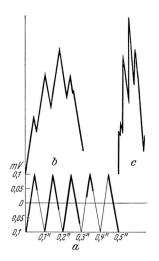

Fig. 5. Sketch. *a*, normal sequence of the α-w with a wave length of 100 σ and with equal amplitudes of the individual waves; *b*, group formation of the α-w caused by a loss of those parts of individual α-w drawn in with a thin line in *a*; *c*, group *c* of Figure 2 (Pernocton narcosis), which has been transferred to the sketch without alteration of its amplitude, but with some shortening of the time scale.

Their duration is 100 σ and their amplitude remains constant at 0.2 mV. If one deletes from these α-w shown in *a* all portions drawn in with a thin line and then puts together the remaining portions of these five waves, one obtains what is shown in part *b* of Figure 5. From the loss of individual portions of the α-w and from the shortening of the period, there results what I called group formation, as it clearly appears in *b*. We are familiar with this group formation from Figures 2 and 3 and can explain its origin in this manner. In part *c* of Figure 5, group *c* of Figure 2 is reproduced at the same amplitude scale, but not at the same time scale, because this would have necessitated a difficult redrawing of the curve. One immediately recognizes the considerable resemblance with *b* which would lead to complete identity of *b* and *c* if the time scale were the same and if the fact had been taken into consideration that in reality not all consecutive α-w have the same amplitude, as was assumed in *a*. Any one of different portions of the ascending or descending limbs of α-w of unequal size may be lost and in this manner a great variety of group formations may appear, as shown in Figures 2 and 3. In the present case only a single example was analyzed to explain this group formation in some detail. Thus this group formation represents a shortening of the period of the rhythm and an incomplete formation of the α-w, also a hastened course of the latter, the waves following upon each other prematurely in accelerated sequences[T98] during which some portions of the α-w are lost. While analyzing in detail the records of Evipan and Pernocton narcosis it occurred to me that I had seen similar curves once before, namely in a case of severe *illuminating gas poisoning*. Figure 6 reproduces the finding obtained at that time. This was the case of a 50 year old man who had poisoned himself together with

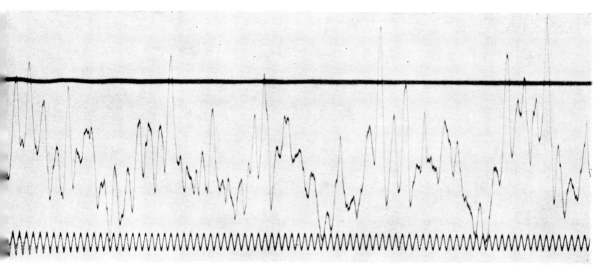

Fig. 6. R.G., 50 years old, deeply stuporous because of severe illuminating gas poisoning, but strong painful stimuli sometimes elicit jerking movements. In the middle: E.E.G. recorded with the oscillograph; at the bottom: time in 1/10ths sec.

his wife because of financial worries. Whereas his wife died, the efforts of our medical clinic succeeded in saving the man's life. At the time of the recording he was still deeply stuporous, occasionally however he showed jerking movements in response to painful stimuli, but could not be awakened by any means. The stupor continued for another 4 days after the recording and a severe mental defect persisted. In my fifth report on page 165, I already showed a recording of the E.E.G. of this man and there also, on pages 165–166, I described his history in more detail. The group formation and the high voltage of the α-w are clearly evident in the oscillograph curve of the E.E.G. (The coil galvanometer has been switched off and its mirror writes the black line at the top.) The α-w underwent a very considerable increase in their length to 195–300 σ, an indication that not only the subcortical or thalamic centers, but also the cerebral cortex itself, had been severely damaged. The individual periods of the rhythmic processes in this case measure 0.4–1.25 seconds and thus approach a little more closely the values found in healthy subjects. It became apparent in later E.E.G. recordings of this patient, when he had regained consciousness, that the amplitude of the α-w, recorded with the same sensitivity of the galvanometer, had regressed by more than half. Group formation of the α-w had disappeared, but the considerable increase in their length persisted.

What should be the *physiological* interpretation of the E.E.G. findings in Pernocton and Evipan narcosis? We know that the primary site of action of both drugs is in the brain-stem, probably in the sleep regulating center, in the thalamus itself or in its vicinity. As soon as the anesthetic effect takes place, a considerable amplitude increase occurs and the α-w of the E.E.G. follow upon each other prematurely in accelerated sequences[T98]. This leads to the above mentioned group formation. This change is most easily explained by the disappearance of an inhibitory and regulatory restraint. This inhibition originates from the primary site of action of these drugs, namely from the thalamus, and exerts its action upon the entire cerebral cortex, or rather upon *those* processes in the cortex whose concomitant bioelectrical phenomena are revealed by the E.E.G. We are dealing with a "disinhibition" of this component of cerebral activity. How does this disinhibition arise? Here too we choose the simplest and most probable explanation, namely that it is caused by the disappearance of the mostly subliminal excitatory processes which continuously originate in the body and in the environment and which via the thalamus stream to the cortex, where they exert a continuous inhibitory action upon the cortical processes referred to above. Simultaneously with this disappearance of all sensory[T99] stimuli destined for the cerebral cortex, its motor performance is also eliminated and thus the disappearance of the cortical motor activity merely represents a simple consequence of the elimination of all afferent excitations. We have to assume that the afferent pathways in the thalamus become interrupted because of some unknown influence which originates in the sleep regulating center, or perhaps that they become impassable on account of some kind of disconnection or similar process. As *Clark*[1] indicated in an extensive anatomical study, the thalamus is of special importance because it is connected with all secondary sensory[T99] pathways, with the exception of the olfactory ones. This relationship and the intrathalamic rearrangement and modification of the stimuli conveyed over these pathways, suggest that the thalamus is "the anatomical equivalent of the very threshold of consciousness". The pathways which originate in the cortex and subserve voluntary innervation have no relationship with the thalamus and thus are not switched off or interrupted there under the influence of Pernocton or Evipan etc. As indicated above, I believe that the loss of motor performance can be explained as an inevitable consequence of the disappearance of all the stimuli which stream to the cortex. The postulate of the

---

[1] *Clark, Le Gros*: The structure and connections of the thalamus. Brain, **55**, 406 (1932). Abstract
   in Zbl. Neur., **66**, 230 (1933).

existence of such continuous inhibitory phenomena in the cerebral cortex can be based upon known physiological facts. Thanks to the studies of *Dusser de Barenne* and *Marshall*[T100] we know of such disinhibitory processes in the cerebral cortex of animals. These investigators were able to demonstrate that after isolating a point in the motor area of the cerebral cortex of cats, dogs and monkeys from its surroundings by a ring of novocaine, the excitability of this point underwent a powerful increase which lasted for many minutes. These observations prove, as *Wachholder*[1] rightly emphasized, that continuous mutual damping processes (tonic inhibitions) exist within the central nervous system. In the case of Pernocton and Evipan narcosis, which concerns us here, this disinhibition is exerted upon those material processes of the entire cerebral cortex which are represented by the E.E.G. This disinhibition originates at the primary site of action of these drugs, *i.e.* in the thalamus, and is caused, I assume, by a disconnection of all afferent pathways. The occurrence of disinhibitory phenomena, which is suggested by the changes visible in the E.E.G. such as amplitude increase of the α-w and their premature occurrence in accelerated sequences[T98] leading to group formation, is also supported by the clinical observations made in the course of the administration of Pernocton and Evipan. During Pernocton and Evipan narcosis the cerebral cortex is suddenly cut off from the inflow of all afferent excitations and therefore disinhibition also sets in immediately. This sudden disinhibition leads to an enhancement of excitability which finds its expression in excitatory motor phenomena. Thus in the case of the intravenous administration of Pernocton for the induction of narcosis, motor excitatory phenomena, appearing during and immediately after the injection, are described by a number of observers. For instance *Reck* and *Haack*[2] emphasize that they observed "in nearly all cases at the end of the injection and shortly thereafter transient clonic jerks which varied in intensity and involved the limb muscles and sporadically also the facial muscula-ture"; they add: "in our experience the clonic jerks were all the more intense, the faster the injection had to be given". However, they were not completely absent even with a slower injection. Observations made in my clinic are in agreement with these findings. Quite similar are the reports on motor excitatory phenomena occurring immediately after intravenous administration of Evipan[3]. This increased excitability of the cortex caused by disinhibition also explains the post-narcotic states of agitation observed by many investigators after administration of Pernocton. *Wachholder* ap-propriately pointed out that probably also many epileptiform convulsions have to be attributed to disinhibitory phenomena. I believe that the heightened excitability of the cortex caused by the exclusion of afferent stimuli provides a plausible explana-tion for the epileptiform attacks in all the cases of severe illuminating gas poisoning, which I had the opportunity to observe personally. Indeed Figure 6 distinctly shows the amplitude increase and the group formation of the α-w and thus, in addition to considerable lengthening of the α-w, exhibits those changes which were interpreted

---

[1] After *Kurt Wachholder*: Die allgemeinen physiologischen Grundlagen der Neurologie, 4th Part. Fortschr. Neur., **5**, fasc. 1/2, 69 (1933).

[2] *Reck* and *Haack*: Pernocton. Allg. Z. Psychiatr., **91**, 417 (1929).

[3] *Stefan, H.*: Klinische Erscheinungen mit Evipannatrium usw. Münch. med. Wschr., **1933**, 808.

as disinhibitory phenomena, even during the profound stupor caused by severe illuminating gas intoxication. If in addition to this disinhibition of the cortex a further as yet unidentified precipitating event occurs, then an epileptic discharge sets in, which likewise has to be included among the motor sequelae of disinhibition. In the waking state of healthy people the continuous damping action of all stimuli streaming to the cerebral cortex can be easily demonstrated on the α-w of the E.E.G. I already mentioned in my first studies on the E.E.G. that pain and distraction by sensory stimuli disturb the recording of the E.E.G. and I stressed that the best E.E.G.s with well developed and large amplitude α-w are obtained while the experimental subject lies in a darkened room which is shielded as far as possible from all noise and while he lets his mind go blank[T101]. I also reported that the pattern[T20] of the E.E.G. is altered in a characteristic fashion by mental work, and came to the conclusion that inhibitory influences are present in all such instances. All sensory stimuli exert a damping effect upon the α-w of the E.E.G. As I again emphasized in my fifth report, the degree of damping corresponds to the degree of concentration of attention. When a task requiring great attention is performed as e.g. when a subject holds a wire within the loop of a steel spring and is enjoined to avoid contact between the two, the few α-w, whenever they still occur, become very flat. In the waking state this damping effect of all sensory stimuli streaming continuously to the cortex from the body and from the environment, manifests itself in the form of a certain *medium* amplitude of the α-w. Thus the events in the E.E.G. which had been known to me for a long time fit well with the disinhibitory phenomena in the E.E.G. observed in Pernocton and Evipan narcosis, and the latter actually confirm the explanation given previously for those earlier observations.

The changes in the E.E.G. occurring during Pernocton and Evipan narcosis which in my opinion have to be considered as disinhibitory processes, also throw some light upon the manifestations of *brain sleep*, which evidently is also induced by the sleep regulating center. It is probable that in this case too, no cortical inhibition occurs, contrary to what had been surmised by *von Economo*, but rather a cortical disinhibition. A whole series of phenomena can readily be interpreted as disinhibitory processes of the psychophysical cortical activity, such as the isolated clonic jerks which are frequently observed when a subject falls asleep, the process designated by *Hoche* in his excellent book on "The Dreaming Ego"[1] as the law of multiplication, the illusions and hallucinations of dreams and others. The psychophysical cortical activity is relieved from the inhibitory pressure to which it is subjected in the waking state by the constant inflow of stimuli from the body and the environment. The well known fact that epileptiform seizures (and this not only in genuine epilepsy, but also in focal lesions of the cerebrum) occur predominantly during sleep, fits well with this view. In the presence of predisposing conditions these seizures are precipitated by the additional factors created by the disinhibition of the cortex which occurs during sleep.

How do the observations made on the E.E.G. in Pernocton and Evipan narcosis

---

[1] *Hoche, A.:* Das träumende Ich. p. 77, Jena, 1927.

agree with my *working hypothesis* to which I referred above? They apparently contradict it. If this contradiction cannot be resolved, then of course this working hypothesis, as any such assumption which cannot be reconciled with the facts, has to be abandoned! However, it seems necessary to me to submit all relevant aspects to more precise scrutiny. In Pernocton and Evipan narcosis we found, in spite of complete loss of consciousness, strikingly high voltage α-w, which became smaller upon awakening from the narcosis. A first assumption one could make would be that the severe alterations of the α-w are incompatible with the appearance of phenomena of consciousness. These alterations consist of increased amplitude and distortion of individual α-w, and these changes are furthermore associated with shortening of the periods in the rhythmic sequence[T102] of these altered α-w. Another interpretation, however, appears to me more probable, when I review all the facts which I collected in the course of nine years. In my sixth report I explained that the continuous, automatically ongoing, psychophysical cortical activity which finds its expression in the E.E.G., is *only* associated with phenomena of consciousness when the local activity exceeds a certain magnitude, which corresponds to *Fechner's* internal threshold, and when simultaneously, generalized inhibition of the entire psychophysical cortical activity takes place. Later I expressed the opinion that the generalized inhibition is probably of *foremost* importance for the appearance of phenomena of consciousness. At this point I must make it clearer than I did in my last reports, that *generalized* diminution in voltage of the E.E.G. is not caused by *every* sensory stimulus towards which attention is directed, but is only elicited by strong and unexpected stimuli, as already reported in my second communication. There I explained that no distinct alteration in the E.E.G. is noted when the same stimulus is frequently repeated. Further investigations led me to the conclusion that the inhibition which originates in the cortical center of activity created by the stimulus, differs in intensity, spread and duration according to the strength of the stimulus and to the overall mental state at that moment. One has to assume that not only the excitation, but the inhibitory effect as well, are *confined locally*, and only with strong and unexpected stimuli does this inhibitory effect spread to involve the entire psychophysical cortical activity. Indeed it is well known that pain is capable of making one deaf and blind[T103]. *A priori* there is little likelihood that because of every evanescent, but nevertheless perceived impression, the entire automatic psychophysical cortical activity should be suspended each time. It is furthermore probable that what is of critical importance for the occurrence of phenomena of consciousness is not the actual amplitude[T104] of the psychophysical activity of the active center, but the *specific* fact that a perhaps only slight local increase of this activity *contrasts* with that of the surrounding areas as a consequence of the inhibition which, as one has to assume, is most intense in the immediate vicinity of the active center and progressively diminishes towards the periphery with increasing distance from the latter. Thus an amplitude difference is produced between the psychophysical activity in the active center and the most strongly inhibited immediate surroundings; a gradient develops, a *potential difference* which becomes equalized again. *I believe that what corresponds to this process of equalization is the psychical event!* Therefore it is not the absolute amplitude of the local psychophysical activity exceeding a certain limit that constitutes *Fechner's* internal threshold, but a certain magnitude of amplitude difference between the local psychophysical activity and that of its immediate surroundings. There are various reasons which over the years have led me to such a concept. It should be clearly understood that these are only the physiological prerequisites which render possible the occurrence of phenomena of consciousness. They cannot explain the miracle which we shall never be able to elucidate, namely that a material cortical process can actually become associated with phenomena of consciousness.

According to my concept, particularly strong local increases in psychophysical activity are by no means necessary for the occurrence of phenomena of consciousness; the local process only has to *stand out* distinctly from the continuous psychophysical cortical activity taking its regular course! The psychophysical activity then has to undergo only a slight local increase or may even remain unchanged. The mere fact of being surrounded by a corresponding zone of inhibited territory is sufficient to produce a very vivid sensation just the same. This concept together with the assumption of an inhibition which arises in the momentary center of activity and is limited in its intensity, spread and time course, also easily explains another fact which I repeatedly emphasized: during mental work, only a *decrease* in potential is observed in the E.E.G., which is an expression of inhibition, and *no* amplitude increase occurs; also during mental work of relatively long duration such potential decreases recur from time to time. I illustrated this in Figure 4 of my sixth report. One has to assume that very different areas of the cerebrum are active sequentially and in part also simultaneously during mental work, as *e.g.* when one solves a difficult problem of applied arithmetic. Thus from time to time here or there a center of activity is formed, from which inhibitions spread to involve limited areas. Their intensity and spread are probably significantly influenced by the degree of concentration of attention. If one records from the forehead and the occiput, then certainly a center of activity here and presently another one there, but each always surrounded by a larger ring of inhibited nerve cells, will be located at any given time between the recording points. In the E.E.G. which reflects the state of activity of all cortical elements located between the recording points of the electrodes, one finds inhibitory phenomena in the form of a decrease in potential at one time, but at another one finds no change during mental work[T105]. This lack of change may sometimes be caused by an intervening pause in the activity. It could, however, also have another cause: even though a center of activity is now situated somewhere along the line which connects the two electrodes, its small amplitude increase is nevertheless insufficient to produce in its surroundings a decrease in potential great enough to manifest itself visibly in the sum total of the electrical phenomena appearing in the E.E.G. The increase of psychophysical activity in the excited center and the decrease in potential in its immediate surroundings may cancel each other to the extent that no change can be demonstrated in the α-w of the E.E.G. It is also not very probable that there should be a very considerable local increase in psychophysical activity during mental work. It would probably only be possible to demonstrate this if the electrodes by chance were to record from the active site itself and in addition were to lie well inside and sufficiently removed from the area of inhibition surrounding it. I came to this conclusion only very gradually and after a long struggle; it has finally delivered me from many doubts which for years emerged time and again.

If we accept the above concept of the physiological conditions for the appearance of phenomena of consciousness as a basis for our considerations, we come to the conclusion that during Pernocton and Evipan narcosis, conscious phenomena cannot occur because no possibility exists for the development of an amplitude[T104] difference within the psychophysical activity which is everywhere enhanced and which exhibits an excessively accelerated course[T98]. A certain damping of the psychophysical activity must first be re-established by stimuli flowing in again from the body and the environment. As a consequence of this there must be a diminution of the amplitude of the α-w, group formation must cease and the rhythmic sequence of the α-w must occur at a slower pace. Under these conditions, because the local excitation is inevitably coupled with an inhibition, a potential difference can arise within the psychophysical activity and hence phenomena of consciousness can appear. I therefore believe that I must keep on adhering to the working hypothesis put forward in 1930, according to which the α-w of the E.E.G. represent bioelectric concomitants of those material processes which one calls psychophysical, because *under certain conditions* they are associated with phenomena of consciousness. The interpretation of the findings obtained during Pernocton and Evipan narcosis which is given above, only tells us something about the *conditions* under which the psychophysical processes become associated with phenomena of consciousness and confers a precisely definable meaning upon this term which had been formulated earlier in such a general way. Of course, in making the assumption of a potential difference within the automatically ongoing psychophysical cortical activity I do not believe I have solved in any definitive way the riddle of the physiological prerequisites for the development of phenomena of consciousness. I believe, however, to have brought it closer to our understanding and I hope through the E.E.G. "to approach still further that which is inaccessible"[1]. *Planck*[2], with reference to one of *Lessing's* well known sayings, aptly stated that it is not the possession of truth, but the successful struggle for it which determines the scientific investigator's happiness!

---

[1] *Rückert, Fr.*[T106]: Die Weisheit des Brahmanen, 14th edition. Nr. 43, p. 264. Leipzig, 1896.
[2] *Planck, Max*: Wege zur physikalischen Erkenntnis, p. 146. Leipzig, 1933.

IX

On the Electroencephalogram of Man

Ninth Report

by HANS BERGER, Jena

(With 7 figures)

(Received September 14, 1934)

[Published in Archiv für Psychiatrie und Nervenkrankheiten, 1934, 102: 538–557

In a short paper in "Naturwissenschaften"[1] Mr. *Tönnies* reports on results which he obtained in several subjects by using a unipolar technique of recording electrical potentials from the human skull. On this occasion he also discusses the E.E.G. described by me[T27]. His paper contains some inaccurate statements about my investigations which demand a brief rectification. Mr. *Tönnies* repeats the erroneous statement, which he had already made earlier, that I had recorded the E.E.G.[T27] from the "intact scalp" of man. This I had done only a few times at the very beginning of my investigations and later only on very special occasions, *e.g.* in newborn infants. Through *Gildemeister's* excellent studies I was familiar with the electrical properties of the human skin which are extremely difficult to evaluate. I also feared that distortions of the curve could occur through the intervention of the psychogalvanic reflex phenomenon and I therefore many years ago changed over to a recording technique with needle electrodes. These are made of pure silver; except for their tips they are covered with baked varnish and their points have a silver chloride coating which is newly made before each recording. In persons with skull defects these needles are inserted under local anesthesia and advanced as far as the dura. When the skull is intact they are pushed forward until their tips lie underneath the periosteum, for it is known from *Fleischl von Marxow's* studies in 1883 that in the dog the electrical potentials generated in the cerebral cortex can also be recorded without difficulty from the bone divested of its periosteum. From Mr. *Tönnies'* report one could perhaps gather that I immediately undertook the investigation of patients without having carried out suitable controls in healthy individuals. I first recorded a whole series of normal E.E.G.s (in 57 healthy subjects and in 75 persons with skull defects in whom the operation dated back for a considerable length of time), before I dared to approach the investigation and interpretation of pathological states. With my

---

[1] *Tönnies*: Naturwiss., fasc. 22/24, June 1, **1934**, 411.

method of bipolar recording with needle electrodes from the bone of the skull, I was quite capable of defining a normal curve. If now Mr. *Tönnies*, as he states in his report, believes that he has obtained different results, this can be attributed to various causes. First, this could be the result of a different recording method, namely the unipolar one; it could perhaps also be related to the fact that the location of the indifferent electrode on the skin of the ear is not quite indifferent electrically or fails to remain so during recording. I have just referred to the variable electrical properties of the skin which are difficult to evaluate. An additional factor which in particular must be taken into consideration when the electrodes are located on the ears, is that several skin muscles have their insertion on the external ear and in different individuals are developed to a very variable degree. Furthermore the very powerful muscle masses of the temporalis and masseter muscles, etc. lie close to the ear. However, in the light of my lengthy investigations another fact appears almost more important to me: this is the extreme sensitivity of the E.E.G. towards all disturbances which consist of stimuli arising from the environment or from the body. I therefore record the E.E.G. with the experimental subject resting comfortably on a couch with eyes closed; furthermore he is placed in a darkened room from which noise is excluded as far as possible. Of course under these conditions the recording instruments have to be located in another room to which the connecting wires lead. I do not know to what extent Mr. *Tönnies* has taken these factors into consideration in his recordings. Furthermore I wish to point out that, in the E.E.G.s of six of the seven experimental subjects whose records are reproduced in Figure 1 of his report, the frequencies of 8–11 hertz can be recognized when accurate measurements are made. These are the frequencies which I had designated as the principal oscillations or alpha waves (α-w). Thus in six of seven experimental subjects the α-w as I described them are present. Two curves show differences, namely No. 2b, which appear to me to be distorted by muscle currents and No. 6 which is perhaps influenced by emotional factors. Finally, Mr. *Tönnies* reports on a direct recording from the human cerebral cortex. This recording was carried out in a patient who lay on the operating table and from whom a tumor had just been removed from the brain under Avertine narcosis. The Avertine narcosis is said to have been over; however, at the same time it is stated that the patient's responsiveness to verbal commands returned only a quarter of an hour later, *i.e.* a quarter of an hour *after* the recording of the E.E.G.! It hardly needs to be emphasized that this recording not even remotely corresponds to the physiological and psychological conditions stipulated by me. On the other hand, I wish to point out that as early as 1931 in my third report (Figure 30)[1], I had published recordings taken from the cortex and from the white matter of the human cerebrum which had been obtained under unobjectionable physiological and psychological conditions and which demonstrated that the principal oscillations originate in the cortex itself. When carrying out such investigations in man one must take into account not only the physiological and anatomical conditions, besides the physical ones, but especially also all the psychological aspects, because man after all is not a physicochemical

---

[1] Arch. f. Psychiatr., **94**, 58 (1931). [This book p. 130]

apparatus however complex, but a *psychophysical entity*! I entirely agree with Mr. *Tönnies's* conclusion that it is impossible to obtain results of *localizing* value from the unopened skull of man. *Caton*, who discovered the bioelectric currents of the *animal* brain, as well as other investigators who followed him, used these observations to determine the approximate location of the sensory centers on the exposed surface of the cerebral cortex. *Kornmüller* and *Fischer* were later able to show that the current oscillations which occur upon illumination of the eyes are confined to the anatomically sharply circumscribed region of the striate area. But *Kornmüller* also obtained the result, which is however contested by other investigators, that the continuous bio-electrical currents of the animal cerebral cortex differ according to the anatomical structure of the area of the cortical surface from which one records. He designated these currents as area specific currents. These continuous currents, first found in 1912 by *Kaufmann*, also occur independently of all external and, as far as one can determine, internal stimuli as well. The E.E.G. of man which I described[T27] corresponds to *Kaufmann's* resting currents and therefore, when recorded with my technique, would represent the sum of *Kornmüller's* area specific currents, provided conditions in man are the same as *Kornmüller* assumed them for the animal. In effect, however, as repeated investigations have shown, the situation with regard to the E.E.G. is as follows: wherever we record with the *bipolar* technique under the experimental conditions which I indicated, we obtain in one and the same human subject an E.E.G. which, with regard to its principal oscillations which I designated as α-w, is always the same. This remains true whether we record from a skull defect located anteriorly or posteriorly, on the right or on the left side, from the dura, from the cortex as indicated above, or finally from the bone of the skull. Although the α-w display a certain characteristic range of variation between 8 and 11 hertz, they can always be demonstrated in a healthy subject. In one and the same person their amplitude varies according to the distance between the recording electrodes. The farther apart these are, the larger the potential; more specifically, the latter increases approximately in proportion to the inter-electrode distance.[1] For the accessory oscillations which I had earlier also described as oscillations of second order in accord with *Neminsky's* reports, I used the designation beta waves (β-w) which is a collective term designated to include a variety of waves, as the frequency analyses[T55] carried out by Dr. *Dietsch*[2] have unequivocally shown. They contain not only oscillations of 30 σ, as I originally indicated and later corrected, but all kinds of frequencies. *Dietsch* subdivided the oscillations into categories labelled C_1 to C_7. In this classification, C_1 corresponds to the principal oscillations, those which I named α-w; C_3 corresponds to the β-w as I originally defined them. A representation of his results in the form of a graph allows one to rapidly survey the characteristics of the individual waves, as is shown in Figure 1. It is noteworthy that the amplitude of C_2 oscillations can increase up to 1/4 of that of the principal oscillations, but from C_3 on all oscillations reach only 1/10–1/30 of the amplitude of the principal oscillations. This also confirms that the principal oscillations are the most significant component of the E.E.G. As emphasized

---

[1] 5th Report. Arch. f. Psychiatr., **98**, 231 (1932). [This book p. 151]

[2] *Dietsch, G.*: Pflüger's Arch., **230**, 106 (1932).

above, I was able earlier to demonstrate that the α-w originate in the cortex itself, whereas recordings from the cerebral white matter exhibit the various wave types subsumed under the collective term of β-w. Earlier I had also observed and reported that the α-w are absent from the E.E.G. recorded from a portion of the human cerebral cortex which had been functionally inactivated by pressure, while the β-w still persist;

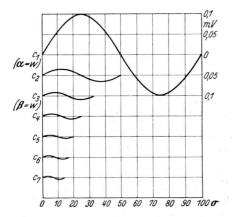

Fig. 1. Single oscillations of the E.E.G. presented in the form of a graph according to the results of Dr. G. *Dietsch's* frequency analyses[T55].

also in chloroform narcosis when the α-w disappear, the β-w persist, just as they do during the loss of consciousness which outlasts an epileptic seizure. These observations, together with other considerations, had prompted me earlier to make the following assumption: the specific function of the cortex finds its visible expression in the principal oscillations, the α-w, of the E.E.G.; accessory oscillations, on the other hand, because they can always be recorded from living cerebral tissue even when the latter is *unable* to function, correspond to the vital processes[T24] of the tissue which occur independently of its specific function. According to the view I held at the time, they represent concomitant phenomena of the nutritional and other processes; the most varied components of the nervous tissue (neurofibrils, glia, blood vessels, etc.) are probably involved in their genesis. I readily admit that one could hold other views with regard to the origin of the accessory oscillations and that one could maintain that the oscillations which differ in their frequencies may be generated by different nerve cells or perhaps may originate in different cortical layers, as *Kornmüller* and others surmise. Certainly the answer to these questions would depend upon animal experiments in which perhaps graded thermocoagulations would have to be used as *Dusser de Barenne*[1] has done in his brilliant investigations on the significance of the giant pyramidal cells. In my studies I refrained from a more detailed investigation of the β-w precisely because of their composite character and also particularly because one can very easily mistake incompletely reproduced muscle currents conducted from a distance for such waves, as *I myself* had done on occasion. However, I also readily admit that local differences of the *accessory* oscillations of the E.E.G. in various recordings of the human brain could well have escaped my notice, because

---

[1] *Dusser de Barenne*: Pflüger's Arch., **233**, 529 (1933).

until now for reasons stated I concentrated my attention predominantly upon the principal oscillations, *i.e.* my α-w, on which I carried out extensive measurements. They are always found when one observes the appropriate precautions and because at the beginning I entered completely "unexplored territory", I confined my investigations to these principal oscillations, for I knew with certainty that they originate in the human cerebral cortex; also, if only because of their slow time course, they could hardly be confused with muscle currents. These principal oscillations indeed give us information on the activity of the cerebral cortex and also present us with the opportunity of making observations of clinical value. Thus, *e.g.* in epileptic dementia in which characteristic mental changes exist, we always find the same alteration of the α-w, as I have repeatedly emphasized. Marked anatomical alterations of the cerebral cortex such as marginal gliosis and other changes can be observed in this condition. This parallelism between *mental* behavior, *anatomical* findings and alteration of the *physiological* processes of the E.E.G., in addition to many other considerations, support my assumption that alterations of the E.E.G., *i.e.* deviations from its norm, may give clinically useful information. In my eighth report I also showed what important conclusions concerning states of narcosis can be deduced from the E.E.G. findings. These observations made on the cerebral cortex itself are in complete agreement with the clinical findings. We have to assume that two possibilities for the development of loss of consciousness exist: one caused by cessation of the activity of the cerebral cortex as in chloroform narcosis, the other caused by continuation of the activity of the cerebral cortex in an altered and disinhibited form brought about by a disconnection of cortical activity from the regulating and restraining center in the thalamus. I have followed up these questions with further investigations.

Speck[1], in excellent experiments which he conducted on himself and in which he breathed air with a low oxygen content, found that with an O_2-content under 8% he rapidly developed disturbances of mental performance. If the experiment was continued for a longer period of time, he lost consciousness. Similar reports on psychological observations during balloon flights at high altitudes are available: with an O_2-content of about 10.5% disturbances of mental activity appear[2]. Because of the great practical importance which aviation has assumed, a voluminous literature has developed which deals in detail with the psychological aspects of these problems. These are of utmost importance for the investigation of aviators. A whole series of fitness tests for airplane pilots has been worked out which include the measurement of the capacity to withstand the effect of air with a low oxygen content. During the war, the Americans used a very simple procedure to select individuals suitable for high altitude flying. They proceeded in the following manner: the subject breathed in and out of a bag with a capacity of 5 liters; a CO_2-absorbing device was inserted between the bag and the mouthpiece used for breathing. Thus the effect of pure

---

[1] *Speck*: Physiologie des menschlichen Atmens, pp. 107, 109, 117 and following pages. Leipzig, 1892.

[2] *Schrötter*: Handbuch der Sauerstofftherapie. Edited by *Michaelis*, p. 238 and following pages. Berlin, 1906.

oxygen want could be observed. The subject's fitness for high altitude flights was determined from the length of time he was able to endure this procedure and from the measurement of the residual oxygen content of the bag. This test procedure was designated in brief as the bag method. By using this method, *McFarland*[1] carried out very interesting psychological investigations in a series of experimental subjects. These demonstrated that with an oxygen content of 11.4%, choice reactions began to deteriorate. With 9% there occurred loss of memory and severe disturbances of attention, and with 8.87% simple sensory and motor responses also became disturbed. An oxygen concentration of 9% in the inspired air is probably the *limit* up to which hypoxia for man is still without hazard; at 8% loss of consciousness occurs very rapidly. In my own investigations I decided to use the bag method and turned for advice and help to our biochemist, Professor *Schulz*, who referred me to the *Dräger Company*. This company supplied me with an excellent apparatus which differed from the American system only insofar as a mask was used instead of a simple mouthpiece. The American method required that the nose be closed by pinching and this, according to my experience, was bound to disturb the E.E.G. Between mask and bag an exchangeable cartridge for carbon dioxide absorption was inserted. A special analysis to determine the amount of residual oxygen in the bag was not necessary, because what mattered to me were not quantitative determinations, but only *those* alterations which appear in the E.E.G. upon inhalation of oxygen-poor air. First I carried out an experiment on myself in which I was lying on a couch with the mask on my face and breathed in and out of the bag while my laboratory assistant watched me. I could stand it for about 5 minutes and then removed the mask because the situation became unbearable and I also became slightly obtunded. One of my physicians, Dr. W., of whom earlier I had already recorded excellent E.E.G.s which I had also published, after having received detailed explanations on the purpose of these investigations from me, declared himself willing to serve as an experimental subject, particularly since he was also greatly interested in these experiments. First a preliminary experiment was again carried out. He breathed for 5 minutes and 30 seconds into the bag, and then removed the mask by lifting its lower rim from the face because he experienced marked dyspnea and began to feel obtunded. Because the two preliminary experiments went well, I proceeded without hesitation to the performance of the principal investigations in which Prof. *Hilpert*, as always before, helped me[2]. Dr. W. was lying comfortably on a couch in a supine position. After application of the electrodes for the recording of the E.C.G. from both arms and after insertion of the needles in the left forehead and the right occiput for the recording of the E.E.G., the mask was put on and Dr. W. breathed while I watched him. The room was in semi-darkness, Dr. W. had closed his eyes and in a separate recording room the E.E.G. and the E.C.G. were continuously being recorded by Mr. *Hilpert* at a recording speed somewhat slower than usual. At first Dr. W. was breathing

---

[1] *McFarland, Ross A.*: Arch. of Psychol., Nr. 145. December 1932.

[2] In addition to Mr. *Hilpert*, who for 10 years has supported me by word and deed in the performance of these investigations, I also owe a debt of gratitude to Dr. *Lemke*, Dr. *Wicke* and Dr. *Winter* for their assistance.

regularly; gradually his respiration became deeper and more labored. I observed him while holding a watch with a second hand and taking notes continuously. Six minutes had passed and he was breathing very strenuously, when I suddenly noticed that a tremor developed in his legs. I called him; he did not respond in any way. I immediately tore the mask off his face and found that he was completely uncon-scious. The excitatory motor phenomena in his legs disappeared immediately, but only after one minute, which appeared interminable to me and during which pulse and respiration were good, did consciousness return! When I reproached him for not having removed the mask as in the preliminary experiment, he said that he had wanted to do so, but then had forgotten; he thought that he must have lost conscious-ness very suddenly. Fortunately Dr. W. suffered no ill effects from this by no means harmless incident. It showed me, however, how dangerous such experiments are and made me lose the courage to repeat them. While all this happened in my presence, Mr. *Hilpert* unsuspectingly continued to record and thus a very valuable observation resulted which I shall discuss now with the aid of a few illustrations.

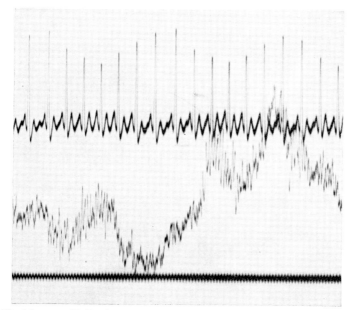

Fig. 2. Dr. W., 25 years old. During the third minute after he began to breathe in and out of the bag. At the top: E.C.G. recorded from both arms; in the middle: E.E.G. recorded with chlorided silver needles from the forehead and occiput; at the bottom: time in 1/10ths sec.

Figure 2 shows a small segment of the continuous record during the third minute after the beginning of the experiment. The pulse is already somewhat acceler-ated; it shows 100 beats per minute. The respiratory frequency measures 14 breaths per minute. The amplification of the E.E.G. was deliberately kept low so that during continuous recording the light spot would not go off the recording surface too easily. Figure 3 shows a small segment of the record from the 6th minute. The pulse has gone up to 120 beats per minute. Respiration has become deeper, but not faster. Because of the strenuous breathing the E.C.G. is markedly distorted. However, the E.E.G. still shows no changes. The records taken at the beginning of the 7th minute show a very irregular respiration and, in addition, a change in the E.E.G. which begins very suddenly and consists of considerable amplitude increase of the principal

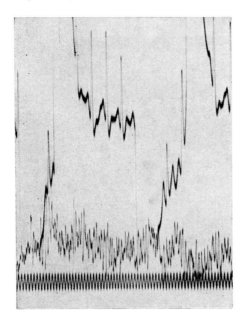

Fig. 3. Dr. W., 25 years old. During the sixth minute after he began to breathe in and out of the bag. At the top: E.C.G. somewhat distorted by the strenuous respiratory movements; in the middle: E.E.G.; at the bottom: time in 1/10ths sec.

oscillations with group formation. Subsequently this change is replaced for a few seconds by the usual E.E.G. pattern. Finally, amplitude increase and group formation become predominant. This was the time, when alerted by the tremor of the legs, I called Dr. W. and realized that he was unconscious, whereupon I immediately tore off the mask. Figure 4 shows a record taken 22 seconds *after* removal of the mask while breathing was quiet, the pulse markedly accelerated to 120 beats per minute and consciousness was completely lost. The alterations of the E.E.G. are clearly visible here. The principal oscillations of the E.E.G. (α-w) have become clustered in groups of 0.44 second length and have considerably increased in amplitude, changes which thus unequivocally display the manifestations of disinhibition. The analysis of the remainder of the record shows that the length of these groups changes from 0.44 to 1.0 second. This change disappears one minute after the removal of the mask simultaneously with the return of consciousness. Thus in O_2-deprivation we find, contrary to our expectations, no *gradual extinction* of cortical function, as one could have expected on the basis of the psychological findings; but just as in Pernocton and Evipan narcosis, one finds a *sudden* onset of *disinhibitory phenomena* in the cerebral cortex which here, just as there, suggest a sudden active disconnection[T107]. The signs which, in addition to the unconsciousness of sudden onset, also drew my attention to the seriousness of the situation were the slight excitatory motor phenomena, the trembling of the legs, which are frequently also encountered in Pernocton and

Evipan narcosis, just as they were seen here. They must be interpreted as the clinical expression of disinhibitory phenomena. We therefore have to assume that the disconnection occurs in the same center where it does in Pernocton and Evipan narcosis and in illuminating gas intoxication as well. However, whereas in Pernocton and Evipan narcosis the disconnection is brought about by the presumably excitatory

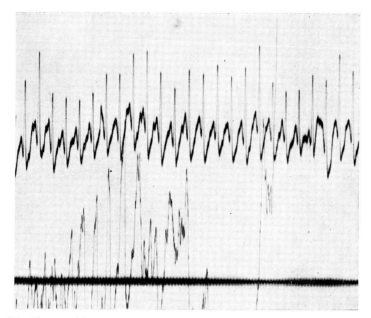

Fig. 4. Dr. W., 25 years old. Twenty-two seconds after removal of the mask, unconscious! At the top: E.C.G.; in the middle: E.E.G.; at the bottom: time in 1/10ths sec.

action of the barbiturates circulating in the blood, in the present instance, as in illuminating gas poisoning, one must attribute it to the lack of oxygen in the blood.

It is necessary to discuss these processes in somewhat more detail, to the extent of my ability to do so. As *H. Winterstein*[1] explained it so well and *Pflüger* had already suspected, acid products of incomplete oxidation first accumulate in the central nervous system when a sudden lack of oxygen develops in the blood. Among these acid products, lactic acid[T108] seems to play the major role. According to *Winterstein's* reaction theory of the regulation of respiration, acid metabolites of this kind originating in the respiratory center itself, exert an excitatory action upon it, because this center is particularly sensitive to such acid products. One has to assume some similar mechanism for the brain-stem center which regulates the events in the cerebral cortex. Here, too, the acid metabolites which are not removed by oxidation because of the lack of oxygen exert an excitatory action and lead to a disconnection, and thereby to a disinhibition of the cerebral cortex. In the light of

[1] *Winterstein, H.*: Allg. Z. Physiol., **6**, 315 (1906). — Naturwiss., **11**, 625 (1923). *Winterstein, H.* and *Frühling, G.*: Pflüger's Arch., **234**, 187 (1934).

Hess[1] excellent observations, which suggest that the onset of sleep in his experimental animals corresponds to a process of *excitation*, I envisage that such a disconnection in the area of the thalamus in the present case is also an *active* process and thus represents an excitatory effect. One is therefore tempted to assume that in Pernocton and Evipan narcosis the disconnection, and therefore the loss of consciousness, is also caused by an *excitatory* action exerted by the barbiturates which circulate in the blood and come into contact with this center. In illuminating gas poisoning it is of course the lack of oxygen in the blood which leads to the formation of acid metabolites and hence to their excitatory action. These observations also raise biochemical questions of great practical importance. To pursue them further a degree of competence in this field would be required which by far exceeds my knowledge.

It appeared probable that the loss of consciousness of the major *epileptic seizure* is caused by the same process and that in this instance too disinhibitory phenomena are involved. I already reported earlier that the loss of consciousness which *outlasts* a major epileptic seizure is certainly *not* caused by disinhibitory phenomena. In my fourth report (Figures 10–13)[2] I showed that a loss of α-w of the E.E.G. is found in these cases similar to what is seen in chloroform narcosis, and that similarly with the return of consciousness the E.E.G. gradually regains its usual aspect characterized by large amplitude α-w. I was not successful in making observations on the major epileptic seizure with simultaneous recording of the E.E.G., in spite of numerous attempts made in subjects who suffered from frequent attacks. Movements interfere with the satisfactory recording of the E.E.G. Most of the time they cause the needles to be displaced or even to be pulled out, so that for the time being I refrained from further attempts at recording during major epileptic seizures. However, from *O. Foerster's*[3] reports which have been verified by many investigators, we know that in an epileptic patient hyperventilation can very easily lead to an attack. *Kornmüller* observed in the animal that the processes in the cerebral cortex which he and *Fischer* designated as "convulsive currents" are facilitated by hyperventilation. In a number of epileptic patients in whom hyperventilation was known to precipitate attacks, I recorded the E.E.G. during hyperventilation. I shall demonstrate two records here. They were obtained in a 33 year old female patient who suffers from genuine epilepsy but who till now definitely has shown no mental defect or epileptic dementia of moderate or even slight degree. In addition to the E.C.G., recorded from both arms, respiration is also registered with *Alfred Lehmann's* pneumograph fastened around the chest, and finally the E.E.G. is recorded. Figure 5 shows a recording taken during normal respiration. With hyperventilation continued for some time, the E.E.G. shows a clear change as shown in Figure 6. The α-w increase in amplitude and merge into separate groups of 0.3–0.5 second duration. These are the changes which we find, albeit in a more distinct form, when the cerebral cortex

---

[1] *Hess, W. R.*: C. r. Soc. Biol. Paris, **107**, 1333 (1931). — Die Methodik der lokalisatorischen Reizung und Ausschaltung subcorticaler Hirnabschnitte. Leipzig, 1932.

[2] Arch. f. Psychiatr., **97**, 18 and following pages (1932). [This book pp. 144 and 145]

[3] *Foerster, O.*: Pathogenese des epileptischen Anfalls. 16th Meeting of German Neurologists, Düsseldorf 1926. — Dtsch. Z. Nervenheilk., **94**, 15 (1926).

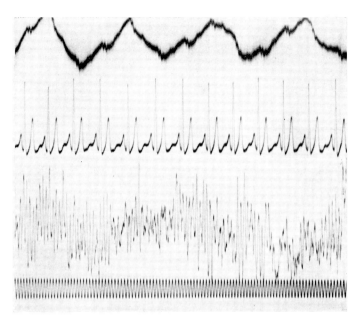

Fig. 5. Miss St., 33 years old. Genuine epilepsy without intellectual defect. At the top: thoracic respiration recorded with *A. Lehmann's* pneumograph; below it: E.C.G. recorded from both arms; below it, E.E.G. recorded from forehead and occiput with chlorided silver needles; at the bottom: time in 1/10ths sec. Normal respiration!

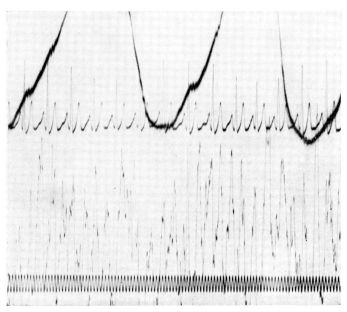

Fig. 6. Miss St., 33 years old. Genuine epilepsy without intellectual defect. At the top: thoracic respiration; below it: E.C.G.; below it, E.E.G.; at the bottom: time in 1/10ths sec. During hyperventilation, several minutes after its onset.

is disinhibited. Trials of hyperventilation repeatedly carried out in other epileptics, while simultaneously respiration, the E.C.G. and the E.E.G. were recorded, gave the same result in those cases in which a seizure was sometimes precipitated by hyperventilation. It therefore seems certain to me that in genuine epilepsy, hyperventilation can lead to disinhibition of the cerebral cortex. In other instances in patients suffering from genuine epilepsy, transient losses of consciousness could be observed under the influence of hyperventilation, or extremely mild attacks if overbreathing was continued. Figure 7 is the record of a patient suffering from frequent epileptic seizures but who has shown no mental deterioration to date. In this patient hyperventilation usually induced a major epileptic seizure within 2 minutes. However, for

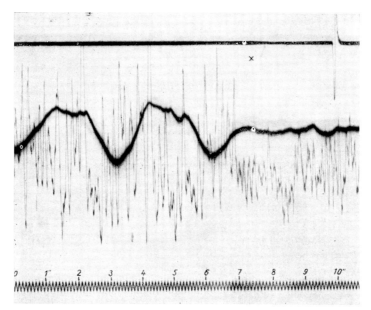

Fig. 7. Miss Z., 21 years old. Genuine epilepsy without intellectual defect. Thoracic respiration recorded with *A. Lehmann's* pneumograph; E.E.G. recorded from forehead and occiput with chlorided silver needles; time in 1/10ths sec. Hyperventilation. At "×" no response upon being called!

technical reasons, as already stated above, it was never possible to record the E.E.G. during such an attack. The figure shows a record taken in this patient during hyperventilation. Only respiration and the E.E.G. are recorded. In the E.E.G., we observe again the strikingly high voltage α-w and their marked group formation, phenomena therefore which indicate disinhibition of cerebral cortical activity. Then suddenly respiration stops. Just before this it could be shown by calling the patient that she had lost consciousness, but no fully developed seizure occurred. Such a seizure, however, developed shortly thereafter. Thus here we find in a seizure which has not come to full development, that consciousness was lost during the disinhibition of the cortex. However, I would like to point out immediately that with the arrest of respiration, one finds a considerable drop in the amplitude of the α-w of the E.E.G. These observations definitely suggest that at the beginning of a major epileptic seizure a disinhibition of the cerebral cortex sets in, and that the loss of consciousness, just as in the unconsciousness of Pernocton and Evipan narcosis and in oxygen deprivation, takes place during the *time* of this disinhibition. In the light of the findings obtained in Pernocton and Evipan narcosis we must assume that here too the disinhibition originates in that center in the region of the thalamus which had been mentioned earlier. Numerous observations suggest that a very intimate relationship exists between epilepsy and this region. *G. Specht* in his excellent discussion of the problem in *L. R. Müller's* "Lebensnerven"[1] refers to the many reasons which support the assumption of a significant involvement of the vegetative nervous system in the seizures of genuine epilepsy. With regard to this question he particularly emphasized the great importance of "the rich variety of patterns in abortive seizures and particularly of the epileptoid states as defined by *Binswanger*". *Specht* surmises that a central region from which consciousness could, as it were, be turned on or off, would probably have to be localized in the vicinity of the vital vegetative mechanisms, *i.e.* in the diencephalon. If one makes such an assumption, the respiratory and vasomotor concomitants of the epileptic seizure can easily be explained. *Karplus*[2] showed that when in an animal the region of the hypothalamus is stimulated, a cry is elicited. *Hess* found in his experiments that in cats upon stimulation[T109] involuntary defecation, micturition and epileptic seizures occurred. All these observations suggest that indeed the area of the third ventricle must be most intimately related to the manifestations accompanying the major epileptic seizure. My observations suggest involvement of the same area and lead to the concept that phenomena of disinhibition appear in the cerebral cortex at the onset of the major epileptic seizure. The anemia of the cerebral cortex observed in man by *O. Foerster*, his pre-paroxysmal vascular spasm, cannot be regarded as the *cause* of the loss of consciousness which occurs at the onset of the epileptic fit, because dilatation of the cerebral cortical vessels has also been observed in the human epileptic seizure. Above all, however, in animal experiments, many investigators have observed that a considerable dilatation of the pial and cortical vessels occurs at the onset of the epileptic attack. Thus the pre-paroxysmal vascular spasm can only represent a frequent, but by no means a necessary concomitant of the major epileptic seizure. It is, however, obvious that this vascular spasm and disturbances of the cerebral circulation in general may be of the utmost importance for the evolution of the attack. In particular, as *Spielmeyer* appropriately emphasized, one must probably regard the anatomical changes in genuine epilepsy as consequences of these disturbances of circulation. A disinhibition of the cerebral cortex elicited from the thalamic center, however, is the *initiating* process of the major epileptic seizure. This disinhibition leads to unconsciousness which may cause a sudden fall. But this does not account for the other phenomena of the major epileptic seizure. Otherwise any disinhibition of the cerebral cortex, *e.g.* in Pernocton and

---

[1] *Müller, L. R.*: "Die Lebensnerven", 2nd ed., p. 550. 1924.
[2] *Karplus*: Wien. klin. Wschr., **1930**, 622.

Evipan narcosis or in oxygen deprivation etc., would necessarily have to lead to an epileptic seizure in each instance. Thus an *additional* factor must be involved. The vascular spasm initiated from the same thalamic region could conceivably play a role in this respect. Its absence in all animal experiments, however, seems to me to militate against such an explanation. Another phenomenon observed in the major epileptic seizure of man is the transient arrest of respiration, which of course could also be induced from the thalamus. In disinhibition of the cerebral cortex as such, *e.g.* in Pernocton and Evipan narcosis, in oxygen deprivation etc., we do *not* find an arrest of respiration. This *is* something new that is added to the disinhibition and indicates that the process, at least in its further evolution, is not limited to the originally involved center. This arrest of respiration could well be the cause which, subsequent to the disinhibition, induces the development of the epileptic seizure.

On the basis of the observations on the effect of hyperventilation I assumed that disinhibition of the cerebral cortex occurs at the beginning of the major epileptic seizure. This agrees well with a number of clinical observations. In the case of sleep we must also assume that disinhibitory processes occur in the cerebral cortex, as I had already stated earlier. Thus one may find some explanation for the relationship between the major epileptic seizure and sleep. The so-called sensory auras which sometimes appear at the onset of the major epileptic seizure and consist of hallucinations and illusions involving various sensory modalities, often recurring in a stereotyped manner, can also be interpreted without difficulty as disinhibitory phenomena. The very ancient observation, already reported by *Galen*, that during the sensory aura the occurrence of the major seizure sometimes may be prevented by applying a tourniquet around the involved limb, can be explained by the assumption that a very energetic stimulus may be able to break through the disinhibition which sets in at the onset of the attack. A sudden inhibition opposes the developing disinhibition. Two further observations corroborate the concept proposed here: status epilepticus can be interrupted by chloroform, an agent which eliminates the α-w of the cerebral cortex and thus makes any cortical disinhibition impossible. Conversely it has recently been observed that Evipan, in accordance with the cortical disinhibition caused by this agent, easily precipitates epileptic attacks in children during brief narcosis. Because the center located in the region of the thalamus plays such a crucial role in the disinhibition of the cerebral cortex at the onset of the major epileptic seizure, it is quite understandable that the course of the latter is associated with such a great variety of vegetative disturbances which are controlled by the region of the third ventricle. The disinhibition at the onset of the seizure associated with the suddenly developing unconsciousness which may cause the patient to fall, is followed by respiratory arrest and the tonic stage. As repeatedly mentioned above, it is for technical reasons impossible to follow the course of the major epileptic seizure in E.E.G. records. However, many observations, especially those made during short absences associated with trismus, and thus with a tonic convulsion, as well as the one shown in Figure 7 above, suggest that in *this* stage the α-w are lost or exhibit only a very small amplitude. This is a sign that the cortex is either not functioning or that it is subjected to strong inhibitory pressure. Following *Fischer's* report, I published in my seventh communication[1] an incidental observation on the subsequent stage of the seizure which is characterized by clonic jerks. Instead of the individual α-w, very large waves with an average duration of 360 σ could be demonstrated which probably resulted from complete fusion of several α-w. In the light of *Fischer's*[2] studies we must assume that these "convulsive currents" arise everywhere in the cerebral cortex and not only in the motor region, but that in the latter they elicit excitatory motor phenomena appearing in the form of clonic jerks. *Karplus*[3] made the observation that following section of the corpus callosum in animals the clonic jerks which are evidently of cortical origin continue to occur simultaneously on both sides of the body. This is further proof that the coordination of activity of the two hemispheres is regulated from a deeper center which presumably is located in the thalamus. The phenomena occurring in the E.E.G. during the clonic stage again suggest the presence of disinhibition, but now the well known group formation has developed into a large wave of uniform appearance. It is possible that the functional derangement caused by the disturbance of respiration and by the change in blood circulation in the cerebral cortex is responsible for producing this altered appearance of the disinhibitory phenomena in the E.E.G. The clonic discharges which gradually subside in intensity are followed by a stage of persisting unconsciousness during which earlier I had obtained E.E.G. records and was able to observe an absence of the α-w. The manifestations of the epileptic seizure to the extent that they were considered here, thus suggest that they are induced from a center located in the region of the thalamus. The cerebrum[T110], like other parts of the central nervous system, represents so to speak the effector organ; through its altered activity the most conspicuous manifestations of the major epileptic seizure are produced. We thus return to the notion that some kind of convulsive center exists in the region of the thalamus. Undoubtedly, however, the function of this center is a purely *physiological* one; from here the cortex is also disconnected under physiological conditions as, *e.g.*, during sleep. In the presence of certain additional factors, however, this physiological process may lead to an epileptic seizure. Among these one must probably include in particular inhibition of respiration and perhaps also disturbances of cerebral circulation. If these factors add their effect, the simple disconnection process changes into an epileptic seizure which thus is ultimately caused by an excitatory process in the thalamic region most likely irradiating to adjacent centers in the same area. In the light of the observations on the E.E.G. the major epileptic seizure, which has been studied in such meritorious fashion by my teachers, *Binswanger* and *Ziehen*, can therefore be described as follows: from the cerebral cortex or any other site in the central nervous system an intense excitation is conducted to the center in the region of the thalamus which regulates cortical activity. This excitation causes a disconnection of the cerebral cortex, which thus becomes disinhibited; loss of consciousness results. The disinhibition of the cortex is followed by maximal cortical inhibition which manifests itself in the form of respiratory arrest, generalized tonic contraction of the entire musculature and in

[1] Arch. f. Psychiatr., **100**, 318 (1933). [This book p. 205]
[2] *Fischer, M. H.*: Med. Klin., **1933**, Nr. 1.
[3] *Karplus*: Wien. klin. Wschr., **1914**, 645.

primary as well as secondary circulatory disturbances. This is followed by renewed disinhibition of the cortex which, having suffered some impairment of function in the meantime, responds to this disinhibition with high amplitude convulsive waves: the clonic stage begins. After the latter has subsided, moderate inhibition of the cortex occurs again, which however becomes associated with signs of cortical exhaustion, the cortex having been completely drained of its reserves during the clonic phase. One could thus reduce this whole process to a very simple formula. A twice recurring alternation between excitation and paralysis takes place within the center in the vicinity of the thalamus which regulates and restrains the activity of the cerebral cortex. These changes become associated with the sequels of similar states in immediately adjacent centers. The principal manifestations of the epileptic seizure could therefore be explained by a twice recurring, to-and-fro oscillation between excitation and paralysis of the diencephalic center, which has become particularly excitable, and by the effects exerted upon the activity of the cerebral cortex resulting from these changes. From the manifestations of Evipan and Pernocton narcosis and from the effect of O_2-deprivation reported above, we also know that this center can very easily be influenced by *chemical* means. In addition to the *ease* with which it can be excited either from the blood stream or from other parts of the central nervous system, we must however assume that in the epileptic there is a certain *weakness* of this center, since it very rapidly fails and in so doing its excitation turns into paralysis. Of course, one could also explain these events by assuming an interaction of two antagonistic physiological centers. However, the assumption proposed here has the advantage of simplicity. Thus it is a *physiological* process which becomes enhanced in this case; a process which also plays a role in other situations, *e.g.* in the partial disinhibition which occurs during sleep. Likewise it is also the normal inhibition to which the brain is subjected during wakefulness, which during the tonic stage of the epileptic seizure reaches an abnormal intensity. This strong inhibition can most easily be explained by assuming that strong stimuli which originate in the body suddenly gain unimpeded access to the cerebral cortex because the center which normally disconnects the cortex has become paralyzed; these stimuli are possibly also the precipitating cause of the respiratory arrest which is apparently so important. For we know that during normal wakefulness also sudden, unexpected and intense stimuli, as *e.g.* a loud noise or a cold stimulus impinging on the skin, and others, are capable of producing an, albeit only brief, respiratory arrest. The major epileptic seizure can be preceded by milder states of disinhibition before a fully developed attack occurs. One can also observe that the double oscillations between disinhibition and inhibition may be followed after the seizure by weaker after-oscillations especially when the attack fails to develop fully. This explanation brings the mysterious event of the epileptic seizure closer to our *physiological understanding*.

     In the waking state, as I have just reiterated, the cerebral cortex is subjected to continuous inhibition of moderate intensity, just as the entire body musculature is under the control of a tonic innervation. This continuous inhibition is most easily explained by assuming that it represents an effect exerted by stimuli continuously flowing into the cortex from the body and from the environment. According to *von*

Economo's investigations the site from which during sleep the cortex is discon-nected[T111] is located in the vicinity of the thalamus. This is an active process which is most easily interpreted by assuming that a conduction block develops along the pathways leading to the cortex. We know that a number of vegetative centers are located in the wall of the third ventricle in the vicinity of the thalamus, as was demonstrated by several investigators. According to the views expressed by *Berze, Reichardt, Veronese, Gamper, Küppers*[1] and others, there are centers located in the brain-stem which exert a considerable influence upon the activity of the cerebral cortex. In particular one has to postulate the existence of a center there which regulates the *tonus of consciousness*, to use *Berze*'s expression. *Foerster*'s and *Gagel*'s[2] interesting observations represent, as it were, the experimental confirmation of this assumption. Phenomena of consciousness and their disturbances can only be ex-plained by an interaction between cortex and brain-stem. In my eighth report I stated that for the appearance of conscious phenomena (which in man are localized exclusively in the cerebral cortex) it is necessary that a potential difference should arise within the ongoing automatic psychophysical cortical activity. Such a potential difference would make a process *stand out* against the background of uniform events. This is neither possible when the cortical activity is completely disinhibited nor when it is subjected to a strong generalized inhibitory pressure. Thus, theoretically, we must consider a third possible cause of *unconsciousness*, in addition to the two which are derived from E.E.G. observations and which are either extinction of cortical activity or cortical disinhibition caused by disconnection. This third cause could be described as the sudden development of a strong, generalized inhibitory pressure exerted on the cerebral cortex. It appears probable that the so-called fainting spells associated with well preserved cardiac activity which sometimes are observed under the influence of overwhelming painful stimuli may be explained on this basis, but for understandable reasons this cannot be proven for man. On the basis of obser-vations on the practice effect, *i.e.* on the manner in which performances which originally are closely linked to mental processes etc., become automatic, *Herbert Spencer, Romanes* and *Herzen* rightly concluded that a certain resistance or, as *Romanes* says, a "ganglionic friction", is a necessary prerequisite for the appearance of phenomena of consciousness. Considerations of a general scientific nature suggest that such an assumption is also quite necessary from a physicochemical and biological point of view. Therefore one would have to assume that a *second* condition for the occurrence of phenomena of consciousness is a resistance opposing the tendency of this potential difference to become equalized. This levelling off probably occurs in an oscillatory manner and requires a minimal time of about 25–50 σ, as suggested by the duration of the principal oscillations of the E.E.G. To this event corresponds the mental process. We can go one step further still and assume that as the potential difference is equalized and in so doing meets a resistance, *electrical* potentials may

---

[1] *Gamper*: Med. Klin., **41** (1931). — *Küppers, E.*: Z. Neur., **78**, 546 (1922). — Klin. Wschr., **1933**, 1009.

[2] *Foerster* and *Gagel*: Z. Neur., **149**, 312 (1933).

be transformed into what *Kurd Lasswitz*[1] *provisionally* designated by the general term of psychophysical energy, his assumption being that the conscious processes are immediately related to this energy. This psychophysical energy is immediately reconverted and leaves behind physiological traces in the form of structural changes of the cortex and of the central nervous system in general. In time, therefore, a continuously progressing restructuring occurs and psychophysical processes are laid down in the brain in material form. Only by the *intermediary* of this psychophysical energy can such structural changes occur and these in turn, when the mental processes recur, can decisively influence new processes[T112]. Thus, as *Lieder* so aptly put it[2], the central nervous system and especially the cerebral cortex undergoes a historical evolution in the course of individual life which cannot be reversed. Therefore, as he pertinently explains, any estimate of the energy expenditure involved in a mental performance would *also* have to take into account the synthetic processes necessary for the appropriate structural alterations which have been acquired in the course of individual existence or perhaps were even in part inherited. Because of this, of course, quantitative measurements will always be unsuccessful.

---

[1] *Lasswitz, Kurd*: Arch. system. Phil., **1895**, **I**, 46.

[2] *Lieder, Franz*: Die psychische Energie und ihr Umsatz. p. 369 and following pages. Berlin, 1910.

X

On the Electroencephalogram of Man

Tenth Report

by Hans Berger, Jena

(With 4 figures)

(Received April 10, 1935)

[Published in *Archiv für Psychiatrie und Nervenkrankheiten*, **1935**, *103*: 444–454]

Recently a number of articles have been published which are concerned with investigations of the electrical potential oscillations originating in the cerebral cortex of man and which arrived at results which appear to be contradictory. In part the differences in the results must certainly be attributed to differences in the methods of recording the potential oscillations, partly however also to other causes. If we first deal with the different *methods of recording*, essentially two have to be taken into consideration: firstly the unipolar and secondly the bipolar recording technique. With the *unipolar* recording method one electrode, the so-called different electrode, is placed on the cerebral cortex, the dura or the bone of the skull, whereas the other, the so-called indifferent electrode, is located in an area which is, as much as possible, devoid of current. For instance, a number of investigators use the region of the ear for this purpose. In a *bipolar recording* both electrodes are placed on the cerebral cortex, the dura or the bone of the skull. The principles of physics which must be considered in relation to these recording methods can easily be deduced from Figure 1. With *unipolar recording*, electrode *a* is reached by current oscillations which are produced by a cone-shaped region located near the point of application of the electrode. The electrode itself lies at the apex of this cone with the current paths increasingly spreading out towards the indifferent electrode for which usually a larger size is selected. It goes without saying that such a recording particularly displays those electrical events which occur in the immediate vicinity of the different electrode *a* and that therefore *this* recording technique is to be recommended especially for localizing purposes. In my first investigations on the electroencephalogram (E.E.G.) I repeatedly tried this unipolar technique for recording from areas of trepanation but later I completely abandoned this recording method again because of the problems which arise from the selection of the site of the indifferent electrode and because of the ubiquity of the E.C.G. With *bipolar recording* the electrical events which occur *between the two electrodes a and b* are displayed (Figure 1). The current

[243]

paths penetrate to a much lesser depth than with unipolar recording; however, they also spread out to the sides in an arc-like fashion and therefore encompass a much larger area. With bipolar recording all electrical processes which originate between the two electrodes are recorded. More specifically, these include not only those which occur along the direct line connecting the two electrodes, but also those

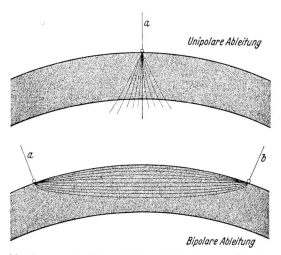

Fig. 1. Paths followed by the current with unipolar and bipolar recording from the cerebral cortex.

which originate within an approximately lens-shaped volume. Undoubtedly this kind of recording is less well suited for localizing purposes than for displaying electrical processes within larger or smaller cortical regions and for the detection of relatively small potential oscillations. In all my investigations on the E.E.G. of man reported earlier, I used the bipolar recording technique. In view of this, the findings obtained by *Foerster* and *Altenburger*[1] appear to me to be of great importance. Using the *unipolar* technique they recorded from the cerebral cortex of man during operations performed under local anesthesia and found that electrical potential oscillations can be recorded from the most diverse regions. The larger and slower of these oscillations correspond to those which I had designated as alpha oscillations. This confirms my findings obtained with bipolar recordings which showed that when one records from the dura of skull defects in the most varied locations, one always obtains the *same* E.E.G. which exhibits large alpha oscillations of 90–120 σ and smaller, more rapid oscillations. In these records only the *amplitudes* of the potential oscillations differed, depending upon the distance between the electrodes *a* and *b*. The voltage increased approximately in proportion to the distance between the electrodes and thus to the number of nerve cells lying between them. The finding that potential oscillations can be recorded from the dura of the *cerebellum*, which I illustrated in Figure 9[2] of my first report, was also confirmed by these two investigators who took records *directly*

---

[1] *Foerster* and *Altenburger*: Dtsch. Z. Nervenheilk., **135**, 277 (1935).
[2] *Berger, Hans*: Arch. f. Psychiatr., **87**, 545 (1929). [This book p. 52]

from the cerebellar cortex. I had emphasized then that the large oscillations in the cerebellar curve occur less frequently than in the E.E.G. of the cerebrum and it appears to me that this is also the case in the curve shown in *Foerster's* and *Altenburger's* Figure 10. In my second report[1] I had also stressed that the alpha oscillations of the E.E.G. are absent in *pathologically altered cerebral tissue*, a finding which these two investigators as well as *Tönnies*[2] document with beautiful illustrations. The potential oscillations recorded by *Foerster* and *Altenburger* directly from the cerebral cortex with the unipolar technique also confirm my view that in man one obtains everywhere the same E.E.G. from areas with completely different architectonic structure and that the situation apparently differs from that reported for animals by *Kornmüller* and *Tönnies*. *Foerster* and *Altenburger* also demonstrated that in man, relatively strong current oscillations occur in the sensory centers under the influence of the appropriate sensory stimuli. I consider these observations to be very important. Such oscillations had been known to occur in the animal since *Caton's* work in 1874. *Foerster* and *Altenburger* were also able to demonstrate a similar change in the motor region and in particular they made the extremely interesting observation that during a movement[T113] the same increase in potential oscillations can be demonstrated simultaneously in the cerebellar cortex! With my bipolar recording taken from the dura, from skull defects or from the bone of the skull, I never succeeded in demonstrating that an *increase* of potential oscillations occurs under the influence of sensory stimuli, but without exception I found a *decrease*. Only in association with the isolated clonic jerks, which occurred in the muscles of the right hand of a patient suffering from dementia paralytica, was I able to record fairly large potential oscillations from the region of the mid-portion of the left central convolutions which had been located with the aid of the cyrtometer[T81]. These oscillations preceded the momentary jerks. In that study I used a bipolar recording from the skull with needle electrodes placed 4 cm apart and in contact with the bone[3]. As I stated before and as I have emphasized time and again in my numerous reports, I never saw in man the increase of potential oscillations within a sensory center which is known to occur in animal experiments. I know of such increases in potential oscillations from animal experiments carried out by others and also from a very few isolated successful experiments which I personally performed many years ago. The reason why I failed to record such potential increases in man is simply that the human sensory centers, because of their location, are inaccessible to recordings from the dura, especially to those taken with the bipolar technique. On the other hand I have observed time and again that the *potential decreased* to about 1/5th of the preceding amplitude under the influence of the most varied sensory stimuli to which attention is directed, and that this was associated with a disappearance of the alpha oscillations. I have been able to demonstrate these changes in many records. *Foerster* and *Altenburger* did not observe such a decrease in potential with direct unipolar recording from the human cerebral cortex even under the influence of sensory stimuli. This could be due to the unipolar recording technique

[1] *Berger, Hans*: J. Psychol. u. Neur., **40**, 160 (1930). [This book p. 75]
[2] *Tönnies, J. F.*: Dtsch. Z. Nervenheilk., **135**, 288, Fig. 2.
[3] *Berger, Hans*: Arch. f. Psychiatr., **100**, 314 (1933) Fig. 12. [This book p. 202]

which displays predominantly the electrical events at the site of the different electrode, whereas with the bipolar recording one is capable of surveying the electrical events of a much larger area. A local excitation is associated with a decrease in potential *outside* the involved sensory area, as can also be concluded from many animal experiments reported by several authors. Thus one has to look outside the involved sensory center for this potential decrease which occurs under the influence of the sensory stimulus. This decrease in potential encompasses much wider areas than the increase in potential, when one records with the bipolar technique which, as mentioned, reveals all electrical processes occurring between the electrodes *a* and *b*. The regions in which a decrease in potential occurs are much larger than the circumscribed area in which the potential is increased. Therefore in the summation curve of the E.E.G. in a *bipolar* recording the result is a potential decrease. Figure 4 of *Range's*[1] work clearly shows that with unipolar recording a considerable potential decrease in response to a stimulus can sometimes also be demonstrated in the cerebral cortex of the rabbit. The disappearance of the alpha oscillations of the E.E.G. described by me[T27], which occurs under the influence of the most diverse sensory stimuli and during mental work, has been documented with beautiful curves by *Adrian* and *Matthews* in a major study in "Brain"[2], so that this fact as such can hardly be disputed any longer. Earlier, in the light of the then available animal experiments, I had already discussed the E.E.G. changes which occur under the influence of sensory stimuli and during mental work and which had caused me great surprise. I had explained then that in a bipolar recording of the E.E.G., the circumscribed local increase in potential is masked by the inhibition which manifests itself in a potential decrease and which is much more extensive than the local excitation coupled with it. Thus these findings with bipolar recording of the E.E.G. are, in my opinion, quite in agreement with those of *Foerster* and *Altenburger* and do not contradict them, as these gentlemen have also pointed out. One could, however, consider yet another explanation for the failure to demonstrate a potential decrease in *Foerster's* and *Altenburger's* studies. This could be related to the overall external circumstances under which the records were taken in the cases reported by them. Their patients lay on an operating table and a surgical intervention was about to be performed or had perhaps already been performed. These patients were in an abnormal emotional state and their attention was probably absorbed by a variety of events, with the effect that the concomitant phenomena of *attention*[T114], — and this in my opinion is what the inhibitory processes represent — did not become clearly manifest. I also demonstrated earlier that the E.E.G. undergoes a considerable change under the influence of emotional excitement. This change assumes the specific form of a shortening of the alpha oscillations sometimes to as much as half their value, *i.e.* to less than 50 σ. Furthermore pain and an uncomfortable position as well as other distracting events etc. can cause very considerable alterations in the E.E.G., so that the process of inhibition and therefore the decrease in potential manifests itself only very fleetingly or not at all[T115]. Under

---

[1] *Range, R. W.*: Psychol. u. Neur., **46**, 364 (1935).

[2] *Adrian* and *Matthews*: Brain, **57**, 355 (1934).

such conditions the alpha oscillations recede; the secondary oscillations, which I also designated as beta waves now stand out more distinctly. They are composed of at least seven different short types of oscillations of variable amplitude[1] and under certain circumstances can also *simulate local differences in the E.E.G.!* Extreme caution is in order when one interprets the curves, as I have learned from eleven years of experience, and in particular much consideration has to be given also to the *psycho-physical* conditions under which the E.E.G. has been recorded. I shall presently show that even excellent physiologists have made the most serious errors when they failed to take into account precisely these psychophysiological factors.

Adrian and *Matthews* in their studies on the E.E.G. of man, which I have mentioned before, came to the conclusion that the electrical potential oscillations which they found, originate in the cerebral cortex itself. Their observations were in agreement with my own. However, they made the erroneous assumption that these potential oscillations originate in the *occipital lobe*. In 75 subjects with decompressive trepanations, I always obtained the same E.E.G. from skull defects situated in the most diverse locations, when I recorded from the dura with the bipolar technique. I never noticed that the alpha oscillations of the E.E.G. obtained when recording from the dura of defects in the posterior part of the skull were of particularly high amplitude. Moreover, from the differences in amplitude of the potential oscillations recorded within or in the vicinity of a skull defect caused by a war injury, it is not necessarily permissible to draw a definite conclusion as to the *site of origin* of these electrical processes, as *Adrian* and *Matthews* have done, particularly not in the manner in which these two investigators have attempted it (see Figure 6, p. 362 of their report in "Brain"). It is actually impossible to know whether underneath the areas of the *skin* from which the records were taken, the *cerebral cortex* was healthy or pathologically changed, whether the dura was abnormally thickened or the lepto-meninges altered, or whether perhaps even a cyst was present. Yet these may well be the reasons why one obtains potential oscillations of different amplitudes from different recording sites. I have just emphasized that no alpha oscillations of the E.E.G. can be recorded from pathologically altered cerebral cortex, and this has been confirmed by the studies of *Foerster* and *Altenburger* and also by those of *Tönnies*. For recordings from the dura within skull defects and for the few recordings which I had obtained directly from the cerebral cortex, I used exclusively subjects in whom I had satisfied myself *by my own personal observation* that healthy cerebral tissue was present in the area of the skull defect. I did this at the time of the decompressive trepanation performed by Prof. *Guleke* several weeks prior to the recording. I also recorded from defects which did not extend beyond the region of the frontal lobe and on these occasions I obtained very excellent E.E.G.s. In my first report, in Figure 5[2], a bilateral needle electrode recording of the E.E.G. is shown which was obtained in a 19 year old girl in whom a bilateral decompressive *Cushing*-type trepa-nation had been performed by Mr. *Guleke* because of a pituitary tumor. The needles

---

[1] *Berger, Hans*: Arch. f. Psychiatr., **102**, 541 (1934) Fig. 1. [This book p. 228]
[2] *Berger, Hans*: Arch. f. Psychiatr., **87**, 541 (1929). [This book p. 49]

used as electrodes were placed on the right and left side on the dura near the superior and anterior limit of the decompressive trepanation. In my third report[1], in Figures 1, 2, 15 and 16, I showed E.E.G.s which had been obtained from a man who, as described there, had a skull defect in the frontal region. One needle electrode recorded from the dura over the most anterior part of the right, the other from the dura over the most anterior part of the left frontal lobe. Here too, at a site far remote from the occipital lobe, an excellent E.E.G. was seen. If, however, one should not consider even *these* recordings as conclusive, then I wish to refer to Figures 1–5 in *Foerster's* and *Altenburger's* study which unequivocally demonstrate the alpha oscillations of the E.E.G. in a *unipolar* recording obtained from the frontal cortex. In this case it is, I presume, no longer possible to make the assumption that these oscillations originate exclusively from the occipital lobe, especially if one takes into consideration the statements on the course of the current paths in unipolar recordings which were made above. *Adrian* and *Matthews*[T116] were led astray by a fact which also greatly preoccupied me in the beginning, namely the powerful influence of eye opening or closure upon the alpha oscillations of the E.E.G. In my earlier studies, especially in my second communication, I reported on this in detail. As proof for their notion that the E.E.G. originates in the occipital lobe and is related to visual function, *Adrian* and *Matthews* cite their finding that it was completely absent in three subjects who had been blind for a long time[T117]. Such an observation, if it were correct, would naturally be of the utmost importance for the interpretation of the E.E.G. From the beginning I had the greatest doubts with regard to these findings, because among the 300 people in whom I had recorded E.E.G.s over the years, there were several who were blind. Thus *e.g.* the above mentioned 19 year old girl in whom a bilateral *Cushing*-type decompressive trepanation had been carried out because of a pituitary tumor, had been blind for several months and nevertheless, as shown in Figure 5[2], presented a typical E.E.G.! Likewise I had recorded excellent E.E.G.s earlier on repeated occasions in other individuals who had lost their eyesight. Admittedly, these were people who had only been blind for a few weeks or at the very most a few months, so that the objection could be raised that because of the brevity of time, an appropriate readjustment might not as yet have taken place in the cerebrum. When I was confronted with *Adrian's* and *Matthews'* definite statements, I did not consider my earlier observations to be conclusive. I therefore grasped the opportunity to investigate blind individuals in whom, as in the cases examined by *Adrian* and *Matthews*, vision had been lost for many years. Like these investigators I studied three blind people[3] in whom total loss of vision had been present for 15, 17 and 18 years. I succeeded in demonstrating the E.E.G. in all three of them and thus *Adrian's* and *Matthews'* statement that the E.E.G. is lacking in blind people is inaccurate. In a 31 year old man, H.H., who completely lost his vision 15 years ago

---
[1] *Berger, Hans*: Arch. f. Psychiatr., **94**, 16 (1931). [This book p. 95]

[2] *Berger, Hans*: Arch. f. Psychiatr., **87**, 541 (1929). [This book p. 49]

[3] As in all my investigations on the E.E.G. performed to date, Prof. *Hilpert* this time too assisted me by word and deed, for which here also I extend to him my cordial thanks. I also thank Dr. *Lemke* for his faithful assistance.

because of a shotgun charge fired at close range and who earns his living as a piano tuner, I found an E.E.G. as shown in Figure 2, when observing the necessary precautionary measures during the recording. One sees fairly high amplitude alpha

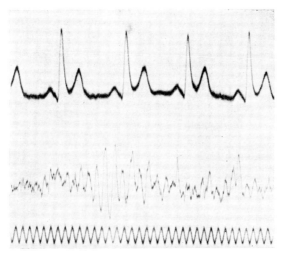

Fig. 2. H.H., 31 years old, completely blind for 15 years. At the top: E.C.G. recorded from both forearms. In the middle: E.E.G. recorded with silver needles from the left frontal and the right occipital quadrants of the head. At the bottom: time in 1/10ths sec.

oscillations with a duration of 110 σ. I must, however, readily admit that it was by no means easy to clearly demonstrate these alpha oscillations in a blind person and it appears entirely understandable to me that *Adrian* and *Matthews* arrived at erroneous results. I recorded from the forehead and occiput with silver needles which, after insertion under local anesthesia, were advanced until their tips were located beneath the periosteum of the skull. In a second blind man, H.A., who was 51 years old and was entrusted with examining fine metal parts in a large factory, I was also able to demonstrate the E.E.G. perfectly well in a recording taken from the forehead and the occiput. This man had lost his left eye through an injury as a child when he was 5 years old and had the misfortune of having his right eye destroyed by gunshot in the war 18 years ago. Much more important and simpler was the demonstration of the E.E.G. in a third blind individual, 40 year old A.F., who works as a bookbinder. Seventeen years ago he had lost both eyes through an injury by shell fragments and at the same time he had become markedly deaf in the right ear. As already mentioned above, it is not so easy to obtain a perfect demonstration of the E.E.G. in blind individuals. In the blind man from whom Figure 2 was obtained, a good demonstration of the E.E.G. became possible only in a second sitting, which had been scheduled 8 days after the first. — What are the reasons responsible for the failure of the English investigators? As I have already emphasized, emotional processes, pain or sensory stimuli which originate from the body or from the environment influence the E.E.G. and can interfere with its demonstration. If we first consider the purely psychological reasons, we recognize that the experimental subject's anxiety markedly interferes with the recording of the E.E.G. The blind individual does not know what happens to him and is apprehensive or at least somewhat distrustful during the recording, in spite of all assurances to the contrary, precisely because he is unable to see what takes place around him. Furthermore his attention is directed towards all events in his environment about which he can only obtain information by means of his organ of hearing. In the blind, the coupling of sensory phenomena to those of attention is completely different from that existing in subjects who are in full possession of their sensory capacities. In full possession of his senses, *man is a "visual being"*. The processes of attention are most intimately connected and entwined with visual function: the process of directing one's attention to an event is closely correlated with focussing of the eyes and with accommodation. Indeed, this goes so far that even the facial expressions of thinking are associated with gaze being directed into the distance and with relaxation of accommodation. Attention, voluntary and involuntary, is firmly connected or, if I may say so, coupled with the visual process. Closure of the eyes in general therefore signifies that voluntary attention is switched off, provided the subject does not particularly intend to or is not induced by some inner attitude to direct his whole attention towards auditory stimuli. In the blind, however, this is completely different. Attention can no longer be connected, as it was in the days of health, with the organ of vision which is now lost. Attention is now connected with auditory and tactile stimuli, and especially when the sense of touch becomes inadequate because of distance, the blind is exclusively dependent upon his sense of hearing. Closure of the eyes in the blind therefore is not sufficient to switch off attention because evidently no change with regard to environmental stimuli is thereby achieved; the two principal senses, the organ of touch and especially the ear, still remain intensely active. It is therefore necessary to carefully avoid any *auditory stimulus* when one records the E.E.G. in a blind individual, who incidentally must know exactly what is going to happen to him and whose full confidence one must have. In my opinion it is for these psychological and physiological reasons that *Adrian*'s and *Matthews*' recordings were unsuccessful. Particularly instructive and conclusive in this respect is the E.E.G. recording in the third blind individual, A.F., described above. He had two glass eye prostheses and was deaf in the right ear. The man had known me for a long time; I had his full confidence and he willingly consented to undergo the investigation. During the very first recording he exhibited an E.E.G. as shown in Figure 3. As a precaution I had him turn halfway on his side and lay his head on his good left ear, which in addition was stopped with cotton wool, so that for practical purposes hearing too was essentially eliminated. The figure shows a normal E.E.G.; its alpha oscillations have a duration of 120 σ. This recording of the E.E.G. in the blind, which had been prompted by *Adrian*'s and *Matthews*' disagreement, is extremely interesting insofar as it again demonstrates the great importance which *mental processes*, the emotional tone and distraction by unintentional stimuli have with regard to the pattern[T20] of the E.E.G. of man. The

E.C.G. which I always recorded simultaneously with the E.E.G. is very useful for the detection of emotional excitement and also allows one to check that the subject who is being examined remains still. Because in every examination I obtain a record at least 6 meters in length, it is *e.g.* very easy, but well worthwhile, to determine the momentary pulse rate. I also have the greatest misgivings with regard to the recording

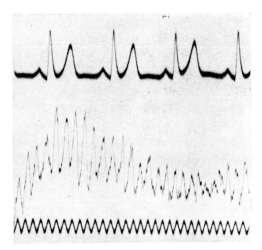

Fig. 3. A.F., 40 years old. Completely blind for 17 years. At the top: E.C.G. recorded from both forearms. In the middle: E.E.G. recorded with silver needles from the left frontal and the right occipital quadrants of the head. At the bottom: time in 1/10ths sec.

of E.E.G.s on the operating table unless one is carrying out very simple investigations. The unusual position, the expectancy of the operation and the influence of the most varied stimuli from the completely unfamiliar environment have to be taken into consideration when interpreting the experimental results. These are factors whose significance can often not be evaluated. Therefore my opinion also differs entirely from that of *Adrian* and *Matthews* with regard to the interpretation of the E.E.G. reproduced by them in Figure 16 of their study, which had been obtained with direct bipolar recording from the cerebral cortex of the parietal lobe. I actually believe that the E.E.G. obtained *before* the operation is the normal one, because the brain in the course of time had largely adapted to the existing pressure and to the altered circulation, in spite of the visible congestion. In favor of this is the fact that the alpha oscillations have a normal duration of 100 σ. *After* the operative intervention which caused severe changes which necessarily appear at recording sites in the vicinity of the operative area, but also in more remote regions, *Adrian* and *Matthews* obtained a pathological, uninterpretable E.E.G. *They* consider this E.E.G. to be normal; however, in the light of my experience this is certainly not the case. I wish to mention this only parenthetically! I indicated above that in persons who had been blind for many years the coupling of the processes of attention to sensory stimuli is different from that seen in normals and this is a factor which complicates the recording of an E.E.G. in these subjects. That this interpretation is correct also becomes apparent from the following observation on *deaf-mutes*. In a deaf-mute, attention is even more intimately connected with the visual process than is the case if someone is in full possession of his sensory capacities: I only draw attention to the lipreading of words and the continuous visual attention which every intelligent deaf-mute exhibits as a most striking feature. From deaf-mutes whose confidence the investigator has earned, one

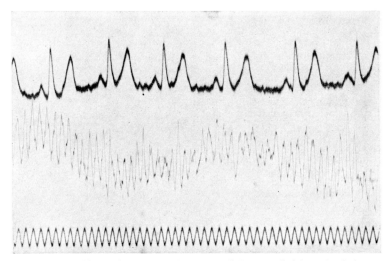

Fig. 4. W.S., 20 years old. Deaf-mute. At the top: E.C.G. recorded from both forearms. In the middle: E.E.G. recorded with silver needles from the left frontal and the right occipital quadrants of the head. At the bottom: time in 1/10ths sec.

therefore immediately obtains excellent E.E.G.s, as soon as visual attention is eliminated by eye closure. Figure 4 was obtained from a 20 year old cobbler, W.S. Having developed normally as a child and after having learned to speak, he suffered severe meningitis when he was about two years old. This led to complete deafness. He completely lost the ability to speak and later received special instruction for deaf-mutes. He is an intelligent and very lively young man. In Figure 4 one sees high amplitude alpha oscillations with a duration of 100 σ. — On the basis of my own investigations I must therefore resolutely disagree with the assertion made by *Adrian* and *Matthews* that the E.E.G. is absent in the blind. When observing the necessary precautionary measures, the E.E.G. has been unequivocally demonstrated by me in three blind individuals in whom vision had been lost for 15, 17 and 18 years. On the basis of my own investigations and in view of *Foerster's* and *Altenburger's* results, I disagree with the statement of the English investigators that the E.E.G. originates exclusively in the occipital lobe. The E.E.G. originates *everywhere*[T118] in the cerebral cortex and constitutes a directed wave of activity of the cortex as I demonstrated particularly in my sixth report[1]. In the E.E.G. a *fundamental function*[2] of the human

[1] *Berger, Hans*: Arch. f. Psychiatr., **99**, 568 (1933). [This book p. 185]
[2] Naturwiss., **1935**, Fasc. 8, 124.

cerebrum intimately connected with the psychophysical processes becomes visibly manifest. This is clearly demonstrated by the above discussed close relationship of the E.E.G. with processes of attention, which represents the most important psychophysical function. I therefore also consider it more correct to retain the term E.E.G., which I coined as the discoverer of these potential oscillations in man, rather than to exchange it for the term which *Adrian* and *Matthews* have chosen and by which I felt greatly honored[T119]!

XI

On the Electroencephalogram of Man

Eleventh Report

by HANS BERGER, Jena

(With 7 figures)

(Received February 1, 1936)

[Published in *Archiv für Psychiatrie und Nervenkrankheiten*, **1936**, *104*: 678–689]

In my ninth report I discussed in some detail the question of the so-called beta waves (β-w) of the electroencephalogram (E.E.G.). The reports which have since been published by several investigators who have taken up the study of this problem, however, make it necessary that I re-state my position on this question, because these accounts of the β-w reflect two different points of view. *Firstly* it is emphasized that, in addition to the β-w of 20–125 hertz which I described, there are some which are considerably faster. For the β-w I originally assumed an average length of 30 σ, and only the frequency analyses[T55] carried out by *G. Dietsch*[1] have taught me that the term β-w, as defined by me[T120], represents a *collective* term including waves with completely different frequencies[T121] and amplitudes. Figure 1 may

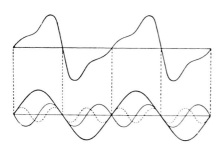

Fig. 1. Breakdown of a composite oscillation (top) into three single sinusoidal oscillations (*Fourier* analysis).

help to convey to those unfamiliar with these studies some idea of the kind of resolution obtained with such frequency analyses. With the aid of this figure it is easy to visualize and to comprehend the essence of such a Fourier analysis. Frequencies of cerebral oscillations up to 1000 hertz have been reported by other investigators; however, it is said that the upper limit most often lies around 600–700 hertz[2]. To date

---

[1] *Dietsch, G.*: Pflüger's Arch., **230**, 106 (1932).
[2] *Rohracher, Hubert*: Z. Psychol., **136**, 308 (1935).

I have not found frequencies above 125 hertz. I admit, however, that this could be attributed to the instrumentation which I use, because my oscillograph and also my coil galvanometer do not reproduce oscillations above 200 hertz. Yet earlier I had the same experience with the *Edelmann* string galvanometer, even though this instrument recorded muscle currents of all frequencies. I am surprised by the statement that when these very rapid oscillations appear during mental work their amplitude should exceed even that of the alpha waves (α-w). These changes coincide with the disappearance of the α-w observed by myself, *Adrian* and *Matthews* and others. I never made this observation in recordings that were free of technical flaws. All this arouses my suspicion that muscle currents have none the less been recorded together with the rapid oscillations which appear to be of cerebral origin. For instance, even with the oscillograph which I used, one can easily record very rapid oscillations which by far exceed the α-w in amplitude, if the subject has the habit of clenching his teeth firmly during the "facial movements of thinking". This causes muscle currents to arise in the temporalis muscle and these are recorded together with the E.E.G. In any case, one must be extremely cautious when using the highly sensitive oscillograph in order to avoid inadvertent contamination by artefacts[T14]. In this context I wish to refer to *Jacobson's*[1] beautiful investigations. He demonstrated that during imagining, recollecting or in the course of concrete and abstract thinking, action potentials appear in *those* muscles which would come into play if the appropriate words were whispered or spoken aloud, even though this is not actually done. One is tempted to think of such sources of artefacts when observing the high amplitude and high frequency oscillations which are said to be of cerebral origin, this all the more so since in man a frequency of muscle action currents of up to 530 hertz has been found, and in the animal experiments in the dog, a frequency even reaching 1250 hertz[2] has been recorded. Still, the frequencies of even these most rapid oscillations of alleged cerebral origin remain very far below those of the electromagnetic oscillations of the human brain reported by *Cazzamali*[3], on which I do not dare to pass judgment because I never carried out any investigations relating to these.

Another interpretation of the β-w given by investigators who have repeated my studies implies that only the α-w of 9–12 hertz are of cerebral origin and that *all* oscillations which I included under the collective term of β-w represent *experimental artefacts*[T10], or have to be attributed to muscle or other currents. I am of the opinion that *this* view too is erroneous. One finds α-w *and* β-w also in the E.E.G.s recorded directly from the human cerebral cortex. Thus the β-w are certainly of *cerebral* origin. Whether they originate in the cortex *itself* is another question. Figure 30 in report III which shows a record taken with the coil galvanometer from the cortex and the hemispheral white matter exhibits β-w, but no α-w in the record obtained from the white matter. Therefore it is possible and even probable that β-w are also generated outside the cerebral cortex. In any case they are of cerebral origin and do not represent muscle currents. In the course of time I made two further observations

[1] *Jacobson, E.*: Abstract Zbl. Neur., **56**, 498; **58**, 178; **61**, 539 and 540.
[2] *Tabulae Biologicae*, Vol. 2, p. 365 and 366.
[3] *Cazzamali, Frd.*: Abstract Zbl. Neur., **77**, 311 (1935).

which prove that the β-w are of cerebral origin and also provide the opportunity to complement earlier reports. Figure 2 shows an E.E.G. recorded with silver needles directly from the cerebral cortex in a 37 year old man suffering from dementia paralytica in whom a cerebral puncture had been carried out. Such a recording excludes muscle currents with certainty. Yet, in addition to the large oscillations of

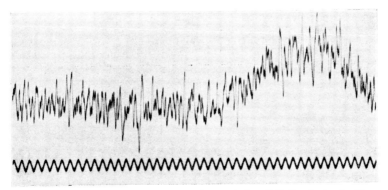

Fig. 2. W.H., 37 years old, suffering from dementia paralytica. E.E.G. obtained with needle electrode recording from the cortex of the left frontal and right parietal lobes. Time in 1/10ths sec.

the E.E.G., one clearly sees smaller oscillations which I included under the collective term of β-w. Their cerebral origin therefore appears to me proven just as it was by the earlier recording from the cortex and from the hemispheral white matter. As mentioned, this E.E.G. was obtained from a man suffering from dementia paralytica. The most prominent clinical features at the time of the recording were acute mental symptoms, consisting of marked euphoria with delusions of grandeur. Earlier in my third and fifth communications I had already reported on findings obtained in such patients. I emphasized in my third report that in patients suffering from *dementia paralytica* in whom the illness had become arrested after malaria treatment, pathological alterations are absent from the E.E.G., sometimes even when considerable mental deterioration has occurred. In cases of general paresis with mental disturbances of acute onset, a pathologically altered E.E.G. was found most of the time before malaria therapy had been carried out. Mainly an irregularity of the α-w was observed. In the curve reproduced in Figure 27 of my third report, the α-w vary in length from 105 to 200 σ. Later, in my fifth communication, I reported on the results of my studies on 29 patients suffering from dementia paralytica and there too I stressed that an *uneven* length of immediately successive α-w appeared to me to be characteristic for general paresis. At the same time I indicated that in dementia paralytica shortening of the α-w may also occur in addition to the increased length of these waves, which is found in all kinds of cortical damage. However, I did not dare to make any more precise statements to this effect, since according to *Dietsch's* frequency analyses[T55], the β-w have a much greater range of variability than I had hitherto assumed. If we take a closer look at Figure 2, we find in a segment selected at random, successive α-w of 50, 50, 50, 50, 50, 110 and 110 σ, in another segment α-w of 50, 50, 50, 110, 60,

110, 110, 110, 90, 90, 50 and 150 σ. Thus we find, just as in earlier instances, a striking lack of uniformity in the length of the successive α-w, but they are also unquestionably *shortened*. One could think that these short high amplitude waves represent β-w. Their amplitude and particularly the fact that smooth transitions in their length from 50 to 60, 90, 110 and 150 σ are found, in my opinion militates against this possibility.

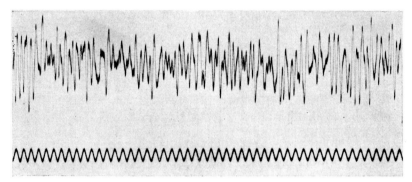

Fig. 3. C.S., 38 years old, suffering from dementia paralytica. E.E.G. obtained with needle electrode recording from the cortex of the left frontal and the right parietal lobes. Time in 1/10ths sec.

Thus indeed in the acute stage of dementia paralytica a shortening of the α-w also occurs. I made a second similar observation, which is shown in Figure 3. This also is an E.E.G. recorded during a cerebral puncture from the frontal lobe and the region of the parietal lobe of a 38 year old man suffering from dementia paralytica. It is again immediately evident that β-w are present exactly as in the needle electrode recording of Figure 2. Thus these β-w are certainly of cerebral origin. The only question that remains is whether they are of *cortical* origin. This E.E.G. too confirms the striking lack of uniformity of the α-w which is found in patients suffering from dementia paralytica at the time of the acute clinical manifestations of the disease. Several segments of this E.E.G. display consecutive α-w of 50, 70, 100, 80, 90 and 100 σ, or elsewhere α-w of 100, 50, 50, 100, 50, 60 σ. When scrutinizing a large section of these recordings, one finds α-w of 45, 50, 55, 60, 70, 80, 90, 100 and 125 σ; thus one finds again smooth transitions in the length of the α-w from 45 up to 125 σ! Therefore there is no doubt that we are dealing with a *shortening* of the α-w and not with β-w. Thus in the stage of dementia paralytica associated with acute clinical manifestations a *shortening of the α-w also occurs*, as I had already suspected earlier. I would like to interpret this as a *sign of irritation*. I am confirmed in this opinion by the observation that the shortening disappears if a clear-cut remission occurs in these patients after malaria treatment. Figure 4 shows an E.E.G. recorded in the same patient about three months later after termination of a course of malaria therapy and of the appropriate follow-up treatment. We see here a regular E.E.G. with an average length of the α-w of 90 σ. This record was taken from the forehead and occiput with silver foil electrodes in the manner which I had described earlier. It is evident that with this method one can also obtain an excellent recording. In the course of my investigations, after I had learned to recognize and to avoid all sources of artefact[T14], I returned more and more often to the technique which originally I had used exclusively and which consisted of recording with *silver foil* electrodes from the forehead and the occiput. It is the least disturbing method for the subject being examined. It can therefore be used without hesitation in every case and when

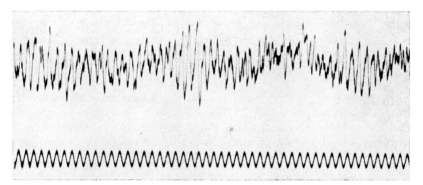

Fig. 4. C.S., 38 years old, suffering from dementia paralytica. Record taken three months after that shown in Figure 3. E.E.G. recorded from the forehead and occiput with silver foil electrodes. Time in 1/10ths sec.

the technique is adequate it yields even more beautiful E.E.G.s than needle electrode recordings.

I already stated before that I interpret the shortening of the α-w as a *sign of irritation* of the cortex. Also I very often found this distinct shortening of the α-w in other patients suffering from dementia paralytica, when I recorded from the bone with needle electrodes or from the skin with silver foil electrodes. This was particularly pronounced in cases of juvenile paresis, as *e.g.* in the 16 year old paretic N., in whom I found α-w of 65 σ. In another case I found α-w of 50 σ and I have also seen shortening of the α-w to 30 σ in a third case. Among other cortical diseases of the brain I found unequivocal shortening of the α-w only in association with extensive lesions of the small cortical vessels which had led to very small circumscribed softenings in the cortex, as demonstrated by the postmortem examination (Professor *Berblinger*). Thus *e.g.* in a 52 year old patient, A.B., who presented with clinical signs for one year, I found α-w of 50 σ in a needle electrode recording taken from the bone. On the basis of these findings too I would indeed like to interpret the shortening of the α-w to less than half their normal length as a *sign of irritation*. This interpretation is in agreement with the conclusions drawn from the variable findings in the different stages of general paresis. Earlier I had also observed a shortening of the α-w under certain *physiological* conditions, as *e.g.* in healthy subjects during emotional states and particularly during anxious agitation. This was documented in my sixth report by E.E.G.s (Figure 1) and recorded observations. Under these conditions, a shortening of the α-w to 55 σ was found. One is also tempted to interpret *this* shortening of the α-w which is physiological as an irritative sign. However, I doubt whether it would be justified to interpret as a sign of irritation the shortening of the α-w which appears during Avertine narcosis (Figure 1 in Report VIII) and which leads to α-w with an average duration of 72 σ. For the present I wish to re-emphasize that this shortening of the α-w during Avertine narcosis is an exceptional finding which at this time cannot be explained. For the interpretation of pathologically altered E.E.G.s my previously expressed view is still valid: namely that only *general disturbances of function*[T42] affecting the activity of the cerebral cortex are revealed in the E.E.G. when it is recorded in the usual way from the skull as a whole. A brain affected by a no longer active disease process which no longer causes general disturbances of function can thus exhibit an entirely normal E.E.G. If, however, general disturbances of function continue, lengthening of the α-w is found which I would like to interpret as a *sign of paralysis of function*[T122]. An evolving process can be associated both with *signs of irritation and paralysis of function* and, correspondingly, depending upon the preponderance of one or the other, shortening or lengthening of the α-w may ensue. This, it seems to me, is the lesson to be learned from the cerebral recordings in the two cases of dementia paralytica and from investigations reported earlier.

In my previous reports, I indicated that considerable lengthening of the α-w of the E.E.G. is found in increased intracranial pressure and particularly also in patients suffering from epileptic dementia or senile dementia. Of course, this lengthening of the α-w has to be interpreted as an indication of an impairment of the activity of the cerebral cortex, or of a paralysis of function, if one wishes to maintain the previously mentioned distinction between signs of paralysis of function and signs of irritation. For the interpretation of these signs of paralysis of function which appear in the E.E.G., I adopted the most probable explanation and considered them to be the visible expression of psychological deficits in general. Likewise in pathological cases, one can generally speaking relate the signs of irritation which appear in the E.E.G., *i.e.* the shortening of the α-w, to phenomena of mental excitation[T123]. As has already been mentioned, phenomena of irritation and paralysis of function can be found in one and the same E.E.G. This is an indication of how complex conditions often are. Thus under these circumstances, any attempt to establish definite correlations between E.E.G. alterations and specific signs of mental excitation or deficit through the analysis of psychopathological signs and symptoms appears to be a hopeless task. The difficulty lies mainly in the psychological sphere, as identical mental signs and symptoms may have very different origins. To make further progress in this matter, it will be necessary to rely on situations which are unequivocal and as simple as possible. Even a sign which appears to be quite elementary, such as disturbance of recent memory, can be simulated to such an extent by other psychopathological disturbances that only the most precise analysis of the individual case may reveal the true circumstances. For a long time therefore I had tried to investigate the electrical activity of the cortex in the famous case of a pure and isolated disturbance of recent memory which *Störring*[1] studied and described so well. Thanks to the kind help received from my colleague *Störring*, this has now become possible[2]. In this

[1] *Störring, G. E.*: Arch. f. Psychol., **81**, 259 (1931).

[2] On this occasion I would like to express my cordial thanks also to Dr. *R. Lemke* and Dr. *W. Lembcke* for their faithful assistance in the performance of my investigations.

33 year old man who had shown complete loss of recent memory for 9 years, I found a completely *normal* E.E.G. when I recorded with silver foil electrodes from the forehead and occiput, as is shown in Figure 5. Thus, as this observation demonstrates, we cannot say that severe disturbance of recent memory, *e.g.* in senile dementia, visibly manifests itself in an increased duration of the α-w of the E.E.G. In this

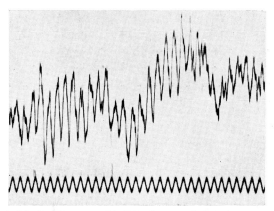

Fig. 5. *G. E. Störring's* Mr. B., 33 years old. E.E.G. recorded from forehead and occiput with silver foil electrodes. Time in 1/10ths sec.

case, as Figure 5 shows, the most severe disturbance of recent memory which can possibly occur is not associated with any alteration of *those* electrical processes which become manifest in the E.E.G. when it is recorded from the skull as a whole. In *Störring's* patient, whose intelligence is not impaired in any way, a general disturbance of function[T42] of the cerebral cortex is now no longer present. Such a disturbance had most likely existed earlier at the time of the acute stage of carbon monoxide poisoning. Perhaps at that time one would have been able to record an E.E.G. similar to the one I showed in Figure 6 of the eighth report and in Figure 13 of the fifth report. Now, however, the general disturbance of function[T124] which had existed at that time has long been compensated and we are confronted with a normal E.E.G. with α-w of 105 σ, like the one found in completely healthy people. This approach therefore does not bring us any closer to the elucidation of the cause of memory loss in this case. Nevertheless we made the important observation that this severe disturbance of cortical activity, namely the complete loss of what is sometimes called the function of laying down engrams[T125], does not find any visible expression in the E.E.G. Accordingly we must certainly be very cautious in our attempts to give precise psychological interpretations to the findings of the E.E.G.!

Does this finding in fact not argue against the working hypothesis which I have invoked repeatedly and which claims that in the α-w of the E.E.G. we are confronted with the material expression of those processes which we designate as psychophysical because, under certain circumstances, they are associated with phenomena of consciousness? I do not believe that the observation that there are no E.E.G. changes when the function of laying down engrams[T125] is lost militates against my working hypothesis, particularly since we do not know at all where and in which cortical layers this function is being performed. On the basis of the views expressed by *von Monakow*, *Berze*, *Kleist* and others, who attribute to the external cortical layers functions which are particularly closely related to mental processes, I had furthermore assumed that the α-w probably originate in this *external zone* of the cortex designated by *Berze* as the "*intentional sphere*". The assumption that the cerebral cortex can be divided into an external and internal zone gained strong additional support through *Bok's*[1] beautiful anatomical investigations. His studies demonstrated that according to cell size and cell density the external and internal principal zones each represent a unit which is independent of the customary division into layers.

Adrian's and *Matthews'* conclusion that the E.E.G. of man originates in the *occipital lobe* would, of course, argue against my concept of the significance of the α-w of the E.E.G. as well as against my assumption that they originate everywhere in the cerebral cortex. The evidence marshalled by these investigators that the E.E.G., or rather the α-w of the E.E.G., are lacking in people who have been blind for a long time proved to be incorrect, as I was able to demonstrate in my tenth report. Thus this argument of the English physiologists has been deprived of a pivotal element of support. In a more recent second report, *Adrian* and *Yamagiwa*[2] nevertheless return to the same view on the basis of measurements of the magnitudes of the deflections and attempt to determine a specific area within the human occipital lobe as the site of origin of the E.E.G. Unfortunately I am unable to repeat the investigations carried out by these two researchers because for this purpose multiple, simultaneous recordings are necessary, each performed with a highly sensitive oscillograph. Nevertheless I would like to stress that conclusive *proof* for their view would, of course, require multiple simultaneous recordings taken not from the scalp, but from the surface of the human cerebrum *itself*, which is obviously impossible. Therefore I can only repeat *those* arguments which I invoked against those of *Adrian* and *Matthews* in my tenth report. The following fact seems to me to argue against their assumption: when one records from the dura with silver needles in cases with bilateral frontal bone defects, one obtains E.E.G.s with beautiful α-w which are just as good as those recorded from any other area of the dura within a bone defect wherever it may be located. Such observations can *e.g.* be made after a *Cushing*-type decompressive trepanation or in cases of post-traumatic skull defects located over the frontal pole. Of course in such instances too, only multiple simultaneous recordings by means of several *calibrated* oscillographs could provide conclusive evidence. Surely, however, as I had already emphasized in my tenth report, the fact that the α-w of the E.E.G. can be obtained with *unipolar* recording from various cortical areas, *e.g.* from the frontal lobe, as *Foerster* and *Altenburger* were able to do, argues against *Adrian's* and *Yamagiwa's* assumption. This observation, I believe, cannot be invalidated by their recordings which were taken from the unopened skull or, more specifically, from the scalp. The following additional facts, however, which argue against an origin of the

---

[1] *Bok*: Z. mikrosk.-anat. Forsch., **36**, 645 (1934).

[2] *Adrian* and *Yamagiwa*: Brain, **58**, 323 (1935).

α-w in the occipital lobe appear to me even more important. When one records simultaneously with two separate galvanometers from the right and left sides of the skull, one obtains essentially the same curve twice. However, in both curves there are always segments which are *not* congruent. In my earlier reports, *e.g.* in my sixth communication in Figures 4 and 5, I published E.E.G.s of a physician which showed

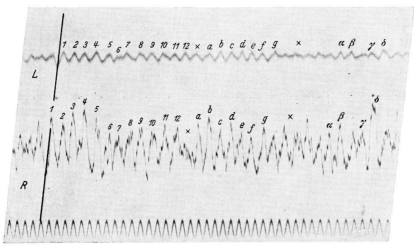

Fig. 6. 46 year old patient suffering from dementia paralytica. At the top: E.E.G. recorded with silver needle electrodes from the left frontal and the left occipital region to the coil galvanometer. In the middle: E.E.G. recorded in identical fashion from the right frontal and the right occipital region to the oscillograph. At the bottom: time in 1/10ths sec. The india ink line connects simultaneous points of the two E.E.G.s. Simultaneous α-w are labelled with identical numbers and letters.

circumscribed discrepancies at point ×. Figure 6 shows such discrepancies in a recording taken simultaneously from the left side of the skull with the coil galvanometer and from the right side with the oscillograph. The curve was recorded in a 46 year old patient suffering from dementia paralytica who presented fairly marked mental deterioration. The α-w show a duration of 135 σ. Because the records of the galvanometers are not in precise vertical alignment, the correspondence of the curves is indicated by a line drawn with india ink. Simultaneous α-w in both E.E.G.s are labelled with identical numbers and letters. At × one finds distinct discrepancies between the two E.E.G.s. If in fact the α-w have their site of origin in the occipital lobe, why then do discrepancies between the curves of the right and left side appear at the points labelled ×? The fact is that these α-w arise locally, and the E.E.G. recorded on the right and that recorded on the left side display potential oscillations which originate from the cortical areas situated between the two electrodes. This is the explanation for the occasional, but ever recurring, discrepancies, even though in general there is a good correspondence between the two curves. This view is also supported by the following fact, which I documented with a curve and which demonstrates the *local* origin of the α-w: within a circumscribed bone defect located over a cortical area which had sustained slight traumatic damage, the α-w measured 130 σ in length, while the record taken simultaneously from the skull as a whole exhibited α-w of 110 σ (Report III, Figure 28, p. 126). By far the most cogent argument in favor of my view, however, is the following: with bipolar recording one finds no α-w of the E.E.G. locally in an area overlying damaged cerebral tissue, *e.g.* in a

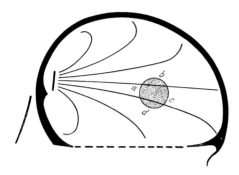

Fig. 7. Diagram borrowed from *Adrian's* and *Yamagiwa's* work, which was designed to illustrate the site of origin of the E.E.G. in the occipital lobe and its spread over the cerebral cortex. In an equally schematic fashion I entered into this diagram a tumor located in the cortex.

cortical area which has lost its function because of pressure exerted upon it, yet these α-w are present in the neighboring intact cerebral cortex (Report II, p. 89). *Foerster* and *Altenburger*[1] reported that with unipolar recording the large potential oscillations of the E.E.G. are completely absent within the area of a tumor. They are found to a lesser degree near the margins of the lesion, but are clearly present in healthy areas surrounding the tumor. An identical observation was reported by *Tönnies*[2]. If one starts from *Adrian's* and *Yamagiwa's* premises and makes use of a drawing presented by these authors, one arrives at the following conclusion, shown in Figure 7. The potential oscillations arising from the centers located in the occipital lobe spread out over the surface of the brain along the lines indicated in Figure 7 and can therefore be recorded everywhere. Now, if a tumor were located in the area indicated in this figure by a dark circle, one should actually expect to be able to record these potential oscillations in the area of the tumor as well. The investigations of *A. W. Meyer*[3] have in fact shown that cerebral tumors, in comparison with normal cerebral tissue, offer less electrical resistance or, what amounts to the same thing, exhibit *greater* electrical conductivity. Therefore there are actually no reasons why one should not be able to record the large potential oscillations in the area of the tumor if these originate in the occipital lobe. *In fact, however, they are missing!* If, contrary to *A. W. Meyer's* observations, one assumes that the tumor nevertheless prevents the spread of potential oscillations arising from the occipital lobe because it may offer a considerable resistance to them, one would have to expect that in a unipolar recording no large potential oscillations should be present *e.g.* at point *c* of Figure 7. But this too does *not* turn out to be the case. These potential oscillations

[1] *Foerster* and *Altenburger*: Verh. Ges. dtsch. Nervenärzte. Munich, **1934**. Report p. 93, Fig. 16–18 and p. 102.

[2] *Tönnies*: Verh. Ges. dtsch. Nervenärzte. Munich, **1934**, 104, Fig. 2.

[3] *Meyer, A. W.*: Dtsch. med. Wschr., **1928**, **II**, 1366.

are present at points *a*, *b*, *c* and *d* in the healthy tissue surrounding the tumor! These observations of a *circumscribed* disappearance of the potential oscillations in the area of pathologically altered cortex demonstrate with complete certainty the *local* origin of the α-w of the E.E.G. and unequivocally militate *against* the assumption of *Adrian* and *Yamagiwa* that the site of origin of these waves is to be found in the occipital lobe! Unequivocally the physiological investigations are complemented in this instance by the experience obtained through the study of pathological cases. The α-w originate everywhere in the cerebral cortex, but the regulation of their sequence is effected from a center located outside the cortex, probably in the thalamus! Though it is composed of action currents of nerve cells differing in so many respects, the E.E.G. represents a *characteristic* curve marvelously woven together into a uniform whole, just as the E.C.G., which reflects the muscle action currents of many elements also, appears as a simple curve with well defined characteristics.

I am, however, willing to listen to other arguments and, as I have emphasized repeatedly, I am prepared to drop my working hypothesis should *facts* be found which *cannot* be reconciled with it. After all, it is the fate of a *working* hypothesis to be replaced by a better one. Fundamentally all of us strive for the same goal: to learn to read the truth in the great book of nature of which man and his brain are but a part.

XII

On the Electroencephalogram of Man

Twelfth Report

by Hans Berger, Jena

(With 20 figures)

(Received December 2, 1936)

[Published in *Archiv für Psychiatrie und Nervenkrankheiten*, **1937**, *106*: 165–187]

Earlier I reported that two completely opposite alterations of the human electroencephalogram (E.E.G.) occur in association with states of unconsciousness. Thus in deep chloroform narcosis and during the unconsciousness which outlasts a major epileptic seizure, one finds that the alpha waves (α-w) of the E.E.G. are absent and that the record appears as a straight line. On the other hand in the unconsciousness of Pernocton and Evipan narcosis, as well as in the acute phase of illuminating gas poisoning and during the unconsciousness caused by oxygen deprivation, one observes a peculiar group formation of incompletely formed α-w of the E.E.G. which follow upon each other prematurely in accelerated sequences[T98], a pattern which I designated as gallop rhythm[T126]. In man these completely opposite conditions are associated with loss of consciousness. I also had the opportunity to study the E.E.G. manifestations accompanying insulin coma, as this method of treatment is used quite extensively in my clinic because of the favorable reports by *Manfred Sakel*[1] on the effect of insulin treatment in schizophrenia. This form of treatment, as is well known, renders the patients deeply comatose when increasing doses of insulin are given. In the course of this treatment epileptic seizures occasionally occur, and this is a sign that the coma must be interrupted immediately; otherwise one should let the patient remain in the comatose state up to about $1\frac{1}{2}$ hours. The E.E.G. of schizophrenics shows no deviation from that of healthy human subjects, provided the recording is not disturbed because the patient is distracted by hallucinations and other influences of this kind. Responses to emotional factors as they are found in healthy people do, of course, also appear in the E.E.G.s of schizophrenics. Figure 1 shows the E.E.G. of A.S., a 17 year old patient suffering from schizophrenia who had

---

[1] *Sakel, Manfred*: Neue Behandlungsmethode der Schizophrenie. Vienna, 1935. — *Duffik, R.* and *Sakel, M.*: Z. Neur., **155**, 351 (1936).

become ill 4 months earlier[1]. In this E.E.G. one sees α-w of an average length of 50 σ. The patient exhibited a certain degree of anxiety during the recording. We see in this shortening of the α-w an effect of the anxious excitation which can also be found in the normal human subject. I already illustrated this in 1933 in Figure 1 of

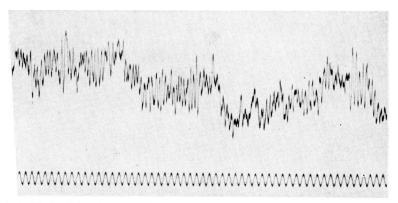

Fig. 1. A.S., blacksmith, 17 years old. Suffering from schizophrenia for four months. Recording with silver needles from forehead and occiput. Time in 1/10ths sec.

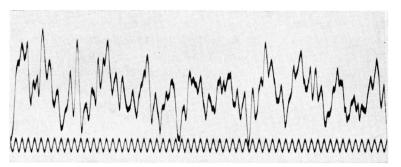

Fig. 2. A.S., blacksmith, 17 years old. Suffering from schizophrenia for four months. *During insulin coma.* Recording with silver needles from forehead and occiput. Time in 1/10ths sec.

my sixth report. During insulin coma with complete loss of consciousness, the same patient exhibited an E.E.G. as shown in Figure 2. Where they are fully developed, some of the α-w are lengthened up to 160 σ and furthermore they show a clear tendency to group formation. These groups have a length of 300 to 650 σ. Exactly as in Pernocton and Evipan narcosis, the α-w are incompletely formed. Additional recordings obtained from other schizophrenics during insulin coma demonstrated that this is indeed a characteristic alteration of the E.E.G. Figure 3 shows the E.E.G. of 16 year old patient E.P., who 4 weeks earlier had exhibited the first signs of psychosis. Although she is in deep insulin coma, the markedly dilated pupils still contract very slightly in response to light. Like Figures 1 and 2 this is a needle electrode recording

---

[1] On this occasion I would like to express here too my cordial thanks to Dr. *R. Lemke* and Dr. *W. Lembcke* for the faithful assistance they gave me in the performance of my investigations!

taken from the forehead and occiput. Again the tendency to group formation appears very clearly; apart from this, however, single, fully developed α-w with a length of 100 to 200 σ are still found. The deeper the coma, the more clearly evident this group formation becomes. Figure 4 represents the E.E.G. recorded with needle electrodes from the forehead and occiput of E.J., a 35 year old woman. This patient had been suffering from schizophrenia for many years and because of the explicit wish of her relatives, insulin treatment was to be attempted. She was in deep insulin coma and her pupils were markedly dilated. She displayed no reaction to pain when the skin

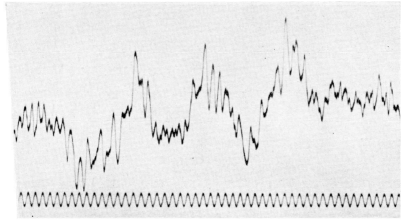

Fig. 3. Miss E.P., 16 years old, suffering from schizophrenia for four weeks. During insulin coma. Pupils still slightly reacting to light. Recording with silver needles from forehead and occiput. Time in 1/10ths sec.

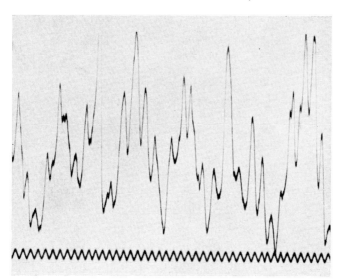

Fig. 4. Mrs. E.J., 35 years old. Has suffered from schizophrenia for many years. During insulin coma. Pupils dilated, hardly reacting to light. Recording with silver needles from forehead and occiput. Time in 1/10ths sec.

of the forehead and occiput was punctured while the needles were inserted even though no local anesthesia was being used. One sees here a pattern which is identical to that which I had previously reported for patients in Pernocton and Evipan narcosis or in deep coma caused by illuminating gas poisoning (see eighth report, Figures 2, 3 and 6!). The characteristic group formation appears with a group length of 0.45–1.3 seconds and with very high voltage α-w. Thus according to the findings in the E.E.G., the unconsciousness of insulin coma has to be included among *those* states in which group formation and gallop rhythm of the α-w are found[1].

In 1933 I already reported that fusion of the α-w of the E.E.G. into high voltage trains of waves occurs in the condition which can be described as a state of impending convulsion in epilepsy (seventh report, Figure 14)[T127]. Furthermore I reported that when localized clonic jerks occur, which may outlast a paralytic attack for days, the E.E.G. shows high voltage wave trains which always precede the individual motor discharges[T128] (*ibid.* Figures 10, 11, 12 and 13). But even without these after-effects which manifest themselves in the form of clonic jerks, one can very clearly recognize the sequelae of a paralytic attack in the E.E.G. Figure 5 was obtained from a 64

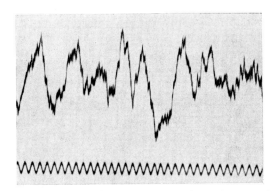

Fig. 5. H.M., civil servant, 64 years old. Suffering from dementia paralytica for years. Record taken in the afternoon following a nocturnal epileptiform attack. Recording with foil electrodes from forehead and occiput. Time in 1/10ths sec.

year old patient, H.M., suffering from dementia paralytica who, 18 hours earlier, had suffered an epileptiform paralytic attack. It represents a record taken with silver foil electrodes from the forehead and occiput of the patient, who was fully conscious and answered questions correctly. The recording was, of course, carried out in a darkened room while the patient had his eyes closed and remained completely still. Again one very distinctly sees the formation of large trains of waves with a length of 300, 350 and even 600 σ. I was able to make such observations repeatedly, and thus we are not dealing with a chance finding in this case. Figure 6 shows the E.E.G. of a 37 year old worker, W.N., also taken with silver foil electrodes. This man has been

---

[1] After completing my investigations I received the study of a Dutch colleague who, as far as I can gather from the German summary, came to the same conclusion. *Franke, L. J.*: Electrische Spanningsverschillen in de Hersenschors van den Mensch etc. Utrecht, 1936.

suffering from dementia paralytica for more than one year. Three days earlier, N. had experienced a severe epileptiform paralytic attack which left in its wake a motor aphasia and a paralysis of the right arm. Again one sees large trains of waves of 150–400 σ, and in between isolated, apparently normal α-w of 90–110 σ, which however markedly vary in amplitude (labelled with *). The irregular aspect of the

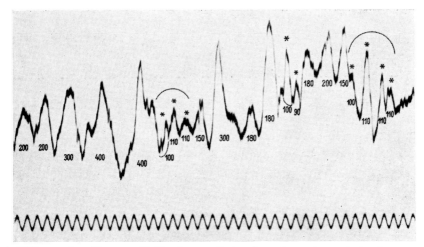

Fig. 6. W.N., worker, 37 years old. Has been suffering from dementia paralytica for more than one year. Three days after a severe epileptiform paralytic attack, leaving as sequelae a motor aphasia and a paralysis of the right arm. Recording with foil electrodes from forehead and occiput. Time in 1/10ths sec.

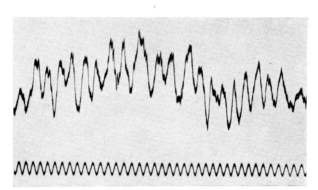

Fig. 7. W.N., worker, 37 years old. Recorded seven days after Figure 6. Ten days after the paralytic attack. Recording with foil electrodes from forehead and occiput. Time in 1/10ths sec.

curve, the unequal length *and* amplitude of the waves become particularly evident here. Ten days after this paralytic attack, when N. was again able to speak and the paralysis of the arm had receded, he showed the E.E.G. reproduced in Figure 7. One finds nearly uniform α-w, which however are prolonged beyond the length found in healthy subjects and on the average measure up to 185 σ.

In my eleventh report I indicated that the β-w also originate in the cerebral cortex itself and that they can be found when one records directly from the human cerebral cortex with needle electrodes. Over the years I have carried out many investigations on the possible pathological alterations of the β-w in a great variety of morbid conditions. In spite of this I have not yet arrived at any clear concept concerning the kind of changes they undergo and the conditions under which these changes occur. This is because the E.E.G. is so sensitive that even in normals it exhibits very great variations and changes in response to a shift of attention, emotional excitement, pain and even unexpected movements. In any given case it may be extremely difficult to determine *what* features have to be attributed to these physiological or psychophysiological states and *which* are those related to the pathological process itself. I had therefore already given up hope of ever making any further progress in this matter and, as I explained previously, I limited myself almost exclusively to a more detailed investigation of the α-w. Nevertheless recent observations have allowed me to make some definite progress and also gave me the opportunity to interpret retrospectively E.E.G.s which had been recorded earlier. In a 66 year old patient, K.S., I found the extremely peculiar E.E.G. reproduced in Figure 8.

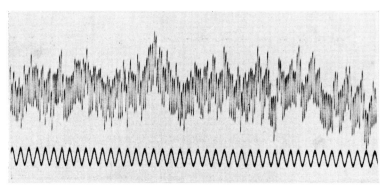

Fig. 8. Mrs. K.S., 66 years old. Three days after onset of motor and sensory aphasia without any other sign of acute brain damage[T129]. Recording from forehead and occiput with silver foil electrodes. Time in 1/10ths sec.

The record was taken with silver foil electrodes from the forehead and occiput and all sources of artefact[T14] had been excluded with certainty. Three days earlier the patient had developed a motor and sensory aphasia without any other signs of acute brain damage[T129]. There were no other signs of paralysis. At the time of recording she was fully conscious and lay completely still in the darkened room with her eyes closed. The E.E.G. consists of strikingly regular waves measuring only 20 σ; at first it was difficult to decide whether these were extremely shortened α-w or, more probably, very high amplitude β-w. However, one can also demonstrate in this E.E.G. some suggestive evidence of α-w with a length of 100–110 σ! On the other hand, in subsequent days the record exhibited very definite regression of the abnormality which led to an approximately normal E.E.G. It was thus possible to determine clearly that these 20 σ waves did in fact represent pathologically altered β-w. Figure 9 reproduces an E.E.G. of the same patient recorded 5 days later than that shown in Figure 8. The patient's condition improved rapidly and markedly during treatment with regular injections of acetylcholine. She understood everything again and regained her ability to speak. The α-w became again more distinct, the β-w were of equal length

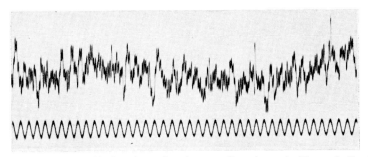

Fig. 9. Mrs. K.S., 66 years old: five days after the recording shown in Figure 8. Condition significantly improved, understands again everything and is able to speak. Recording from forehead and occiput with silver foil electrodes. Time in 1/10ths sec.

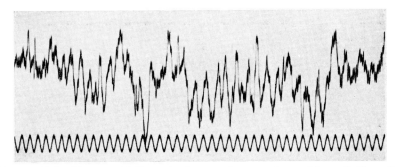

Fig. 10. Mrs. K.S., 66 years old. Record taken on the same day as Figure 9. Recording from forehead and occiput with silver foil electrodes. Time in 1/10ths sec.

to those shown in Figure 8 and were still very pronounced. Figure 10 shows a further amplitude decrease of the β-w and at the same time exhibits beautiful α-w with a length of 110 σ. I believe that this was a case of circumscribed cerebral thrombosis which regressed rapidly under the influence of the vasodilator action of acetylcholine. Restoration of the normal E.E.G. occurred in parallel with the clinical improvement. In this case I cannot doubt that I have encountered a pathological alteration of the β-w. At this point I wish to point out that several French authors[1] drew attention to the fact that in cortical lesions of vascular origin the first, the second and sometimes several of the most superficial layers of the cerebral cortex are almost always spared. Earlier I had seen patterns which I would now like to interpret as resulting from a

---

[1] *Alajouanine, Thurel* and *Hornet*: Abstract Zbl. Neur., **81**, 274 (1936).

pathological alteration of the β-w. I have observed such changes in senile, demented patients with presbyophrenia, in many patients with dementia paralytica, especially in juvenile paretics, furthermore in a man with a very extensive cerebral abscess in the centrum semiovale of the left cerebral hemisphere and also in cases presenting sequelae of severe illuminating gas poisoning. In a 55 year old patient Mrs. M.M., 5 days after an extremely severe illuminating gas intoxication, I obtained with needle electrode recording the E.E.G. shown in Figure 11. Mrs. M. remained unconscious

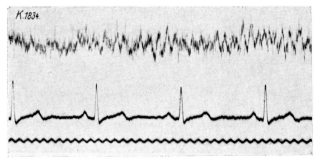

Fig. 11. Mrs. M.M., 55 years old: five days after very severe illuminating gas poisoning. Needle recording of the E.E.G. from forehead and occiput. E.C.G. recorded from both arms with lead foil electrodes. Time in 1/10ths sec.

for 18 hours after the intoxication and had a severe convulsive seizure with tongue biting. After return of consciousness she had still to be catheterized regularly because she was unable to void. Mentally she exhibited most severe disturbances of old and recent memory, so that she was unable to state her age and place of birth, did not know whether she was married and so forth. While the α-w remained preserved, the β-w had considerably increased in amplitude.

Earlier I had already carried out many investigations on the E.E.G. in manic-depressive patients and I reported on these briefly in 1931. For instance, in patients suffering from *melancholia* I was unable to find alterations of the E.E.G. even when they presented with the most severe inhibitory phenomena[T41]. In some instances I found an E.E.G. which was identical to that of a normal subject during rest, as is shown in Figure 12. This E.E.G. is a needle electrode recording taken from the forehead and occiput of a 27 year old patient R.V., who had been admitted to hospital 10 days earlier for treatment of severe melancholia associated with marked mental inhibition[T130]. We see beautiful α-w with an average length of 110 σ, *i.e.* a completely normal picture. Not infrequently one finds in patients with melancholia an E.E.G. as shown in Figure 13. This E.E.G. was obtained from 37 year old patient A.A., who had been admitted to hospital for treatment only 3 days earlier. Mrs. A. is suffering from melancholia associated with anxious agitation. During the recording, however, the patient lay perfectly still with her eyes closed in the darkened room. The E.E.G. shows shortened α-w with a length of 70 σ. We also found such E.E.G.s in healthy subjects who were in a state of emotional excitement. Therefore this

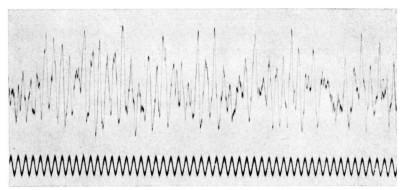

Fig. 12. Mrs. R.V., 27 years old. Admitted to hospital ten days earlier for treatment of *severe melancholia*. Needle electrode recording from forehead and occiput. Time in 1/10ths sec.

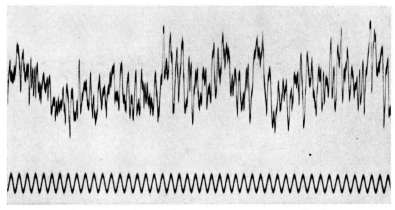

Fig. 13. Mrs. A.A., 37 years old. Admitted to hospital three days earlier for treatment of *severe melancholia*. Foil electrode recording from forehead and occiput. Time in 1/10ths sec.

recording likewise gives results which in no way deviate from normality. It only shows the phenomena associated with emotional excitement which become manifest in the E.E.G. of the melancholic patient exactly as they do in the E.E.G. of the healthy person. I had obtained the same negative results earlier in studies of E.E.G.s recorded in patients suffering from *mania*. I reported on these observations also in 1931. It is, of course, obvious that only certain states of this illness are suitable for the recording of an E.E.G., and all patients who show motor agitation have to be excluded.When one observes these precautions one usually finds an E.E.G. as shown in Figure 14. This illustration is the record of an 18 year old girl J.T., who had been admitted to the clinic for treatment four weeks earlier because of severe mania and who was still in a hypomanic state at the time of the E.E.G. recording. One sees an E.E.G. which could very well have been obtained from a normal person whose attention was distracted by some external events. The reason for this is simply that because of the patient's hypervigilance, a true *resting* curve cannot be obtained. This E.E.G. therefore gives no information about possible changes of cerebral cortical activity in mania. Surprisingly enough I found in a patient who was in the manic stage of cyclic insanity an E.E.G. of a kind which I had never seen before in such patients. Figure 15 shows this E.E.G. recorded from the forehead and occiput with silver foil electrodes. It was obtained from a 43 year old teacher, A.P., who had repeatedly been treated in the clinic because of manic-depressive attacks. She had been readmitted to my clinic for two months because of very severe manic agitation. The E.E.G. was

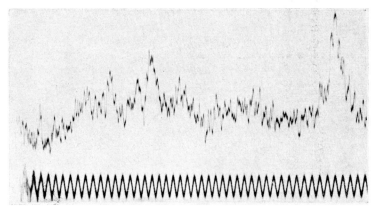

Fig. 14. Miss J.T., 18 years old. Admitted to hospital four weeks earlier for treatment of severe mania; still hypomanic. Needle electrode recording from forehead and occiput. Time in 1/10ths sec.

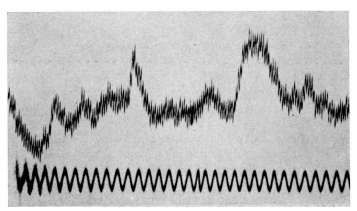

Fig. 15. Miss A.P., 43 years old. Had suffered repeated manic-depressive attacks. Admitted two months earlier because of severe mania; still very agitated. Foil electrode recording from forehead and occiput. Time in 1/10ths sec.

recorded when, judging from external appearances, she had quieted down somewhat, but there was still vivid flight of ideas. During the recording, contrary to all expectations, the patient lay completely still in the darkened room with her eyes closed. The recording, which is 10 meters long, exhibits throughout its entire length the same pattern, which is shown in Figure 15. Because this finding appeared to me so startling and also so important, I again took a record from the same patient two days later.

Once more a curve 10 meters in length was recorded. Exactly the same peculiar E.E.G. was found, consisting exclusively of β-w with a length of 17–22 σ. It goes without saying that this patient had received no drugs within the 24 hours preceding the recording of the E.E.G., as had been the case for all patients from whom an E.E.G. was recorded. This finding prompted me to search for similar E.E.G.s in the manic state of cyclic insanity. I found a similar E.E.G. in 37 year old worker O.R. Three weeks before, R. had been admitted to the hospital for treatment of severe manic agitation. After he had quieted down somewhat while still clearly exhibiting flight of ideas, I obtained an E.E.G. as shown in Figure 16. Here too one observes a

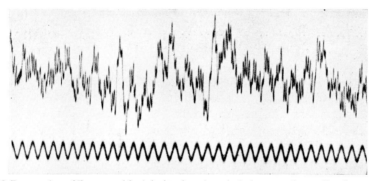

Fig. 16. O.R., worker, 37 years old. Admitted to hospital three weeks earlier for treatment of severe mania; somewhat quieter, but still markedly agitated. Foil electrode recording from forehead and occiput. Time in 1/10ths sec.

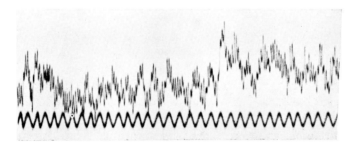

Fig. 17. O.R., worker, 37 years old. Record taken on the same day as Figure 16. Foil electrode recording from forehead and occiput. Time in 1/10ths sec.

marked prominence of strikingly high voltage β-w with an average length of 20 σ, even though in addition α-w of 110–125 σ are also found. Figure 17, which shows the E.E.G. of the same patient, exhibits even more clearly this striking amplitude increase of the 20 σ β-w. Two days later, when the patient had quite unexpectedly become much calmer and had slept for the first time without requiring any drugs, these large amplitude β-w had disappeared! An E.E.G. was found which was identical to that of a healthy person whose attention was aroused. Therefore, these anomalous E.E.G.s do not represent chance findings, but bear some causal relationship to the manic excitation. Here in mania we are dealing with pathologically altered β-w of very definite length, in much the same way as above we observed pathologically altered β-w in cortical thrombosis.

We now have to discuss in somewhat more detail the *sites of origin* of the α-w and β-w of the human E.E.G. At this time I wish to stress again, as I have done repeatedly since 1932, that the term β-w is a collective one which encompasses waves of completely different frequency[T121] and amplitude. Their time course, however, is always faster than that of α-w and under normal conditions they are also always of smaller amplitude. By taking records from the cortex and the hemispheral white matter, I already demonstrated in 1931 that the α-w of the E.E.G. of man originate in the cerebral cortex itself and that from the hemispheral white matter one obtains only small oscillations of a kind which can be found in any living tissue. More recent recordings taken from the cerebral cortex, which I showed in my eleventh report, exhibit α-w and β-w; thus the site of origin in *both* types of waves is in the cortex. Earlier and again in my ninth report published in 1934, I submitted that perhaps the β-w represent concomitant phenomena of the nutritional processes which take place in every living tissue and thus also occur in the cerebral cortex. However, I also referred there to the view held by other investigators who expressed the opinion that the oscillations of different frequencies[T121] owe their origin to different nerve cells, or perhaps to different cortical layers. I emphasized at the time that this problem should be pursued further by means of the research technique of thermocoagulation which had been applied so successfully by *Dusser de Barenne*. Since then *Dusser de Barenne* in collaboration with *McCulloch*[1] has performed excellent investigations on the cortex of the macaque. When recording with the bipolar technique after thermocoagulation of the full thickness of the cortex, these investigators no longer found any electrical oscillations in the region of the altered area. Therefore unequivocal proof has been provided that in the macaque too, the potential oscillations originate in the cerebral cortex itself. The two investigators have, however, reported results of still greater importance which clearly demonstrate the distant effect exerted by a local cortical destruction upon the electrical oscillations of other spatially separate and intact cortical areas. This observation of course is of utmost importance for the whole problem of localization. I am, however, particularly interested in the effects resulting from thermocoagulation of different layers within the thickness of the cortex. *Dusser de Barenne* and *McCulloch* found that when they thermocoagulated the three external layers of the cortex of the macaque in the region of the motor area, the electrical potential oscillations were preserved after the operation, but had a different appearance from the potential oscillations of the intact cortex. Figure 18 shows two illustrations taken from the work of *Dusser de Barenne* and *McCulloch*. At the top are represented the electrical potential oscillations of the intact region of the motor area of the macaque as they appear in a bipolar recording. One sees very large amplitude oscillations with an average length of 90 σ which correspond to the large oscillations of the human E.E.G. which I designated as α-w. The lower picture shows also

---

[1] *Dusser de Barenne, J. G.* and *Warren S. McCulloch*: Amer. J. Physiol., **114**, No. 3 (February 1936).

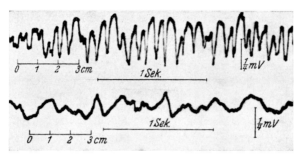

Fig. 18. At the top: bipolar recording of the potential oscillations of the motor cortex of the macaque. At the bottom: the same type of recording taken from the same area after thermo-coagulation of the three external cortical layers. From *Dusser de Barenne* and *Warren S. McCulloch*.

a bipolar recording taken from the same region of the motor area of the cortex of the macaque; however, the three external layers have been destroyed by a thermo-coagulation of precisely specified duration. It is obvious that potential oscillations still occur. These are α-w which have become slower and flatter; they now show a length of 140 σ and are similar to those appearing in the dog during gradual failure of circulation (see fifth report, Figure 10, 11 and 12; 1932!). From this brilliant experiment of *Dusser de Barenne* and *McCulloch* it follows unequivocally, I believe, that the large potential oscillations do *not* originate in the three external layers of the cortex, but that they arise from the internal cortical layers. I am convinced that this finding is of utmost importance. One can probably apply the results of these animal experiments to man, without hesitation. This therefore implies that in man also the α-w do not originate in the external principal zone of the cortex, but in the fourth to the sixth cortical layers. Consequently the further conclusion appears justified that the β-w, which have a completely different length, originate in the different cortical layers[T131] and more specifically that the *shorter* ones among them arise principally in the upper cortical layers. These shorter waves are characterized not only by their faster time course, but also by their lesser amplitude. Therefore it is also very probable that they owe their existence to the smaller nerve cells which are found in the upper cortical layers. These assumptions, which I have made in the light of *Dusser de Barenne's* and *McCulloch's* beautiful animal experiments, do not correspond at all to the view I formerly held on the basis of my own experience! Indeed as early as 1930 I had advanced the working hypothesis that the α-w of the E.E.G. represent the material concomitants of those cortical processes which one calls psychophysical because under certain circumstances they are connected with phenomena of consciousness. However, as mentioned before, I assigned to the β-w a completely subordinate role. Several observations had prompted me to put forward this working hypothesis: There was first the waxing and waning of the α-w in which the length of the periods corresponds to the psychological phenomena known as fluctuations of attention. Furthermore, there was the observation that the α-w are absent in states of unconsciousness, in chloroform narcosis or after a severe epileptic seizure. From the beginning, on the other hand, this view seemed to conflict with the observed

E.E.G. changes which occurred in response to a sensory stimulus towards which attention was directed. However, in view of the impossibility of recording with my technique directly from the human sensory centers, I explained the findings, which differed from those obtained in the animal experiment, by assuming that I was merely observing the *distant effect* of the local increase of the potential oscillations and that this distant effect represents a form of inhibition. The human observation of *Foerster* and *Altenburger*[1] demonstrated that indeed in man also the potential oscillations in the corresponding sensory center recorded with the *unipolar* technique increases in response to a sensory stimulus. My findings were therefore in good agreement with my working hypothesis. The disappearance of the α-w during mental work could also easily be accounted for on the basis of a predominance of the more generalized inhibitory effects over the circumscribed local amplitude increase of the α-w in the momentary center of activity, as I explained in detail earlier. I therefore time and again decided to hold on to this working hypothesis. I also elaborated it still further insofar as, in the light of *Berze's* views, I came to the conclusion that in the E.E.G. I was confronted with the continuous automatic activity of the three external cortical layers or of *Berze's* so-called intentional sphere.

A whole series of reasons, to which I alluded earlier, indicate that the so-called external principal zone of the cortex, which consists of the three external layers, is particularly closely related to mental processes. An additional reason which one could cite is the observation made by *Bielschowsky* and *Rose*[2] that the external cortical layers have a greater oxygen requirement as compared to the internal ones. The third cortical layer especially stands out by its high oxygen consumption. The investigation on the development of neurofibrils carried out by *Aaki*[3] also show that the second and the upper part of the third cortical layer are characterized by late differentiation which is a sign of a highly developed function. In the E.E.G. of man we are confronted not only with the activity of the three external cortical layers, but with that of the *entire thickness of the cortex* and thus with the continuous automatic activity of the external *and* of the internal principal zones, *Berze's* intentional and impressional spheres. My earlier assumption that we are merely dealing with the activity of the three upper cortical layers, *i.e.* with that of the intentional zone, has to be abandoned!

How is this different concept to be reconciled with my findings on the E.E.G. of healthy subjects reported earlier? When attention is directed towards a sensory stimulus, a local increase of the potential oscillations occurs which involves, of course, especially those originating in the impressional sphere, *i.e.* the internal principal zone; these are the α-w. This local increase exerts an inhibitory effect upon the activity of the remaining parts of the impressional sphere. This accounts for the well known decrease in potential, the disappearance of the α-w and the exclusive appearance of the various β-w in the E.E.G. recorded from the skull as a whole or

---

[1] *Foerster* and *Altenburger*: Dtsch. Z. Nervenheilk., **135**, 277 (1935).

[2] *Bielschowsky, Max* and *Maximilian Rose*: J. Psychol. u. Neur., **33**, 73 (1927). — *Rose, Maximilian*: J. Psychol. u. Neur., **47**, 1 (1936), especially p. 22.

[3] *Aaki*: Abstract Zbl. Neur., **74**, 5 (1934).

from circumscribed areas outside the sensory centers. Most often the β-w which appear under these circumstances are of short duration. They originate in the upper cortical layers and indicate that these layers, which constitute *Berze's* intentional sphere, are in a state of readiness for activity. The sensory stimulus towards which attention has been directed is, or at least *can* be, followed by further mental processing; thus the readiness for such processing is provided. *Ectors*'[1] beautiful experiments, however, have shown that in the rabbit too, one finds *no* increase in the voltage of the potential oscillations in response to the most varied sensory stimuli, even in the areas of the corresponding sensory centers. On the contrary, there is a voltage decrease associated with disappearance of the large α-w which are replaced by smaller, brief β-w, as I described it for man as early as 1930. These experiments on the rabbit were carried out with *bipolar* recordings taken directly from the cerebral cortex with electrodes that were 4–5 mm apart. These findings conflict to some extent with the results obtained in animals by *Fischer* and *Kornmüller*, who used *unipolar* recording[2]. They also conflict with the findings of *Foerster and Altenburger* to which I referred above and which were obtained in man, also with unipolar recording. Perhaps this could be explained by the different recording methods which were used. *Ectors*, however, also found that when the physiological stimulus is increased, the decrease in voltage appears not only in the cortical center related to the sensory modality involved, but sometimes occurs everywhere in the cerebral cortex, a finding which likewise coincides completely with my observations in man reported earlier. Finally, this investigator was able to find everywhere in the cerebral cortex of the rabbit the same pattern of potential oscillations, corresponding to my α-w of man[27]. He made these observations in bipolar recordings taken from cortical areas which were completely different in their architectonic structure, a finding which also agrees with my results on the human E.E.G. obtained in recordings taken from the cortex or from the dura of bone defects located in completely different regions of the skull. Moreover, *Travis* and *Dorsey*[3] already reported in 1932 that the same action currents were always found when they recorded from the cortex of the rat, even in areas which differed completely in their structures. Even though the occurrence of a local increase of potential oscillations in the respective sensory center thus again appears doubtful, I nevertheless believe that the voltage decrease which takes place under the influence of a sensory stimulus to which attention is directed, is the effect of an inhibition and results from the loss of α-w and not from their transformation into β-w.

Also during mental work a pattern has been repeatedly found in the E.E.G. which is identical with the one I had published earlier on several occasions. It is again clearly shown in Figure 19. During strenuous mental work the high amplitude α-w disappear almost completely; in their place β-w appear. I recorded numerous such E.E.G.s and was always able to make the same observation, which has been confirmed by all subsequent investigators. Even with *unipolar* recording from the cerebral cortex

[1] *Ectors, Leon*: Arch. internat. Physiol., **43**, 267 (Oct. 1936).

[2] *Kornmüller, A. E.*: J. f. Neur., **44**, 447 (1932). — *Fischer, M. H.*: Pflügers Arch., **230**, 161 (1932).

[3] *Travis, Lee Edward* and *John M. Dorsey*: Arch. of Neur., **28**, 331–338. Abstract Zbl. Neur., **65**, 635 (1932).

of man, *Foerster* and *Altenburger* found no increase of the potential oscillations while an arithmetic problem was being solved. This is in contrast to their above mentioned finding obtained during the influence of sensory stimuli. As I reported earlier, mental work which requires a fair amount of time, *e.g.* the solving of a difficult problem of applied mental arithmetic, is carried out in stages separated by pauses. The periods

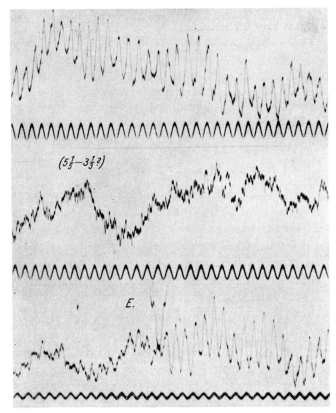

Fig. 19. I.B.[T49], 16 years old. At the top: E.E.G. in the resting state before calculating. Time in 1/10ths sec. In the middle: E.E.G. while solving the problem, $5\frac{1}{5} \times 3\frac{1}{3}$. At the bottom: at E the problem is solved! Needle recording from forehead and occiput.

of work which last 0.5 to 2 seconds alternate with pauses of equal length, as is demonstrated very clearly in a curve shown earlier in my sixth report, which is again presented here as Figure 20. In many E.E.G.s recorded during the performance of mental tasks of varying degrees of difficulty, I have attempted to determine more precisely *which* of the potential oscillations subsumed under the collective term of β-w particularly increase in amount or amplitude. During mental work I found in my daughter Ilse predominantly β-w of 12–20 σ; in my son Klaus these measured 11–18 σ, in my assistant Dr. S. 18–22 σ, in Dr. W. 12–24 σ, in Dr. W.R. 10–20 σ, in Dr. G. 20 σ and so forth. I also compared the amplitude of the β-w which occur during mental work with those exhibited by these individuals in the resting state. It became apparent that

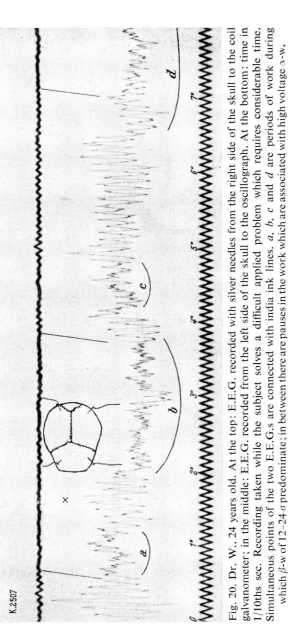

Fig. 20. Dr. W., 24 years old. At the top: E.E.G. recorded with silver needles from the right side of the skull to the coil galvanometer; in the middle: E.E.G. recorded from the left side of the skull to the oscillograph. At the bottom: time in 1/10ths sec. Recording taken while the subject solves a difficult applied problem which requires considerable time. Simultaneous points of the two E.E.G.s are connected with india ink lines. a, b, c and d are periods of work during which β-w of 12–24 σ predominate; in between there are pauses in the work which are associated with high voltage α-w.

during mental work, the β-w of 11–24 σ showed not only a four- to eightfold increase in amount—sometimes 5 brief β-w immediately succeeded each other—but they also increased in amplitude. Therefore, contrary to my earlier assumption, the changes during mental work consist not only of a loss of α-w, which leads to a clearer emergence of the β-w because the latter are difficult to recognize in the presence of high voltage α-w, but in addition, β-w of *definite length* also increase in amount and amplitude during mental work. It is not possible that this merely represents an inhibition of the processes underlying the α-w; a simultaneous increase of *those* processes which are related to the β-w of 11–24 σ occurs. Thus in conjunction with the above cited reasons for the genesis of the β-w in the upper cortical layers, it appears very probable that these brief β-w represent phenomena that are concomitant with mental work itself and are not, as I had previously assumed, the sign of an inhibitory effect exerted from a distance by the centers which are active at any time and changing in location. The activity of the impressional sphere, *i.e.* of the internal principal zone of the cortex which is the site of origin of the α-w, is therefore suspended when mental work is performed, a view which is in accord with our psychophysiological experience concerning the contrast that to a certain degree exists between sensory attention and mental work. Unlike the E.E.G. recorded under the influence of a sensory stimulus to which attention is directed, a record taken during mental work, as *e.g.* the one shown in Figure 20, demonstrates not only a readiness to perform work, but indeed the *actual work* of the intentional sphere. This concept had already been suggested to me in 1932 by several people on the occasion of a lecture given at the Jena Medical Society. *Ohm*[1] in 1933 in a paper in which he takes up the discussion of my E.E.G.[T27] expressed the opinion that the α-w are *transformed* into shorter waves, namely into β-w, under the influence of a perceived sensory stimulus and during mental work. Later the same opinion was expressed by other investigators, such as *Rohracher*, *Brémer* and others[2]. Till now, however, I have always been reluctant to accept this view which at first glance appears most probable. I only refused to accept it because I thought that it could not be reconciled with the animal experiments and with the more recent observations in man which demonstrate that an amplitude increase of the potential oscillations occurs in the corresponding sensory center in response to a sensory stimulus. I believed that in man during mental work, the same changes should occur at the sites which at any given time were actively engaged in this work. Contrary to my expectations, I never found an amplitude increase, but always a decrease in potential, even when I recorded from the dura of skull defects in completely different locations. I explained these findings by assuming that in spite of the very different locations of recording sites, I had up to then never recorded from an active center or from its vicinity, but that I was only observing the distant inhibitory effect emanating from the focus of activity. In contrast to *Ohm* and other authors, however, I still maintain that under the influence of a sensory stimulus or during mental work, no

---

[1] *Ohm, J.*: Gräfes Arch., **129**, 526 (1933), especially p. 546. — Z. Hals- usw. Heilk., **37**, 122 (1934), especially p. 123 and 136.
[2] *Rohracher, H.*: Z. Psychol., **136**, 308. — *Brémer, F.*: C. r. Soc. Biol. Paris, **120**, 1339 (1935); **122**, 464 (1936). Meeting of April 25, 1936.

transformation of α-w into β-w takes place, but that there is inhibition of the α-w together with an increase and greater prominence of β-w. Therefore I now consider the α-w to be the concomitants of the activity of the internal principal zone of the cortex, and I regard certain β-w, those of 11–24 σ duration (42–90 c/sec) as the concomitants of the activity of its external principal zone which is particularly closely related to mental processes.

How are my additional *earlier* observations on the *alterations* of the α-w to be reconciled with my *present* view? The α-w are undoubtedly a principal component of the E.E.G. and therefore of cortical activity in general, which also continues during sleep. My current concept surely is also in agreement with the observation that the fluctuations of attention coincide in time with the waxing and waning of the α-w and that the peak of the waxing phase of the α-w at any given time coincides with the state of inattention, if I may call it that. It is furthermore not surprising that the newborn does not yet exhibit any α-w[T132]. This is so because the entire cortex, the internal and the external principal zones, are still undeveloped and therefore the α-w are missing. The pathological findings obtained earlier also fit into my present concept without any difficulty. I have stressed repeatedly that only general disturbances of function[T42] are revealed in the E.E.G. They manifest themselves through an alteration of the length of the α-w, which become slow, shortened or irregular. General disturbances of function, of course, involve the entire thickness of the cortex and therefore also the area of origin of the α-w, the internal principal zone of the cortex. The absence of α-w *e.g.* in chloroform narcosis is caused by the fact that the action of chloroform extends throughout the entire thickness of the cortex and does not remain limited to the external zone only. The same applies for the severe disturbances of function which appear after an epileptic seizure and which consist of unconsciousness and loss of the α-w of the E.E.G. The same is true for the large trains of waves which appear when a seizure is imminent or for the large potential oscillations which precede clonic jerks. These result from a fusion and from a considerable amplitude increase of α-w; they probably reflect above all the strongly intensified and disinhibited activity of the internal zone of the cortex. The same applies for the disinhibition occurring during Evipan and Pernocton narcosis, during the action of insulin, etc. Increased intracranial pressure, cerebral hemorrhage, a tumor, a skull fracture cause considerable slowing of the α-w; the effect of pressure damages the cortex in its entire thickness. In epileptic dementia too, the entire cortex, and not only the external principal zone, has been impaired in its activity, hence the very striking slowing of the α-w. The irregularity and other changes of the α-w in patients with dementia paralytica can easily be reconciled with my view, because in this disease both deep *and* superficial cortical layers are damaged. The amplitude increase of the α-w under the influence of cocaine or during the excitatory stage of chloroform narcosis is also fully compatible with an origin of the α-w in the deeper cortical layers. The action of these poisons is likewise not confined to a particular cortical layer. These observations suggested that it might be of interest to investigate whether there are drugs or stimulants[T133] which exert an excitatory action confined exclusively to mental activity. One would expect that the effect of such a substance would lead exclusively to an increase in the amplitude of the β-w of 11–24 σ. I believed caffeine or coffee to be such a stimulant and repeatedly I performed experiments to this effect which seemed at first to confirm my assumption. Later, however, I began to have considerable misgivings about making use of the E.E.G.s obtained in this way. Under the influence of two cups of very strong coffee, one indeed obtains in healthy subjects E.E.G.s which correspond to a state of vivid mental activity, provided one waits about 30 minutes to let the caffeine action develop to its fullest extent before starting the recording. However, without exception, the subject denies having achieved a state of complete *relaxation* when asked about this after the recording taken while he was lying in the darkened room with his eyes closed. The caffeine action caused the experimental subject to be continuously pre-occupied with his thoughts even though he appeared outwardly calm. The altered E.E.G. is therefore simply the concomitant phenomenon of a more vivid ideational activity which had been stimulated by the caffeine intake and does not allow one to identify a possible action of the caffeine upon certain β-w. Under the influence of caffeine one is no longer able to achieve relaxation and to stop one's thought activity, so that in fact we cannot prove anything with these experiments. Yet I still believe that the findings in certain manic conditions in fact represent a state of excitation of the intentional sphere associated with an exclusive occurrence of β-w with an average length of 20 σ. These findings agree quite well with the opinion expressed above. I have never seen such E.E.G.s in normal persons in the course of any of the recordings which I have now taken over a period of more than 12 years. Until now I have seen them in this particular form only in manic patients. This finding in mania demonstrates a cortical disturbance of function affecting only the external principal zone of the cortex. Now, however, observations can be interpreted which so far have remained incomprehensible to me. I made such observations in a case of agitated senile dementia and they include the record shown before which had been obtained during severe mental disturbance following carbon monoxide poisoning. In these instances too we are dealing with disturbances that involve predominantly the external principal zone of the cortex and these findings confirm in a certain measure the opinion expressed above. We are now in a position to differentiate between in-dividual parts of the composite potential curve of the E.E.G. and to establish *causal* relationships between alterations of these parts, namely of the α-w and of certain β-w, and the observed *clinical* manifestations. Thus an interpretation of the E.E.G. as defined by me[T27] has become possible to a certain degree! To make a distinction between the individual activities which we encounter in the form of α-w and of certain β-w is of course artificial, for in the normal state a very close coordination of the activities of the two cortical zones is indispensable. It goes without saying that for the *psychophysiological* activity of the cortex continuous coordination of the activities of the external and internal principal zones of the cortex is absolutely necessary. After relinquishing my working hypothesis which I had proposed as early as seven years ago, I now come to the following conclusion:

In the characteristic potential curve of the E.E.G. of man, which is composed of the action currents of the various nerve cell layers and is woven into a homogeneous whole, *the total physiological and psychophysiological activity* of the human cortex finds its visible expression. The α-w of the E.E.G. originate in the internal principal zone of the cortex; they correspond to its continuous *physiological* activity and they show distinct alterations in general disturbances of function[T42] of the cortex. Certain β-w with a length of 11–24 σ, whose site of origin probably has to be sought in the cell layers of the external principal zone, correspond to the *psychophysiological* activity of the cortex; they must be regarded as the material concomitant phenomena of *mental* processes.

A Note of Correction

[Published in *Archiv für Psychiatrie und Nervenkrankheiten*, **1937**, *106*: 508]

In my twelfth report on the electroencephalogram of man in "Archiv für Psychiatrie", volume 106, page 165 [this book p. 267], the figures 8, 9, 10, 15, 16 and 17, as it later became apparent, are distorted by an alternating current which entered the recording apparatus without being noticed! The presumed β-w of the E.E.G. of 20 σ length represent such alternating current oscillations[T134]! Since power for the lighting system is supplied by a direct current and there are no alternating current installations in the building in which the oscillograph is housed, these can only be stray currents. In spite of the screening devices, they unfortunately entered just into the E.E.G.s of *patients* and caused me to draw wrong conclusions. Although before and after each recording of the E.E.G. the oscillograph was found to be free of current, such currents entered into the apparatus only during the recording itself. This may make my error appear in a milder light.

However, on the basis of my numerous other findings I still maintain that in many mental disturbances one finds, predominantly, certain β-w and I hope to be able to publish better documentation of this soon.

I have also not changed my view on the sites of origin of the α-w and of certain β-w, nor have I changed my interpretation of these wave forms given in the twelfth report, even though I readily admit that the documentation published there concerning the significance of certain β-w, as far as it was derived from pathological cases, does *not* rest on solid evidence.

Jena, March 21, 1937   HANS BERGER

XIII

On the Electroencephalogram of Man

Thirteenth Report

by Hans Berger, Jena

(With 6 figures)

(Received April 30, 1937)

[Published in *Archiv für Psychiatrie und Nervenkrankheiten*, **1937**, *106*: 577–584]

In my last report, the twelfth of the series, I explained in detail the reasons for which I had abandoned my earlier working hypothesis concerning the psychophysiological significance of the α-w of the human E.E.G. I came to the conclusion that the α-w arise in the internal principal zone of the human cerebral cortex, and that they are the electrical concomitants of its continuous physiological activity. I also concluded that certain β-w of a length of 11–24 σ, on the other hand, represent concomitant phenomena of the psychophysiological activity of the cortex. In that report I also reproduced several E.E.G.s of patients which, in addition to other arguments discussed there in detail, were meant to lend further support for this view. Later it became apparent that six of these illustrations, namely Figures 8, 9, 10, 15, 16 and 17, were distorted by artefacts[T135] and therefore could not be used as evidence to support the statements which I made in that report regarding the significance of these records. I clarified this matter in a note of correction, which appeared in these Archives[1] and explained that the trains of waves interpreted as β-w of 20 σ in those six figures are alternating current oscillations which entered into the records of those three patients in spite of appropriate precautions. In this note of correction, I also promised to publish more satisfactory evidence in the near future. I was of course very anxious to fulfil this promise *soon*, which shall now be done in this thirteenth report[2]. The recording of E.E.G.s in patients with severe mental illness is always fraught with many difficulties. Success in obtaining a satisfactory E.E.G. depends upon the fulfilment of so many conditions on the part of the subject being investigated, that it is often entirely a matter of chance whether a recording carried out with much diligence will be successful or not. Either the patients do not close their eyes at all, or they open them just at the most inopportune moment; they fail to lie still in the recumbent

---

[1] Arch. f. Psychiatr., **106**, 508. [This book p. 289]

[2] In the performance of these investigations again Dr. *R. Lemke* and Dr. *W. Lembcke* lent me their faithful assistance, for which here too I thank them cordially!

position during the recording; they sit up from the couch or move their head, talk, laugh or weep and, when needle electrode recordings are carried out, they pull out the needles through an unexpected head movement or deliberately.

Very often during insulin therapy of schizophrenia, before the patients reach the actual stage of coma, precomatose states of agitation of variable degree occur

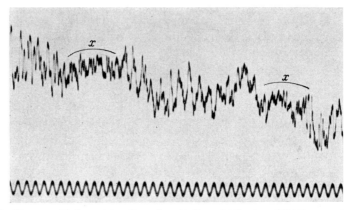

Fig. 1. M.G., 42 years old, in a state of manic agitation. At the top: E.E.G. recorded with silver needles from forehead and occiput. At the bottom: time in 1/10ths sec. At x: increased occurrence of short β-w, which are also clearly recognizable between x and x, where they are superimposed upon the α-w.

during which the mental changes are frequently the most striking features. The satisfactory recording of E.E.G.s during insulin coma itself is easy. I illustrated several such records in Figures 2, 3 and 4 of my twelfth report. However, for the reasons cited above, the recording of an E.E.G. during the states of agitation is seldom successful. In a moderately successful recording taken in a schizophrenic during the precomatose state of agitation, I found an E.E.G. in which short β-w with a length of 19 σ dominate the entire record. In the twelfth report I also stressed how difficult it is to record E.E.G.s in manic patients. I was once exceptionally lucky in recording the E.E.G.s of two such patients. These records are reproduced in my twelfth report. However, they are not faultless, because they were contaminated by an alternating current entering from the outside. Therefore, I show in Figure 1 the E.E.G. record obtained from a 42 year old patient who has suffered from episodes of manic-depressive psychosis since she was 31 years old. This is a needle electrode recording which had been obtained while the patient still showed clear signs of manic agitation. Especially during the periods marked with the letter x, it is evident that short β-w with a length of 17–22 σ predominate. Also between these two parts of the E.E.G., the short β-w also appear quite distinctly and are superimposed upon the easily recognizable α-w. The recording was unfortunately interrupted when the patient, who until then had been lying completely motionless with her eyes closed, suddenly tore out the needle electrodes with her hands while bursting into laughter and got up.

Much more convincing and considerably easier from the point of view of recording is the investigation of the action which certain drugs known for their clinical effects exert upon the different wave types of the human E.E.G. I already indicated in my last report that I was unable to demonstrate unequivocally that one or several cups of strong coffee produce an effect predominantly upon the short β-w,

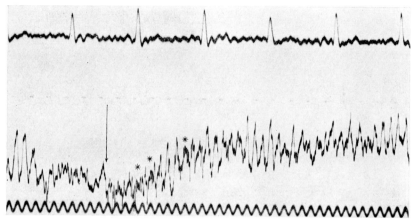

Fig. 2. E.E., 26 years old; 30 minutes after the subcutaneous injection of 0.2 gram of caffeine-sodium-salicylate. At the top: E.C.G. recorded from both arms. In the middle: E.E.G. recorded with chlorided silver needles from forehead and occiput. At the bottom: time in 1/10ths sec. The arrow indicates the onset of the caffeine effect.

as one would expect according to my theory. In that report I also explained why it is impossible to make such observations. However, I did not let the matter rest, and investigated the effect of injections of caffeine, with which I obtained unequivocal results. These, however, must be judged in the broader context of other pharmacological experiments. In a 26 year old man E.E., 0.2 gram[T7] of caffeine-sodium-salicylate was injected subcutaneously into the right arm. A small segment of the E.C.G. and E.E.G. recorded 30 minutes later is shown in Figure 2. The pulse beats 80 times per minute, the E.C.G. is somewhat disturbed by an oscillatory artefact. The E.E.G. recorded with needle electrodes from the forehead and occiput clearly reveals on the right side of the arrow the increased incidence of β-w with an average length of 16 σ. The increase in occurrence of these short β-w is very clear, especially at the points indicated by an asterisk, but elsewhere in the right half of the E.E.G. the marked prominence of the β-w is also evident. During the recording the experimental subject lay completely still with his eyes closed in the darkened room which was only dimly lit by a shaded candle. Figure 3 shows a recording taken from the same subject E.E. at a time when he was not under the influence of any drug. The E.C.G., again somewhat distorted by an oscillatory artefact, shows a pulse rate of 86 per minute. The E.E.G. shows beautiful α-w with a length of 90 σ; β-w are also present but are clearly less prominent in amplitude and amount in comparison with the findings shown in Figure 2. Perhaps one could still doubt whether in this case the

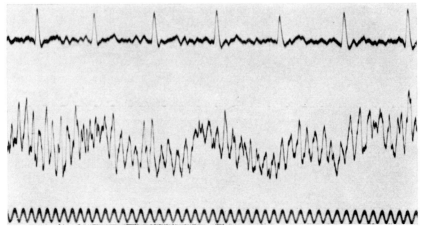

Fig. 3. E.E., 26 years old. At the top: E.C.G. recorded from both arms. In the middle: E.E.G. recorded with chlorided silver needles from forehead and occiput. At the bottom: time in 1/10ths sec.

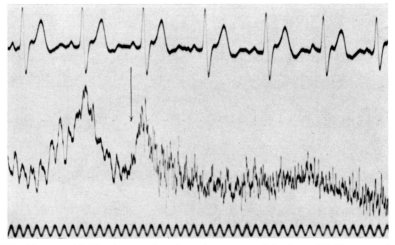

Fig. 4. E.B., 23 years old; 30 minutes after the subcutaneous injection of 0.02 gram of cocaine hydrochloride. At the top: E.C.G. recorded from both arms. In the middle: E.E.G. recorded with chlorided silver needles from forehead and occiput. At the bottom: time in 1/10ths sec. The arrow indicates the onset of the cocaine effect.

increased occurrence of short β-w in the E.E.G. really reflects the stimulating effect of caffeine. These doubts, however, will be dispelled by further experimental results.

We know that cocaine when taken in toxic doses produces states of extreme psychic agitation and motor restlessness. However, these are usually also associated with clouding of consciousness. In 1931 in my third communication, I reported that a dose of 0.03 gram of cocaine hydrochloride induces a slight amplitude increase of the α-w of the E.E.G. which appears clearly about 30 minutes after the injection[1].

---

[1] See Fig. 9 and 10 in Arch. f. Psychiatr., **94**, 32. [This book p. 109]

At that time, however, I recorded curves only with the coil galvanometer which, because of their small size, fail to reveal details of the β-w. A very small but still effective dose of cocaine acts exclusively as a stimulant of mental activity. This stimulating effect has led to the habit of chewing coca among inhabitants of South America and has been responsible for the disastrous abuse of cocaine as a stimulant in civilized countries. Figure 4 shows on the right side of the arrow the effect of a sub-cutaneous injection of slightly less than 0.02 gram of cocaine hydrochloride which had been given 30 minutes before to the 23 year old experimental subject E.B. During the recording the subject lay completely still in the darkened recording room with his eyes closed and thus the recording proceeded quickly and was fully successful. The E.C.G. is shown at the top. The heart beats 86 times per minute; the pulse is hardly accelerated. At the beginning of the segment of the curve shown here, the E.E.G. distinctly exhibits α-w with a length of 100 σ. After the arrow, it rather suddenly undergoes a considerable modification quite similar to, but still more pronounced than that shown in Figure 2 occurring under the influence of caffeine. Short β-w, with an average length of only 13 σ in this case, are densely superimposed upon the α-w and at times replace them completely! We are confronted here with the graphic representation of the stimulating action exerted by cocaine upon mental processes! The effect of cocaine is more powerful than that of caffeine; correspondingly the change in the E.E.G. in comparison with that occurring under the influence of caffeine is much more distinct and therefore more striking.

Furthermore we know that *atropine* is the foremost among those alkaloids which exert a stimulating action upon the cerebral cortex and upon mental processes in particular. In the treatment of the sequelae of epidemic encephalitis, one uses atropine in amounts which by far exceed the maximum dose; however, in these instances atropine is given exclusively by mouth. I frequently recorded E.E.G.s in persons who, because they suffered from the sequelae of encephalitis, received high doses of atropine, but I never obtained E.E.G.s which were altered by atropine alone. Atropine acts more quickly and energetically when it is given by subcutaneous injection to an experimental subject who is not habituated to this drug. Figure 5 shows such a record obtained from the same subject E.E., of whom Figures 2 and 3 were shown above. Figure 2 demonstrated the E.E.G. under the influence of caffeine and Figure 3 showed the normal resting curve. At the top of Figure 5 one sees the E.C.G.; the pulse beats 86 times per minute. The E.E.G. recorded below is markedly altered throughout and shows exactly the same changes as they occur under the influence of caffeine and cocaine, only they are *still* more pronounced and now predominate in the entire segment of the curve shown here and even in the entire record which is several meters long! This record was taken 30 minutes after the experimental subject, who lay with his eyes closed in the completely quiet and darkened recording room, had received a subcutaneous injection of 0.0005 gram of atropine sulfate. Here the characteristic β-w have a length of 11–16 σ and thus correspond in their duration to the β-w which E.E. showed under the influence of caffeine. Only some time after the dissipation of the atropine effect did the E.E.G.s exhibit again the same pattern as that of Figure 3. Therefore under the stimulating action of caffeine, cocaine and atropine, in accordance with the appearance of phenomena of mental stimulation and excitation and in parallel with the gradual increase of these particular effects, we see an increasingly distinct change in the E.E.G. This change is characterized by the presence of short β-w of 11–16 σ which

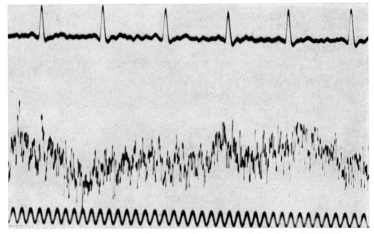

Fig. 5. E.E., 26 years old; 30 minutes after the subcutaneous injection of 0.0005 gram of atropine sulfate. At the top: E.C.G. recorded from both arms. In the middle: E.E.G. recorded with chlorided silver needles from forehead and occiput. At the bottom: time in 1/10ths sec.

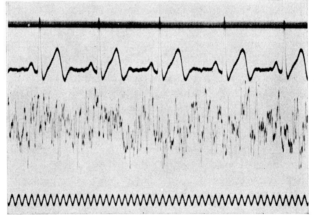

Fig. 6. Mrs. E.D., 32 years old; 45 minutes after the subcutaneous injection of 0.02 gram of morphine hydrochloride. At the top: E.C.G. recorded from both arms. In the middle: E.E.G. recorded with chlorided silver needles from forehead and occiput. At the bottom: time in 1/10ths sec.

dominate the pattern. I explained in my last report why I assume that these β-w belong to the material concomitants of mental processes.

At this point I would like to consider some additional observations. In 1933 in my eighth report[1] I gave a brief account of the phenomena in the E.E.G. which

---

[1] Arch. f. Psychiatr., **101**, 453. [This book p. 210]

are associated with the action of morphine. It is well known that morphine is capable of exerting a frankly *stimulating* effect on people who have become habituated to it or to other opiates and that precisely for this reason abuse may occur, especially among physicians. Figure 6 shows the E.E.G. of 32 year old E.D., who was habituated to opiates. The record was taken 45 minutes after the subcutaneous injection of 0.02 gram of morphine hydrochloride. At the top the E.C.G. is recorded; the heart beats 64 times per minute. The E.E.G. shows an increased incidence of short β-w which exhibit an average length of 13 σ. Furthermore every experienced psychiatrist knows that even scopolamine may sometimes elicit states of agitation, although this drug usually exerts a very powerful depressing action. As early as 1931 I reproduced in my third report[1] an E.E.G. which demonstrates the disappearance of the α-w under the combined action of scopolamine and morphine. Nevertheless I also observed later that an increased number of β-w appear in the E.E.G. in *those* cases in which, exceptionally, scopolamine hydrobromide had induced a stimulating effect. However, most of the time, the records are distorted by movements etc. to such an extent that it is doubtful whether they can be evaluated from a scientific point of view. In addition I would not like to leave unmentioned that when recording the E.E.G. directly from the human cerebral cortex in a 29 year old man who was anesthetized with chloroform, I observed at the beginning of narcosis a group formation of the α-w which also decreased considerably in amplitude. They reminded me of the very different group formation and the gallop rhythm of Evipan and Pernocton narcosis etc. However, as mentioned, the amplitude of the α-w declined continuously at the same time. In 1931 in my third communication[2] I also reported in detail on the usual E.E.G. findings in chloroform narcosis. In any case it became evident from all this that one is well advised, when interpreting the results, to take into account possible individual differences in the action of these drugs.

I believe, however, that the results reported here are in excellent agreement with my assumption that short β-w with a length of 11–24 σ represent the material concomitants of mental processes. Thus these pharmacological findings support my view more unequivocally and more clearly than the results derived from pathological cases. They were recorded while observing all necessary precautionary measures and are free of artefacts[T135]. I therefore believe that I have completely fulfilled my promise made in the mentioned note of correction and that I have done so better than would have been possible by showing only E.E.G.s of mental patients. Because of the results reported here and of the other reasons discussed in detail earlier, I am convinced of the validity of the views expressed in the final sentence of my twelfth report, which reads thus:

Certain β-w with a length of 11–24 σ, whose site of origin probably has to be sought in the cell layers of the external principal zone of the human cerebral cortex, correspond to its *psychophysiological* activity; they must be regarded as the material concomitant phenomena of *mental* processes![T136]

---

[1] Arch. f. Psychiatr., **94**, 33, Fig. 11. [This book p. 110]
[2] Arch. f. Psychiatr., **14**, 37, and Fig. 16, 17, 18 and 19. [This book p. 112]

XIV

On the Electroencephalogram of Man

Fourteenth Report

by Hans Berger, Jena

(With 12 figures)

(Received April 12, 1938)

[Published in *Archiv für Psychiatrie und Nervenkrankheiten*, **1938**, *108*: 407–431]

In my earlier reports in these Archives, I repeatedly referred to the changes occurring in the electroencephalogram (E.E.G.) during a major *epileptic seizure*. After a severe epileptiform seizure I found that the alpha waves (α-w) of the E.E.G. were lost and reappeared gradually with the return of consciousness. I first reported this in 1931 (third report, Vol. 94, p. 132 footnote) and later documented it with illustrations (fourth report, 1932, Vol. 97, p. 18, Figures 10 to 13). The investigations carried out at that time were made with a coil galvanometer which did not permit an accurate reproduction of the beta waves (β-w) because of its low sensitivity. Several years ago I recorded the E.E.G. with the oscillograph after the end of a severe epileptic seizure. At this time I wish to report on these records because they complement significantly my earlier accounts. A 47 year old man, Gl., who suffered from genuine epilepsy formerly had rare attacks, which have recently become more frequent. In this patient I found that after a major attack which by chance occurred just during the recording, the α-w were absent during the state of unconsciousness which outlasted the seizure, but that fast and low voltage β-w could be demonstrated during this time. The record was taken with two galvanometers, a coil galvanometer and an oscillograph, connected in parallel and with needle electrodes from the forehead and occiput. Figure 1 shows the E.E.G. before the attack and Figure 2 shows it after the seizure at a time when the excitatory motor phenomena had completely disappeared and while the patient was unresponsive and lying completely still. A few seconds later Gl. was clear in his mind and his thinking was well organized, but he knew nothing of the attack. However, the E.E.G. of Figure 3, which was then recorded, shows a very interesting finding. Before the seizure the α-w of the E.E.G. had an average length of 125 σ, as is evident from Figure 1 and as can be seen more easily in the coil galvanometer curve. After the severe cerebral discharge the length of the α-w increased to an average of 165 σ and individual waves even showed values as high as 250 σ. As I have always emphasized this slowing of the α-w indicates a severe disturbance of cortical function[T137]. It is found especially in epileptic dementia which generally develops in patients with genuine epilepsy who have had frequently recurring attacks over a long period of time. I reported this first in 1931 (third report) and later documented it with curves. However in this case it is interesting that a single severe seizure was sufficient to elicit, at least temporarily,

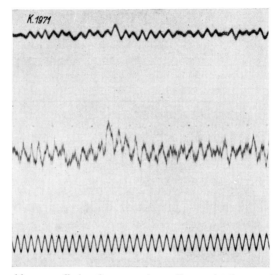

Fig. 1. Gl., 47 year old man suffering from genuine epilepsy. At the top: E.E.G. recorded with the coil galvanometer; below it: E.E.G. recorded with the oscillograph. Both galvanometers are connected in parallel. At the bottom: time in 1/10ths sec. Needle electrode recording from forehead and occiput.

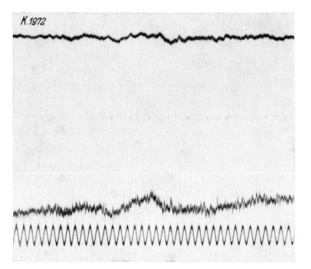

Fig. 2. Gl. during the unconsciousness following a major epileptic seizure which has run its course. The same recording technique and connections as in Figure 1.

these marked alterations in the previously normal E.E.G. This makes it visibly apparent to us that even a single attack does in fact produce severe impairment of cortical activity. Such impairment has been attributed by various investigators, and particularly by *Spielmeyer*, to the disturbance of cerebral circulation associated with the seizure and to the consequences of this disturbance. In this regard I would also

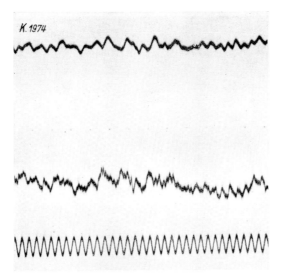

Fig. 3. Gl. a few seconds later than Figure 2. The patient is again clear in his mind and his thinking is well organized. The same recording technique and connections as in Figures 1 and 2.

like to mention that potential oscillations in pathological cases which many investigators have designated as delta waves, are nothing but pathologically slowed α-w. In contrast to other reports I also wish to stress the following point: in 1932 (fourth communication, Vol. 97, p. 147–148), I already reported that great temperature increases during fever, unlike what one might expect, did not cause shortening, but on the contrary a considerable lengthening of the α-w; in one case in which the temperature was 39.6°C the value increased from 100 to 140 σ.

I have always emphasized that I was unable to follow the course of a major epileptic seizure in the E.E.G. First of all, the occurrence of a seizure during the recording of an E.E.G., even in an epileptic with frequent attacks, is an exceptional coincidence. If, however, one is fortunate enough to have this chance of catching an attack, then the powerful excitatory motor phenomena and the muscle currents associated with them mask everything and make it impossible to obtain a satisfactory recording of the electrical potential oscillations of the brain. This gap in our investigations has now been closed by the excellent studies and the beautiful recordings made by *Gibbs* and his coworkers[1]. With a somewhat less sensitive instrument they

[1] *Gibbs, Frederick, William Lennox* and *Erna Gibbs*: Arch. of Neur., **36**, 1225 (1936).

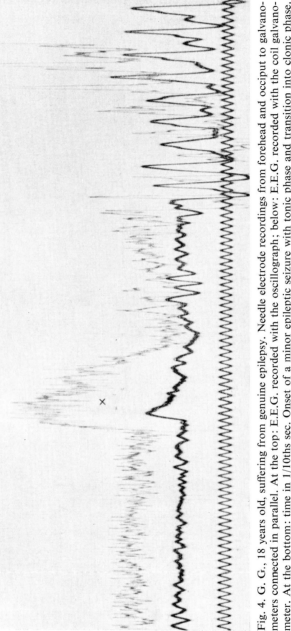

Fig. 4. G. G., 18 years old, suffering from genuine epilepsy. Needle electrode recordings from forehead and occiput to galvanometers connected in parallel. At the top: E.E.G. recorded with the oscillograph; below: E.E.G. recorded with the coil galvanometer. At the bottom: time in 1/10ths sec. Onset of a minor epileptic seizure with tonic phase and transition into clonic phase.

succeeded admirably in recording the electrical concomitants of a major epileptic seizure and they were also successful in demonstrating the local discharges underlying *Jacksonian* attacks. They even had the opportunity to record with needle electrodes from the *cerebral cortex itself* during a major seizure, so that all criticisms raised against these records are no longer valid. Nevertheless there was a small disadvantage in the use of the less sensitive galvanometer insofar as the β-w were not recorded satisfactorily. Very interesting also are the descriptions of larval seizures given by these investigators. These manifest themselves only in the electrical record of the cerebral events, without being apparent externally. On the basis of E.E.G.s recorded during hyperventilation experiments in epileptics I had previously assumed that the epileptic seizure itself is induced by disinhibition of the cerebral cortex and that the sudden onset of unconsciousness falls within the beginning of the period of disinhibition. Till now I have never been able to learn anything definite concerning the condition of the E.E.G. during the tonic stage of the epileptic seizure in man. From the illustrations shown by *Gibbs* and his coworkers it now becomes apparent that rapid and small potential oscillations, *i.e.* β-w, are present during the tonic stage. In an 18 year old patient G.G. who suffered from genuine epilepsy and who in addition to major seizures also had milder, abortive attacks, I made an observation years ago which I dare to interpret only now, after having seen the convincing records of *Gibbs*. The patient had experienced a minor seizure with brief unconsciousness during which also excitatory motor phenomena in the form of slight clonic flexion movements of the left hand were observed. Figure 4 shows the beginning of this minor attack which from beginning to end lasted almost 30 seconds. The E.E.G. is recorded with needle electrodes from the forehead and occiput. The galvanometers are connected in parallel and their sensitivity is thus reduced, which in this case is an advantage. The E.E.G. taken with the oscillograph is recorded at the top. The E.E.G. taken with the coil galvanometer appears in the middle. Time is indicated in tenths of seconds. The mirrors of the galvanometers are not in exact vertical alignment; however, in the E.E.G.s the oscillations corresponding to each other can be immediately recognized. In the right half of the figure one sees the high voltage potential oscillations which correspond to the clonic stage. These oscillations are still well recorded by the coil galvanometer, while the mirror of the oscillograph is deflected beyond the recording surface. This clonic stage is preceded by a segment of curve in which the α-w, which in this patient are prolonged and of high voltage, are replaced by shorter oscillations. In the corresponding oscillograph curve of the upper E.E.G. the predominance of short, high voltage β-w becomes very clearly apparent. At " $\times$ " a fairly large potential oscillation occurs and just at this point, in the descending limb of the oscillation, one sees clearly an increased number of high voltage β-w. Earlier I had had misgivings concerning this record and I wondered whether we were really dealing in this case with β-w of the E.E.G. or perhaps with unintentionally recorded muscle currents. For this reason I had not yet published this finding. I believe that the clearcut records obtained by *Gibbs* and his coworkers which certainly do not contain muscle currents now make it possible to interpret this curve recorded from the surface of the skull. It follows from it that loss of the α-w and the appearance of high voltage β-w must correspond to the tonic stage of the epileptic seizure. In the E.E.G. record shown in Figure 4 we are dealing only with a very mild and abortive attack, and this is the reason why it was possible to record it. The cardiazol treatment of schizophrenia introduced by *von Meduna* now offered the opportunity to elicit epileptiform attacks suitable for the investigation of the E.E.G. at any time, so that

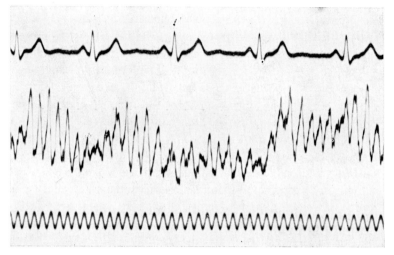

Fig. 5. H. Fl., 25 years old, suffering from schizophrenia. At the top: E.C.G. from both arms; pulse 60. In the middle: E.E.G. needle electrode recording from forehead and occiput. α-w = 115 σ. At the bottom: time in 1/10ths sec.

one no longer had to depend upon their chance occurrence[1]. I therefore took up the study of the E.E.G. during cardiazol convulsions with great expectations, but unfortunately became disappointed. In none of the epileptiform seizures which I recorded did I succeed in obtaining even one satisfactory E.E.G. during the course of a major attack. The suddenly beginning excitatory motor phenomena were always so powerful that they completely masked the cerebral oscillations. Even the coil galvanometer with which I intended to record the E.C.G. from both arms, always recorded the clonic jerks of the arms. The mirror of the much more sensitive oscillograph was always deflected beyond the recording surface, so that nothing was being registered. Only recordings after the attacks were successful, but they showed nothing new and were identical with the findings of absent α-w and the appearance of small, fast β-w shown in Figure 2 of this report. And yet even under these conditions some interesting results were obtained. In a 25 year old schizophrenic, Fl., the E.E.G. recorded before cardiazol injection presented the picture reproduced in Figure 5. The record was taken from the forehead and occiput with needle electrodes while

[1] Dozent Dr. *Rudolf Lemke* again assisted me by word and deed in the recording of all E.E.G.s on which I report in this communication. In addition, Dr. *Werner Lembcke* helped me in the performance of the cardiazol studies. I wish to take this opportunity to thank both colleagues sincerely for their faithful help.

the patient was lying in a darkened room with his eyes closed. At the top the E.C.G. is shown. It was recorded from both arms and shows a pulse rate of 60 per minute. In the middle the E.E.G. is recorded. It exhibits beautiful α-w with an average length of 115 σ. At the bottom, time is indicated in tenths of seconds. After the intravenous injection of cardiazol there was a sudden marked increase in the pulse rate; a severe

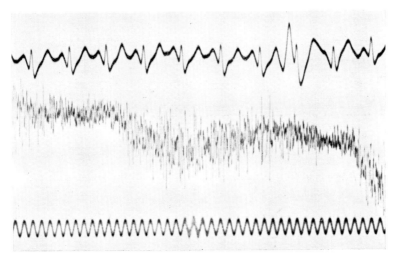

Fig. 6. H. Fl. (Figure 5). During the unconsciousness following a severe epileptic seizure induced by intravenous cardiazol injection and *before* a second and equally severe attack, which followed immediately. At the top: E.C.G., pulse rate 140! In the middle: E.E.G. At the bottom: time in 1/10ths sec.

epileptiform seizure with a tonic and clonic phase developed. Figure 6 was recorded after this severe attack. The E.C.G. is clearly altered, the pulse rate now measures 140 per minute and the E.E.G. also shows severe changes. High voltage β-w dominate the picture. For one second they become a little lower in voltage, then for 1.8 seconds they increase in amplitude and then diminish again. These are the same periodic fluctuations which I had first observed in the E.E.G. a long time ago and repeatedly noticed since then, and which I considered to be the expression of an intrinsic rhythm of the cerebral cortex. This fluctuating amplitude increase of the β-w in this case was the prelude to a second and equally severe convulsive seizure which followed immediately upon the recording shown in Figure 6 and which caused the mirror of the oscillograph to be deflected at once beyond the recording surface. It is probable that the very onset of the tonic stage of this seizure had just been recorded in the E.E.G. at this point. It goes without saying that the state of excitation which becomes manifest by the appearance of these β-w does not inevitably lead to an attack. This becomes particularly apparent from *Gibbs'* beautiful illustrations of larval seizures. We encounter this state of cerebral irritation in still another situation which is illustrated in Figure 7. The 26 year old schizophrenic K.A. had a severe epileptic seizure after an intravenous injection of cardiazol, the recording of which was once again unsuccessful. After the attack he was lying with eyes closed in a state of unresponsiveness and complete exhaustion. The E.C.G. which is altered in comparison with earlier recordings, shows a pulse rate of 150 per minute, whereas before 66 pulse beats per minute had been counted. The E.E.G. is again composed exclusively of β-w which, however, are of somewhat larger amplitude than those usually seen after the end of

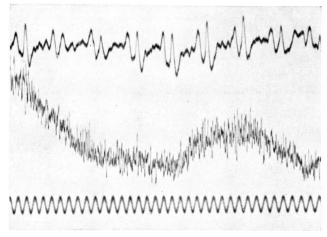

Fig. 7. K. A., 26 years old, suffering from schizophrenia. Still unconscious after a severe epileptic seizure induced by intravenous injection of cardiazol and before a subsequent severe twilight state. At the top: E.C.G. recorded from both arms, pulse rate 150! In the middle: E.E.G. At the bottom: time in 1/10ths sec.

a major seizure (see Figure 2!). This recording was immediately followed by a severe twilight state. The numerous and high voltage β-w here too indicate a *state of cerebral irritation*. These are of course pathological manifestations which should not be equated with the β-w of the normal E.E.G. of the healthy subject.

I reported earlier on the E.E.G. concomitants of absences (brief loss of consciousness *without* motor excitatory phenomena or deficits). I emphasized that during a true absence the α-w disappear and that the E.E.G. is composed of β-w. I later felt obliged to correct my first report on this matter which I had made in 1932 at the meeting of the Middle German Psychiatrists and Neurologists in Chemnitz[1]. There I had stated that during an absence the β-w also increase considerably in amplitude and incidence. I had observed that during what appeared to be a pure absence, excitatory motor phenomena in the form of teeth clenching nevertheless do occur. Muscle currents from the temporalis muscle were therefore recorded together with the E.E.G. and simulated an increase in the amplitude of the β-w (fifth report, Vol. 98, p. 154, 1932). Repeated investigations, however, have convinced me that this occurs relatively seldom and that with some experience one can distinguish the muscle currents from the β-w and thus avoid this error. In pure absences of genuine epilepsy one finds indeed, besides the loss of the α-w, a moderate increase in amplitude

---

[1] *Berger, Hans*: Arch. f. Psychiatr., **96**, 746 (1932)[T 138].

and a considerable increase in frequency of the β-w. These then resemble those β-w seen in Figures 2, 6 and 7 and those in Figure 4 before the appearance of the high voltage convulsive waves. *Gibbs* and his coworkers investigated many epileptics with minor seizures. They report the interesting finding that in such patients they sometimes observed during these minor seizures relatively large potential oscillations

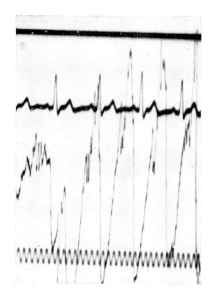

Fig. 8. J. K., 15 year old schoolgirl suffering from genuine epilepsy. At the top: E.C.G. recorded from both arms to the coil galvanometer. In the middle: E.E.G. recorded to the oscillograph from forehead and occiput with silver needle electrodes. At the bottom: time in 1/10ths sec. K. counts aloud while lying in a darkened room with her eyes closed.

which did not reveal themselves either subjectively or objectively in the condition and behavior of the patients. In 1933 in my seventh report, I already pointed out that in epileptics with frequent seizures high voltage potential oscillations are sometimes found even outside the attacks and I called these oscillations an actual visual representation of the *predisposition to seizures*. This assumption was confirmed time and again. In epileptics with frequent attacks such potential oscillations of considerably higher voltage are not at all rare. These oscillations occur repeatedly one after another and not the slightest change can be observed in the patient during this time. Figure 8 shows such an E.E.G. It was obtained from a 15 year old girl, J.K., who since her 9th year of life has suffered from minor and major attacks, twilight states and true absences caused by genuine epilepsy. During the absences which last for only a short time, a loss of α-w and a distinct increase in frequency and slight increase in amplitude of the β-w of the E.E.G. often occur, but certainly not every time. High voltage potential oscillations occurred in K. quite independently of these absences during recording of the E.E.G. with needle electrodes from the forehead and occiput. These oscillations correspond to the changes which *M. H. Fischer*[1] designated as "convulsive currents". Like the high voltage potential oscillations of the E.E.G. which precede the clonic jerks, they result from a fusion of incompletely formed α-w, as I already

---

[1] *Fischer, M. H.*: Med. Klin., **1933,** I.

mentioned in 1934 (ninth report, Vol. 102, p. 239). In Figure 8^{T139} these high voltage potential oscillations have a duration of 600 σ. It is interesting that while these potential oscillations, which are reminiscent of the gallop rhythm of Pernocton and Evipan narcosis, occur (eighth report, Vol. 101, p. 222 and following pages,1933), consciousness is in no way disturbed, as I was able to demonstrate to my own satisfaction by the patient's ability to count aloud without interruption. In K. such high voltage potential oscillations followed upon each other often for as long as 8–21 seconds without any noticeable excitatory motor phenomena or without even the slightest clouding of consciousness. It is probable that the occurrence of these potential oscillations was limited to a circumscribed area, just as had been the case for the high voltage potential oscillations recorded in a patient described in the seventh report (Vol. 100, p. 201, 1933; Figures 10–12). There the high voltage oscillations were recorded from the bone of the skull in the hand area of the precentral convolution; they preceded the individual slight clonic jerks of the fingers which had continued for several days after a paralytic attack and which were also not associated with any disturbance of consciousness. I believe that loss of consciousness occurs only when high voltage potential oscillations appear everywhere in the cortex as a consequence of a *generalized* cortical disinhibition, as it does for instance in Evipan narcosis.

In a direct recording from the cortex, *Foerster* and *Altenburger*[1] made the observation that in cortical seizures localized potential oscillations precede the circumscribed convulsive phenomena. This of course makes one wonder whether during a *voluntary movement* in a normal subject one could perhaps also record somewhat smaller potential oscillations from the calvarium over the corresponding portions of the motor area. I had already performed 40 such experiments in 1932 with completely negative results, even though the records were always taken from the skull in the region of the corresponding central convolution which had been accurately determined with the cyrtometer^{T81}. Needle electrodes 1.5 cm apart and a highly sensitive oscillograph were used for these recordings. More recent experiments also failed; recordings taken while both hands performed simultaneous movements and in which the electrodes were placed on the skull over the hand areas of both central convolutions were equally unsuccessful. It was also impossible to demonstrate any influence of writing movements carried out by a subject with his eyes closed while simultaneous recordings were taken from the skull over the left hand region and over the convexity of the left occipital lobe. The one and only change which occurs in the E.E.G. is that caused by focussing of attention which manifests itself by a disappearance of the α-w and their replacement by β-w. I also made experiments in which records were taken with needle or foil electrodes from the skull as a whole in the course of the most diverse voluntary movements. In these experiments too only the well known concomitants of any increase in the level of attention appeared in the E.E.G. Higher voltage potential oscillations were never recorded, not even an increase of the β-w, even when the contraction of certain muscles, *e.g.* the pressing together of both hands or the *Jendrassik*

---

[1] *Foerster* and *Altenburger*: Verslg. Ges. dtsch. Nervenärzte, Munich, 1934, Ber. p. 96, Figure 7.

maneuver, were performed as vigorously as possible and maintained for a fairly long time. Of course, satisfactory experiments of this kind succeed only with intelligent experimental subjects, who have to be made particularly aware that all associated movements must be avoided, especially those of the head and above all clenching of the teeth, which occurs so readily with any physical effort. It is therefore better that the mouth be kept slightly open during such experiments. When such a posture, *e.g.* of the hands, is maintained for a relatively long period of time, regular fluctuations can be demonstrated in the E.E.G., which again correspond to the intrinsic rhythm of the brain and which reflect fluctuations in the level of attention. Thus if all associated movements of the head etc. are avoided, the performance of a movement causes changes in the E.E.G. only to the extent required by the focussing of attention upon this movement. The normal motor performance *as such* does not manifest itself in the E.E.G. at all.

I have repeatedly recorded the cerebral potential oscillations from circumscribed areas of the intact skull, as I just reported, and even more often from skull defects which had resulted from palliative trepanations. However, for a number of investigations I consider the recording from the *skull as a whole* as more informative, because I believe that the human cerebrum functions as an undivided whole. The E.E.G. reveals a wave of activity which progresses over the entire cerebral cortex in a certain direction, as I repeatedly explained in my earlier reports. The results of animal experiments, *e.g.* those of *Brémer, Ectors, Jasper* and others, also argue in the same direction. *Brémer's* experiments on sleeping cats[1] provide particularly convincing evidence that in animals too the activity of the cerebral cortex is coordinated in such a manner as to make it react as an undivided whole. These experiments demonstrated that if one records with two galvanometers from two completely different areas of the cerebral cortex of the sleeping cat, both regions awaken simultaneously in response to an arousal stimulus. *Pick*[2] was able to show that *e.g.* in animals under the influence of ether, no temperature differences between various points of the cerebrum can be demonstrated. He concludes from this that, at the onset of narcosis, different cortical areas of the cerebrum are *simultaneously* inhibited in their energy yielding activity. One should also mention *Lashley's* interesting observations which were made in a different field. From his experiments in rats he also concluded that in a certain sense the cerebral cortex functions as a whole[3].

From the beginning of my investigations in 1924 I always endeavored to show that even when recorded from the skull or from the scalp, the E.E.G. reveals the potential oscillations of the brain and more specifically those of the *cerebral cortex*. Since 1929 in my numerous publications I have time and again demonstrated this by means of records. In 1931 (third report, Vol. 94, p. 130, Figure 30) in a recording taken from the cortex and from the hemispheral white matter of the human cerebrum,

---

[1] *Brémer, F.*: L'activité électrique de l'écorce cérébrale et le problème psychologique du sommeil. Lecture given in Bologna, October 20, 1937.

[2] *Pick, E. P.*: Klin. Wschr., **1937, II**, 1481.

[3] See *William McDougall*: Aufbaukräfte der Seele, edited by *E. Rothacker*, p. 237, 238. Leipzig, 1937.

I demonstrated again that the E.E.G. as I describe it[T27] originates from the cerebral cortex itself, but that fortunately it can also be recorded from the bone of the skull and indeed even from the scalp. The recording conditions are therefore quite similar to those of the E.C.G. In spite of this it is repeatedly being stated, and this always by the same people, that the proof has not been supplied that the E.E.G. described

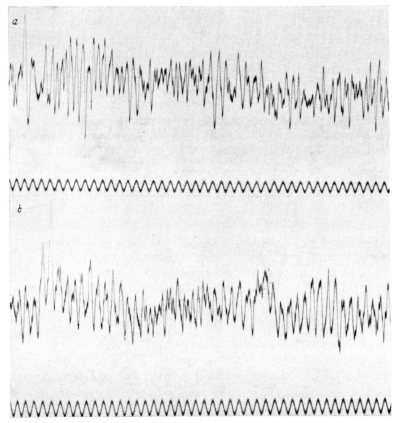

Fig. 9. C. S., 38 years old, suffering from dementia paralytica. (a) E.E.G., needle electrode recording from the cortex of the left frontal and the right parietal lobes. (b) E.E.G. recording with silver foil electrodes from forehead and occiput. Time in 1/10ths sec.

by me[T27] reveals the potential oscillations of the cerebral cortex. For this reason in my eleventh report (Vol. 104, 1936) in Figures 2 and 3, I again published E.E.G.s which had been recorded directly from the human cerebral cortex with needle electrodes. Yet the objection is always being repeated in the same manner. In Figure 9 I therefore demonstrate once more, side by side, the needle electrode recording of the E.E.G. from the cerebral cortex of the frontal and occipital lobes, and a silver foil electrode recording of the E.E.G. from the scalp taken from one and the same individual. These records were obtained from a 38 year old paretic C.S., in whom a cerebral puncture was carried out. Advantage was taken of this opportunity for recording the E.E.G. directly from the cortex. The identity of these two E.E.G.s is evident. Thus if only the unfounded criticism would stop that no proof had been established that the E.E.G. as I describe it[27] is identical with the potential oscillations of the cerebral cortex! This proof has been furnished in numerous investigations, and not only by myself. Also the other contention, first made by *Adrian* of Cambridge, that the α-w of the E.E.G. only originate in the occipital lobe, was refuted not only by me, but by many other investigators as well who used direct and sometimes unipolar recordings taken from the human cerebral cortex itself, so that even *Adrian* himself abandoned this view. Especially the lack of α-w in the region of a tumor which infiltrates the cortex and their presence in the areas bordering upon the tumor, appears to me to constitute particularly convincing proof for my assumption. In my eleventh report (Vol. 104, 1936) I carefully assembled my evidence without anyone so far having even made an attempt to refute it. Recently *Jasper*[1], in multiple simultaneous recordings from various regions of the human skull, also observed that in the occipital lobe α-w are sometimes absent while at the same time they are present in the precentral region and vice versa. This would surely be impossible if the α-w originated exclusively in the occipital lobe and spread from there into other cortical areas. Long ago I repeatedly referred precisely to this fact of the transient disparity of simultaneous E.E.G.s, *e.g.* of those of the right and left cerebral hemispheres, as constituting evidence against an occipital lobe origin of the α-w (the last time in the eleventh report, Vol. 104, p. 263, 1936). In animal experiments *Spiegel*[2] found in the cat persistence of the α-w of the E.E.G. in the frontal lobe which had been totally isolated by surgical transection. Numerous animal experiments by other authors also argue in favor of my view that the α-w originate locally everywhere in the cerebral cortex, so that really this objection too which has been repeated time and again always by the same people, could at last be laid to rest!

Earlier I had a preference for needle electrode recordings from the bone of the skull, but now I have increasingly adopted the technique of *foil electrode recording*. I use very thin pieces of pure silver foil which are only 0.005 mm thick and 7 × 10 cm in size. These are placed upon the forehead and occiput. A piece of flannel only slightly larger in size than the foil and soaked in 20% sodium chloride solution is placed under the foil and an identical piece of flannel covers the silver leaf. An overlying rubber bandage fixes the two foil electrodes to the head and simultaneously prevents drying of the flannel pieces. The location of the foil electrodes is best shown in Figures 10 and 11 which require no further explanation. For the experimental subject this foil recording is much more comfortable than the recording with needles, which cannot be inserted without local anesthesia. Quite a few of the experimental subjects, and especially patients, resist the insertion of needles. They become anxious and distrustful and this prevents a satisfactory recording of the E.E.G. In addition the action of the adrenalin which is added to the novocaine lessens after the needles have been in place for a certain length of time, and instead of the original very marked contraction of the skin vessels, vasodilatation ensues

[1] *Jasper, Herbert H.*: Arch. of Neur., **39**, 96 (1938).
[2] *Spiegel, E. A.*: Amer. J. Physiol., **118**, 571 (1937).

and with it local bleeding easily occurs around the needle tip. This disturbs the recording, quite apart from the fact that after some time the anesthetic action of novocaine also lessens. Pain develops at the puncture site which prevents even more the further satisfactory recording of the E.E.G. It was because of this that some of my investigations were disturbed or completely thwarted, *e.g.* when the object of

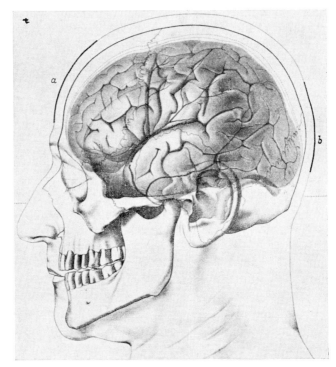

Fig. 10. Location of the silver foil electrodes *a* and *b* over forehead and occiput.

the study was to demonstrate the influence of a drug upon the E.E.G. under conditions in which one had to wait for a considerable time in order to obtain a fully developed drug action. The recording with foil electrodes is first of all more comfortable and therefore normal subjects and patients permit it more readily; it furthermore allows one to take records which can be continued for as long as one likes. In records taken with needle electrodes, which are usually placed at points *1* and *2* of Figure 11, the E.E.G. exhibits the potential oscillations of a long, but narrow ellipsoid region extending between the two electrodes. With foil electrodes however, of which each covers an area of 70 cm^2, one records the potential oscillations of a cortical region which is larger than half the total surface of the human cerebral cortex. Of course, recording with foil electrodes also has its disadvantages, because all interferences and contaminating extraneous currents such as *e.g.* muscle currents etc., appear much more prominently in the record. However, the same applies also to the recording of the E.C.G. with foil electrodes, yet this recording method which is the most comfortable one has not been abandoned because of this. The function which manifests itself in the E.E.G. as a *unitary* process can best be recorded, both in normal subjects and in patients, with the foil electrode method.

That the E.E.G. indeed represents a *unitary process*, follows, I believe, from simultaneous double recordings as I mentioned above and as I had also once discussed

a

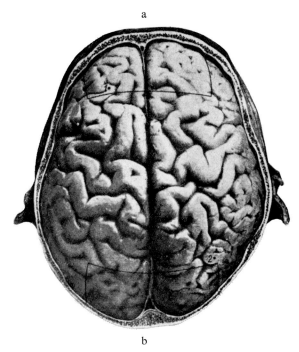

b

Fig. 11. Location of silver foil electrodes *a* and *b* projected upon the cerebral convolutions. *1* and *2*: location of the needle electrodes used for recording from the skull and for direct recording from the cerebral cortex in Figure 9*a*!

it before. The α-w originate locally everywhere in the cerebral cortex; they are, however, controlled from outside. In my third report (Vol. 94) I drew attention for the first time to the correspondence between the rhythms of different cortical areas of the cerebrum. On the basis of the animal experiments of *Travis* and *Dorsey* (1932) and in the light of my own observations on the E.E.G. in Pernocton and Evipan narcosis, I attempted in my later reports to interpret this correspondence by assuming the existence of an extracortical, probably thalamic control of this wave of cerebral activity (sixth report, 1933, Vol. 99, p. 184; seventh report, 1933, Vol. 100, p. 195; eighth report, 1934, Vol. 101, p. 218). Only in this way is it possible to explain why one and the same potential oscillation appears in identical form over both cerebral hemispheres when one records with separate galvanometers from the two sides. Again let me refer to Figure 12. It was obtained from a 57 year old patient, M.Z., who suffered from general paresis and who was already markedly demented. I had explained earlier that particularly in general paresis the α-w which occur in a sequence are much more unequal in length and form in comparison with those of healthy subjects. Such E.E.G.s therefore are particularly well suited for comparative studies. The α-w in Figure 12 show distinct lengthening; they measure on the average 160 σ. They are, however, fairly high in voltage and therefore make it possible, even with a

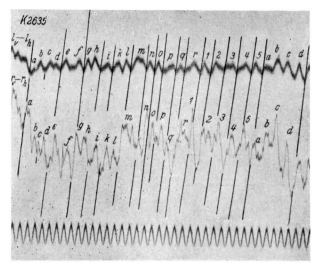

Fig. 12. M.Z., 57 year old patient suffering from dementia paralytica, exhibiting marked mental deterioration. At the top: E.E.G. recorded from the left side of the skull (forehead and occiput) with needle electrodes and the coil galvanometer. In the middle: E.E.G. recorded in the same fashion from the right side of the skull with the oscillograph. At the bottom: time in 1/10ths sec. The galvanometers are not connected together. Because the galvanometer mirrors were not in precise vertical alignment, the points coinciding in time are connected with india ink lines. In both E.E.G.s the α-w which correspond in time are labelled with identical letters or numbers.

less sensitive galvanometer, to obtain a sufficiently clear recording which enables one to make comparisons. The recordings shown here were taken with needle electrodes from the left forehead and the left occiput to the coil galvanometer, and from the right forehead and the right occiput to the oscillograph. Because the mirrors of the separate galvanometers are not in exact vertical alignment, simultaneous waves of the two E.E.G.s are connected with india ink lines. The individual α-w of the right and left hemispheres which correspond to each other are labelled with identical letters or numbers. A detailed comparison of the two curves shows that the individual α-w completely coincide in their time course and that they are as precisely identical in form as it is possible for them to be in recordings taken with two galvanometers of different sensitivity. They only differ occasionally in their amplitude as is often the case with double recordings, particularly in general paresis. Because in general paresis each α-w, as mentioned, differs more or less distinctly from the one preceding or following it, each having its individual form and length, it is particularly easy to demonstrate that the corresponding α-w of the right and left cerebral hemispheres are always identical in form and length. What fills me with wonder time and again is how the cerebral cortex with its 14 billion ganglion cells, extensive as it is and with its rich differentiation of anatomical structure, even though it displays only few local structural variations, is remarkably integrated into an entity which acts as a whole, as is apparent from the E.E.G.

Earlier when discussing the effect of a motor performance upon the E.E.G., I had to consider the influence of the focussing of attention upon the cerebral potential oscillations and had to point out that apart from the latter, muscle activity[T140] as such does not manifest itself at all in the human E.E.G. Time and again it becomes evident that any increase in the level of attention induces marked changes in the human E.E.G. According to the beautiful experiments carried out by *Ectors*, *Jasper*, *Jasper* and *Rheinberger* and others, the conditions in the animal are very similar. Every investigator of the E.E.G. is immediately struck by the fact that the record of one and the same human subject looks quite different, depending upon whether he keeps his eyes open or closed, and that the change in the condition of the eyes almost immediately elicits the appearance of the corresponding change of the E.E.G. This indeed was the point of departure for the erroneous assumption that the α-w were related to vision, that they originated in the occipital lobe and that they were lacking in blind individuals. I refuted this assumption in earlier reports. Man is after all a visual creature and his attention is therefore most intimately connected with vision. This can be shown most strikingly in children who for reasons to be discussed below exhibit the best resting curves if they do not happen to be apprehensive. The child's attention is still particularly strongly connected with visual function and therefore the change in the E.E.G. upon eye opening is particularly pronounced. Any kind of mental work also changes the E.E.G. in the same way, a fact which I have repeatedly emphasized and which has been confirmed by all subsequent investigators. The assumption that this alteration of the E.E.G. is induced by the motor concomitants of mental work, subsumed under the concept of the "facial movements of thinking", must also be discarded, because a motor performance as such, as I have reported before, fails to influence the E.E.G. Rather, as in any focussing of attention, there is a different setting or a *shift* in cortical activity[T141] inasmuch as this activity appears in the E.E.G. Other investigators have contended that *congenital mental deficiency* manifests itself in the E.E.G. I already disputed this notion during the discussion at the 11th International Congress of Psychology in Paris in 1937. The E.E.G. of an adult mental defective does not differ from that of a normal individual who is in full possession of his mental capacities, provided one is not dealing with very defective idiots or with forms of mental retardation associated with focal cerebral and especially cortical lesions. The commonly encountered mental defectives, and also imbeciles, *i.e.* those without focal manifestations, have completely normal E.E.G.s. In these cases there is no general disturbance of function[T42] of the cerebral cortex of the kind which usually finds its expression in the E.E.G. However, there has been a loss or lack of certain cortical mechanisms[T43], if I may use this expression, which the healthy growing child only acquires partly through his own efforts[T142], but for which an inborn structural basis must also be present. One may even observe the peculiar fact that mental defectives in general exhibit better resting E.E.G. curves than intelligent persons. When I wanted to demonstrate beautiful E.E.G.s to colleagues who were interested in such recordings, I particularly liked to use a certain imbecile[T143]. This is an interesting fact which is worthwhile discussing in more detail. It can easily give rise to a false concept if one designates as "*resting record*" the E.E.G. obtained in a darkened room from an individual whose eyes are closed, who is mentally as relaxed as possible and is shielded from all external and, as far as possible, internal stimuli as well. The potential oscillations do not correspond at all to a pause during which cerebral activity is interrupted by a period of rest, but they are indicative of the *continuous automatic cortical* activity which is undisturbed by external or internal stimuli. Or, if the corresponding state is viewed from the psychological point of view, this just described resting state corresponds to the undisturbed passive course of ideation[1]. When through associative connections mental images follow upon each other as they do in a dream or in a state which we can experience introspectively, when we doze[T144] with eyes closed, then this corresponds precisely to what we have called the subject's resting state. In such a state we let ourselves drift along with the stream of our conscious processes and are as it were merely spectators of the mental events taking place in ourselves. This is a certain *passive* state which in general also goes along without any signs of fatigue. I therefore do not wish to call an E.E.G. recorded during such a state, a resting E.E.G., as I have done till now, but would prefer to call it a *passive* E.E.G. for the sake of brevity and in order, I hope, to prevent misunderstanding. The E.E.G. during increased attention or mental work differs very markedly from this type of record, as was already emphasized above. The α-w are lacking more or less completely and the record is made up of β-w of 11–24 σ when attention is increased and mental work is performed. The more difficult and strenuous the mental work and the more intense the concentration of attention, as is the case, *e.g.*, while one makes a precise observation, the more pronounced are the changes in the E.E.G. During mental work which continues for a relatively long time, periodic fluctuations become apparent in the E.E.G. with a transient return of the α-w. If we interpret these observations from a psychological point of view, we can say that the condition which correlates with this altered E.E.G. is one in which we experience a feeling of activity. I would therefore like to designate this E.E.G. also for the sake of brevity as the *active E.E.G.* If this condition lasts for a relatively long time, we have a distinct feeling of fatigue. In this state we intervene in the passive course of ideation and continuously scrutinize it. Without exception this represents an active conscious process (a paying of attention, mental work, thinking in the proper sense of the word). From the psychological point of view this process is associated with the appearance of the well known fluctuations of attention occurring during mental work which are correlated with the fluctuations of the E.E.G. Man can certainly not remain passive when internal or external stimuli affect him. Among the internal stimuli we must include the thoughts which arise spontaneously within the stream of consciousness and captivate his interest. This is precisely why children,

---

[1] See *Th. Elsenhaus*: Lehrbuch der Psychologie, edited by *F. Giese*, 3rd edition, p. 301–318, 1937.

primitive people and also mental defectives are particularly well suited for the recording of beautiful "resting records" and why they generally yield more beautiful E.E.G.s than intelligent experimental subjects, unless the latter have had special psychological training. In general an intelligent and mentally active person has much more difficulty to let himself be driven passively for a long time by the stream of his thoughts. Therefore we most frequently encounter mixed E.E.G.s which are composed of passive and active parts and in which sometimes the one, sometimes the other part predominates.

An E.E.G. predominantly composed of α-w is a sign of undisturbed automatic cortical activity and the α-w are the concomitants of this activity. *Rohracher* and *Gemelli*, however, are of a completely different opinion. They see in the α-w the concomitant phenomena of a *vegetative process*. Earlier I had also considered such a concept. This was at the beginning of my investigations, when I was not yet as convinced of the cortical origin of these strikingly regular potential oscillations as I became later. Furthermore at that time I did not yet have any positive proofs for their origin in the *cortex itself*. Now, however, since their cortical origin is proven, I feel that such an assumption is unjustified, as I already explained in the discussion in Paris in 1937. There are indeed people in whom the α-w are completely missing, even in prolonged E.E.G. recordings repeated time and again. The α-w are absent in these individuals not because they do not have any α-w, as has been assumed prematurely and erroneously by many investigators, but because certain psychological factors prevent their appearance. I only wish to draw attention to the fact that experienced investigators on the basis of repeated recordings taken in different subjects reported that the blind do not show any α-w, a contention which I was able to disprove without difficulty. I cannot quite understand how vegetative processes, which are essential for life, could be suppressed for a long time by mental influences and not merely abolished for the short periods which *Rohracher* found in his experimental subjects. The relative independence of the course of the α-w from the respiration, which is so important for all vegetative processes, as well as the independence from the cerebral circulation also militates, in my opinion, against *Rohracher's* assumption. Furthermore, in man the α-w diminish markedly in amplitude during sleep, according to the few investigations which I carried out on this subject. Other investigators in a much larger material found that during sleep the α-w may be completely absent. Surely during this period of recovery of the brain, vegetative processes should become more manifest than ever. I concede that one could interpret the disappearance of the α-w in chloroform narcosis as being related to some vegetative process. Nevertheless I fail to understand why these vegetative processes should be so intensely enhanced as one would have to postulate them to be in the case of Evipan and Pernocton narcosis, illuminating gas intoxication, and also in the case of oxygen *deprivation*! I therefore believe that I must reject *Rohracher's* and *Gemelli's* view. I know that in doing so I am in agreement with many investigators who studied both the human and animal E.E.G. As I have explained in detail elsewhere, I completely agree with the other view proposed by *Rohracher*, namely that the β-w of the E.E.G. which are found during mental work represent its physiological[T145] concomitants. But even with regard to *this* matter, my opinion differs on *one* point from that of *Rohracher* and of *Gemelli*. In my numerous recordings of E.E.G.s during mental work I hardly ever found β-w with a frequency above 50 hertz, although I had the means of recording without difficulties frequencies of up to 200 hertz. *Rohracher* observed β-w of up to 1000 hertz and even up to 2000 hertz, according to *Gemelli*. Recently *Franke* and *Koopmann*[1] also reported to have found β-w of up to 500 hertz. However, I have my doubts about all these reported findings, because these investigators observed such high frequencies of the β-w in E.E.G.s which they recorded from the scalp. Thus contamination with muscle currents, which may exhibit such frequencies, cannot be completely ruled out, especially since mental work is accompanied by widespread muscle currents not only in the face, but also in the muscles used for speech. I believe that only *direct* recording from the *cortex* could prove that β-w may exhibit such high frequencies. During cortical recordings of this kind I did not observe any frequencies above 50 hertz. *Jasper* indicated in his most recent report that in man he found potential oscillations with a frequency of up to 48 hertz. In all animal experiments when direct recordings were taken from the cortex itself, no frequencies above 60 hertz were found by *Ectors, Brémer, Jasper* and many others. Surely *Rohracher*'s statement would therefore require verification by *direct* recording from the *human cerebral cortex*. *Adrian* believes that the same nerve cells generate at one time the α-, at another time the β-rhythm. As I already explained in Paris I cannot adhere to this view. Certainly in the human E.E.G. we do not observe that at one time the α-rhythm *alone* appears in the passive E.E.G., and that at another time the β-rhythm *alone* occurs in the active E.E.G. Rather the situation is such that in the normal waking human subject the α-rhythm is always necessarily associated with the β-rhythm and only the latter can occur *alone* in a relatively pure form in the active E.E.G. In view of the division of labor which we must assume to exist everywhere, and also in the central nervous system, it is surely much more likely that potential oscillations which differ as much in their amplitude and time course as do the α-w and β-w of the human E.E.G., are generated by different nervous elements. *Brémer* who with his excellent animal experiments prepared the way for the interpretation of the E.E.G. as I describe it[T27], arrives at a similar concept when he states that the rapid potential oscillations probably must be attributed mainly to the smaller nerve cells in the upper cortical layers. *Adrian*[2] made the extremely interesting observation in monkeys, which *Brémer* confirmed in cats, that when a sensory organ is stimulated adequately, one can record from the cortex a *double* response to the stimulus: first, a large diphasic wave occurs which appears only in the corresponding cortical nerve center, and secondly, a more or less pronounced increase in the frequency of the continuous cortical potential oscillations takes place which can be observed everywhere in the cerebral cortex even in areas far removed from the activated sensory center (*Adrian*'s "afterdischarge"). *Brémer*[3] added an equally important observation to those made by *Adrian*. He found that in the cat

[1] *Franke* and *Koopmann*: Z. Neur., **162**, 259 (1938).

[2] *Adrian*: J. of Physiol., **88**, 127 (1936).

[3] *Brémer, F.*: C. r. Soc. Biol. Paris, Meeting of January 30, **1937**.

during deep sleep the large diphasic wave ("la réaction primaire") continues to occur in the corresponding cortical sensory center in response to adequate stimulation, but that the general increase in frequency ("la réaction secondaire", the "after-discharge") disappears. In man I was the first to observe the generalized response of the cerebral cortex which is related to this "afterdischarge" seen in animal experiments. This response appears in the E.E.G. following *all* sensory stimuli to which attention is paid and consists of a disappearance of the α-w and their replacement by β-w. I assume that the α-w disappear because they are inhibited everywhere. In the animal experiments this afterdischarge disappears during deep sleep. In man during deep sleep no mental processes follow upon a stimulus: the *mental activity* which is induced by a stimulus during wakefulness and which constitutes the response of the self to this stimulus is, of course, lost during sleep. Thus I actually see in *Brémer's* results a *further* experimental confirmation of my assumption that the cerebral cortex functions as a whole as far as *mental processes* are concerned and that precisely the β-w, and not the α-w, are the concomitant phenomena of mental activity! I therefore believe that the α-w of the E.E.G. of man are concomitant phenomena of the automatic physiological cortical processes and that certain β-w with a length of 11–24 σ represent material concomitants of the processes of consciousness. I have expressed this view in several reports. Starting from the beautiful thermocoagulation experiments of *Dusser de Barenne* and *McCulloch* I had assumed that the α-w originate in the three deeper cortical layers of the human cerebral cortex and that the shorter among the β-w, including the briefest ones, probably arise in the three superficial layers of the cortex. *Dusser de Barenne* has now amended his earlier report on the results of these thermocoagulation experiments. If in these thermocoagulation experiments on the cortex of the macaque one waits for a few weeks after the operation before recording the potential oscillations of the cortical areas which have been reduced to the three deepest layers, it can be shown that the same E.E.G. can be recorded from both the experimentally reduced and the intact cortex. *Dusser de Barenne* and *McCulloch* attribute the alteration of the E.E.G. in the acute thermocoagulation experiment to the disturbances caused by the operation itself and not to the loss of cells. In the opinion of these investigators, different recording conditions are created in the acute thermocoagulation experiments first of all because one records through the killed surface and secondly, because acid products originating in the necrotic layers diffuse into the deeper layers and reduce their activity. Nevertheless I believe that this change in the interpretation of these experiments does not in any way alter the fact that the reduced cortex exhibits both in the acute *and* in the chronic thermocoagulation experiment *large oscillations* which correspond to the α-w of my E.E.G.[T27]. *To me* this was and remains the only important fact. Whether the E.E.G. recorded immediately after thermocoagulation did or did not contain short oscillations like my β-w[T27] is irrelevant and could also not be determined with certainty by simple inspection of the records, but only by a frequency analysis[T55] of the curves. I never denied that β-w could also originate in other than the three superficial cortical layers. I have only assumed that the brief and briefest β-w of 11–24 σ indeed most likely originate in the three upper cortical layers. *Dusser de Barenne's* recent assumption that the large potential oscillations in the monkey, which correspond to my α-w[T27], originate in all cortical layers is based on strychnine experiments. I cannot accept these results obtained under pathological conditions as crucial evidence and I cannot acknowledge without reservations that it is possible to extrapolate from them to the E.E.G. of normal human subjects. Moreover, one may also consider the possibility that functional restitution may account for the fact that some months after thermocoagulation the same E.E.G. can be recorded both from a mutilated area of cortex consisting only of the three deepest cortical layers and from the neighboring intact cortex. In spite of all this I still consider it most likely that the *different* wave types of the E.E.G. originate from *different* nerve cell types or different nerve cell layers of the human cerebral cortex. The large and relatively slow α-w probably originate from the large pyramidal cells of the deeper cortical layers, whereas the briefer and briefest β-w which are also generally very low in amplitude probably have their origin in the small and the smallest nerve cells of the three upper cortical layers. Of course I cannot prove this, but many arguments which I assembled elsewhere support this view. I also continue to believe that the α-w are a concomitant phenomenon of the continuous automatic physiological activity of the cortex; β-w of 11–24 σ represent material concomitants of psychophysiological processes. I am strengthened in this belief by the results of studies carried out by many other investigators and not the least by the findings obtained in animal experiments. This assumption suggests itself as the most plausible one to an investigator who has recorded many E.E.G.s in normal subjects and in patients under the most varied conditions. Previously I had already indicated that my α-w and β-w[T27] bear no relationship to the electromagnetic oscillations which according to *Cazzamalli* emanate from the human brain. It is out of the question that the α-w and β-w of my E.E.G. exert any effect at a distance; they cannot be transmitted through space. Upon the advice of experienced electrophysicists, I refrained from any attempt to observe possible distant effects[T146]. In Germany, as elsewhere, considerable ingenuity and great sums of money have been spent precisely to perform such experiments which have yielded negative results, as I have learned from people knowledgeable in this field. I wish to emphasize this particularly at this point, because views similar to those expressed by *Cazzamalli* were recently propounded by *Franke* and *Koopmann*. This could again lead to expensive and fruitless experiments. In this connection, however, I would again like to draw attention to a certain point which I have repeatedly mentioned in the past. When mental work is performed or when the type of activity designated as *active conscious activity* becomes manifest in any way as, *e.g.*, upon the transition from the passive to the active E.E.G., a considerable *decrease* in the amplitude of the potential oscillations of the human brain occurs in association with this shift in cortical activity.

Translator's Notes

T1 For bibliographic references the format used by Berger was retained. This format does not follow a consistent pattern and no attempt was made in the translation to make Berger's bibliographic references conform to a standardized form.

T2 The term "injury currents" is used here to translate the German word "Längsquerschnittströme", which, in the literal sense, is untranslatable. The term could be loosely translated as "currents of longitudinal and cross sections" and in its physiological meaning is synonymous with "injury currents".

T3 Without referring to Beck's and Cybulski's original paper, it is impossible to know what is meant by "the simplest mental states". The relevant passage in Beck's and Cybulski's paper reads as follows: "This fact becomes easily understandable if one assumes that the electrical phenomena in the cerebral cortex correspond to the simplest mental states, namely to the sensations, possibly also to the images evoked by them".

T4 In the text the Russian names are spelled as they are customarily transliterated into English. In the bibliographic citations, Berger's original spelling according to the rules of German transliteration of Russian is retained. Although this introduces some discrepancy in spelling between text and bibliographic references, there was hardly any other choice, since many of the cited original works of the Russian authors had been written in German and were published in German scientific journals. Therefore even in the original publications the authors' names had been spelled according to the rules of the German transliteration of the Russian language.

T5 The German word used in the original text is "Tonstiefelelektroden", which cannot be translated accurately into English; "boot-shaped clay electrodes" is as close a paraphrasing of the original term as appears possible. These were non-polarizable electrodes made of cotton embedded in clay and protruding from a glass tube filled with zinc sulfate. The latter made contact with a zinc wire and established the connection with the galvanometer. These electrodes were in common use in the 1920s.

T6 The German word for "insert" is "Einsatz". According to Tönnies (personal communication received from Prof. R. Jung, Freiburg), this probably refers to a "coil carrier".

T7 In giving dosages of drugs, Berger uses only numbers with no indication of weight (*e.g.* 1.5 Veronal). In German speaking countries this was common usage and the numbers refer to grams.

T8   The phrase "in the circuit" was added in the translation for the sake of clarity. It does not appear in the German original. This also applies to other similar instances later in the text and the legends to the figures.

T9   The German term translated by "continuous cerebral current oscillations" is "ständige cerebrale Stromschwankungen". Berger uses this term frequently. It refers to what today one would call "the background activity of the E.E.G." The problem in translating Berger's original term arises from the German word "ständig", which in this context refers to a continually recurring event (*i.e.* the current oscillations) and for which "continuous" seems to be the English term approximating most closely the original German one.

T10   The literal translation of the German word "Versuchsfehler" would be "experimental error" and not, as given here, "experimental artefact". It is certain, however, that Berger uses the word "Fehler" here and elsewhere in the sense of "artefact". Since this translation seemed to render Berger's meaning more intelligible for the contemporary reader, it was adopted throughout this volume.

T11   The question mark at the end of this sentence also appears in the original German text, where it is equally uncalled for from a grammatical point of view. Berger may have taken the liberty of using it in order to emphasize his ever questioning attitude concerning the problem he discusses here.

T12   "Magnification" is the literal translation of the German word "Vergrösserung". In this case it refers to a purely optical method of increasing the deflection of the galvanometer beam. There was certainly no amplification involved.

T13   The word "shorter", and not "smaller" as one would logically expect from the context, also appears in the original German text.

T14   The literal translation for "Fehlerquellen" would be "sources of errors" and not "sources of artefacts". For justification of this translation, see translator's note T10.

T15   "Privatdozent" (or "Dozent") in German speaking universities is a member of the academic teaching staff with the rank roughly corresponding to that of a lecturer or assistant professor in universities of the English speaking world. "Privat" in this case refers to the custom that he receives no salary for his teaching activities from the university, but has the right to collect a portion of the students' fees.

T16   The word "amplitude" has been added in the translation for the sake of clarity. Berger only mentions "fluctuations" ("Schwankungen"), without making it too clear to what phenomenon this term is applied. Figure 4, however, shows that he refers to fluctuations of amplitude.

T17 "Assistant physician" is a literal English translation of the German term "Assistenzarzt". The position of an "Assistenzarzt" in German speaking countries roughly corresponds to that of "resident" or "assistant resident" in English speaking countries.

T18 In translating this sentence, the temptation was great to replace "impressions" by "stimuli", which would be more in accordance with modern English usage. Berger's choice of the word "Eindrücke" ("impressions") however almost certainly is deliberate, for he does use the word "Reize" ("stimuli") elsewhere. It is probable that what the word "impression" connotes to him, and what "stimulus" does not, is the fact that the former implies an involvement of atttention or conscious perception, whereas the latter does not necessarily carry these implications.

T19 When speaking of the "cerebral curve", Berger in this instance does not refer to the E.E.G., but to the record of the vascular responses which he had studied at the turn of the century.

T20 The literal translation of the phrase "pattern of the curve" would be "course of the curve" ("Kurvenverlauf"). The meaning of this phrase in the latter form would, however, remain unclear in English. Although "pattern" is a paraphrase, rather than a strict translation of the original German term, it appears justifiable to use it in this and other similar instances.

T21 The original text says only "against a localization". The words added in the translation serve to clarify an otherwise somewhat obscure sentence.

T22 The German word "geradlinig" literally translated means "straight" or "running in a straight line". From the context, it is obvious that the word "smooth", used in the translation, renders Berger's intended meaning more accurately.

T23 Berger undoubtedly refers here to the line labelled β in Figure 6 and which runs horizontally across the composite curve of α-w and β-w, labelled α–β.

T24 The term "vital processes" was used here to translate the German term "Lebensäusserungen", which literally means "expressions of life" or "manifestations of life". Berger seems to use this term to describe in a general way the fundamental biological processes common to all living tissues such as metabolism, respiration etc. This becomes evident from the subsequent sentence in which by "special function" he obviously implies the specific neuronal functions of brain tissue which are peculiar to it and which, in contrast to the "vital processes" ("Lebensäusserungen"), it does not share with other living tissues.

T25 The German term "Dissimilation" has been retained in the English translation, although in English it is little used in the sense employed by Berger here. *Dorland's Illustrated Medical Dictionary* (24th ed.) defines "dissimilation" as follows: "The act or process of dissimilating. The reverse of assimilation." The same dictionary defines "dissimilate" as "to decompose a substance into simple compounds, for the production of energy or materials that can be eliminated". This is precisely the meaning Berger had in mind, as is brought out clearly by the subsequent sentence. The argument he presents here is explicable in the light of his notion that in the nervous system, metabolic energy is a source of "psychic energy" and that the latter can be measured indirectly through extrapolation from physical measurements of other forms of energy released by the nervous tissue of the brain. (See introductory chapter.)

T26   See T10 and T14.

T27   Berger indeed speaks of "my α-w" ("meine α-w") or later, on some occasions, of "my E.E.G." This phrase presents somewhat of a problem in translation. In German it does not sound quite as possessive as in its literal English translation. On the other hand, a freer translation, such as "the α-w described by me" or some similar phrase sounds a little too detached. The course followed was to translate the phrase literally, as in the present instance, whenever this seemed possible without producing an awkward or equivocal English sentence. Whenever a less literal translation seemed preferable, a phrase such as "described by me" was used instead of the possessive "my".

T28   The literal translation would be "my E.E.G." See T27.

T29   The sentence should probably read "... even though the needle electrodes *inserted in the region of the parietal eminences* are connected to the more sensitive galvanometer". The words in italics, however, do not appear in the original text.

T30   This sentence is ambiguous in the original text. Strictly speaking "its" refers to "segment". The word "segment" is not followed by "of the record" in the original text. It is probable, however, that Berger had the E.E.G. record in mind and not merely the segment marked with a cross in Figure 5.

T31   Berger leaves the meaning of "Cp" unexplained. It probably stands for "cortex parietalis".

T32   The original German text does not specify that the findings are "post mortem", but within the context in which it appears the German word "Befund" would most likely be interpreted in this sense.

T33   The original German text speaks of "results of time measurements in connection with the influence of sensory stimuli" ("Ergebnisse der Zeitmessung bei der Einwirkung von Sinnesreizen"). It proved impossible to find a satisfactory literal English translation of this phrase and it became therefore necessary to paraphrase this passage.

T34   The original text mentions only "magnitude of the heart beat" ("Ausgiebigkeit der Herzschlägen") without reference to the E.C.G. However from the relevant passage in the first report, it is evident that what Berger had in mind was the amplitude of the deflections of the E.C.G.

T35 The original text says "E.E.G." instead of "E.C.G.", but this must be a printing error.

T36 The German term used by Berger is "Narkotika", which is nearly synonymous with the English term "general anesthetics". However, Berger also includes scopolamine among this group of drugs. In his time this alkaloid was frequently used as a potent sedative in agitated psychotic patients. Thus Berger applies the term "Narkotika" also to a group of drugs which today one would not describe as general anesthetics, but which have in common with these, their ability to induce sleep or sleep-like states. For this reason it was felt that in this context "sleep-inducing drugs" would be the most appropriate English translation of the term "Narkotika".

T37 The original text says "E.E.G." instead of "E.C.G.", but this is undoubtedly a printing error.

T38 What Berger obviously means is that the amplitude increase of the α-w had been observed already before the needles had been pulled out. Nevertheless it was decided to follow faithfully the original text in the English translation.

T39 Literally translated the sentence would read "... one can by no means consider as normal all E.E.G.s recorded from a skull defect in a patient with a palliative trepanation". It is almost certain, however, that Berger does not wish to refer to a single patient, but to patients with palliative trepanations in general. In German, unlike in English, the singular term is acceptable in such a case and can be used to convey the general meaning.

T40 The term "encephalogram" used here refers to an air encephalogram (pneumoencephalogram).

T41 German: "Hemmungserscheinungen". The inhibition referred to here is used to describe a slowing of mental functions as seen in depression and carries no neurophysiological implications.

T42 The German term used by Berger is "allgemeine Betriebsstörungen des Gehirns". It probably is impossible to translate this term accurately into English. "Allgemein" commonly corresponds to the English word "general", but it also may connote the meaning of "unspecific" and the two meanings in German are not as clearly separate as they are in English. In the present instance "general" probably renders Berger's intended meaning more accurately than "unspecific", although the latter may also be implied to some degree. The term "Betriebsstörungen" raises a further problem in translation: "disturbances of function" which is the translation chosen here, fails to render all that is implied by the original German word. "Betrieb" is not synonymous with the English word "function", but implies a multiplicity of activities integrated into a more or less coherent whole, as are *e.g.* the various activities that make up the total operation of a factory. The term "Betriebsstörungen" seems to refer to a disturbance in the mutually interlocking aspects of such activities, rather than to disturbances of individual functions.

T43 "Mechanisms" paraphrases, rather than accurately translates Berger's original term "Apparate". The use of the literal English translation "apparatus" (plur.), however, would result in a rather incongruous English sentence.

T44 "Overall activity" is the English translation chosen for "der gesamte Betrieb"; for the problems raised by this term see T42.

T45 The original legend erroneously says "Trepanation on the left side".

T46 German "Gesamtbetrieb", see T42.

T47 The English translation of this French quotation is as follows: "that the electromotive investigation of the brain makes it possible for us to study accurately the fundamental material conditions of psychophysiological processes".

T48 Berger wrote a short introduction to Dietsch's paper published in *Pflüger's Archiv*. He was interested in comparing the amplitudes of the E.E.G.s in different subjects, but realized that such amplitude measurements would only be meaningful if the resistance of the electrodes applied to the head were known. He explains that initially he had measured the resistance with a telephone attached to a bridge circuit and from Dietsch's subsequent comments it becomes apparent that the source of alternating current was provided by an inductorium delivering a current with much too high a frequency. Geheimrat Wien, who was a professor of physics at the University of Jena, considered this method unsatisfactory and asked his assistant, Dr. Dietsch, to develop an adequate method of resistance measurement. Dietsch describes this method in his paper. He measured the impedance of the head by applying to it an alternating current within the frequency range of the E.E.G. (5.7–20.3 c/sec). A contact rotating on a plate resistor provided a quasi-sinusoidal low frequency alternating current. A bridge circuit was used to measure the impedance of the subject's head to which this sinusoidal alternating current was applied. Depending on the electrodes and frequencies, values ranging from 740 to 14,400 ohms were found. The average impedance for the frequencies found in the E.E.G. was 10,000 ohms. The emf of the source generating the E.E.G. was calculated to be about 6×10^{-5} volts. This corresponds to a current strength of 6×10^{-9} amperes, which was in good agreement with the deflections (2–3 mm) obtained with the previously used mirror galvanometer, which operated as a current and not as a voltage measuring device. The earlier impedance measurements obtained with a telephone bridge circuit, however, were not in accordance with these figures. Had they been correct, one would have expected an 8 mm deflection with the galvanometer, a value which was never observed.

In a later publication, Dietsch analyzed these problems in more detail (DIETSCH, G., Zur Messung des Wechselstromwiderstandes am Schädel des lebenden Menschen, *Pflüger's Arch. ges. Physiol.*, **1932**, *230*: 499–508) and established that when he used chlorided silver needles, 95% of the resistance was contributed by the latter. Compared with this, the resistance of the tissues became negligible. He concluded that the emf of the E.E.G. can be calculated with a fair degree of accuracy only when the electrode resistance is that high.

T49   The legends of the original Figures 1, 5, 8 and 9 give the initials "J.B." instead of "I.B.", but this must be an error, as is evident from the text in which the subject's first name is given as "Ilse" (Berger's daughter). The same applies to the legend of Figure 2 of the 7th report and probably to the legend of Figure 19 of the 12th report.

T50   "Cp" probably stands for "cortex parietalis" or for "(gyrus) centralis posterior".

T51   "Functional compensation" was chosen as the translation for the German term "funktionelle Ausgleichung", even though a more literal translation of this term would be "functional equalization". From the remainder of the sentence, however, it appears more likely that the chosen translation is the more appropriate one.

T52   The inconsistency between the numbers in the text and those in the legend to Figure 7 also appears in the original.

T53   The English translation of this French quotation is: "One would have to show either that the psychic phenomena can only appear by causing the disappearance of a proportional quantity of the kinetic or potential energy... the brain ought to become cooler or its electrical potential ought to diminish!". It is of interest that Berger introduces this quotation by emphasizing how much his own views are at variance with those expressed by Armand Gautier, whom he cites here. In fact Berger's own reasoning, at least in his earlier years when he studied brain temperature, was very much like that expressed by Armand Gautier. (See introductory chapter.)

T54   The word "specific" was added in the translation. The German text speaks only of "Funktion" without any further qualifying adjective. In the context of this sentence, however, the German term "Funktion" implies a notion of specificity which would be lost in the English translation without the added adjective.

T55   The original German term used by Berger is "kurvenanalytische Untersuchungen" which cannot be translated accurately into English. It is however clear that he referred to what in today's E.E.G. terminology is called "frequency analysis". Dietsch carried out these frequency analyses by applying Fourier's theorem to the records obtained by Berger. These studies were published in *Pflüger's Arch. ges. Physiol.*, **1932**, *230*: 106–112. The frequency analysis was carried out manually from the raw data. The records were magnified 30 times by projecting them with an epidiascope upon a large sheet of drawing paper. They were then redrawn with a pencil. The disadvantage of this method was that the thickness of the tracing was also magnified 30 times (to about 2 mm). This introduced a source of error into the measurements, especially with regard to the points of intersection of a steeply rising curve with the ordinate. The fundamental period of the recorded oscillations was subdivided into 24 intervals of equal length. The segments of the curve over this interval were treated as straight lines and their values were integrated and then summed over all 24 intervals. By this laborious method, Dietsch analyzed some normal and some pathological E.E.G.s and found that the harmonic content of the latter was far greater than that of the former. The normal E.E.G. showed frequencies up to the 7th harmonic, whereas for the pathological E.E.G.s the range extended to the 11th harmonic. The patients, whose records were chosen, were suffering from epileptic dementia, dementia paralytica and skull fracture.

T56   Pyrifer was a commercially available injectable pyrogenic solution obtained from killed, non-pathogenic bacteria and was used to induce fever artificially for therapeutic purposes.

T57   The original phrase used by Berger is "rein mechanisch bedingt" ("purely mechanically"). Since the meaning of "mechanisch" in German is a little broader than that of "mechanical" in English, it was decided to paraphrase this term in the English translation in the hope of having thereby rendered Berger's intended meaning more faithfully.

T58   The word "recording" was added in the translation. The original text says only "at the two sites" ("an beiden Stellen").

T59   The original German text is as follows: "Die Schwankungen des E.E.G. werden aber nicht durch die Blutbewegungen im Gehirn hervorgehoben". It is almost certain that "hervorgehoben" ("emphasized") is an error and should read "hervorgerufen" ("caused"). For this reason the latter translation was chosen.

T60   In this legend and those of the subsequent Figures 10, 11 and 12, the literal translation of the German would be "respiration stopping" (German "Atmung aussetzend"), but in view of the fact that the cervical cord had been transected, it seems evident that respiration had actually stopped.

T61   The original text mentions only that "the heart beats are considerably larger ("ausgiebiger") than under normal conditions", without referring to the E.C.G. curve. It is obvious from Figure 12 that Berger's statement is based on the amplitude of the deflections of the E.C.G. (See also T34.)

T62 The phrase "in this case" was added in the translation to make clear that Berger, when speaking of the very low energy expenditure of the cerebral cortex, is referring only to the case of idiocy under discussion here and not to the metabolism of the cerebral cortex in general. That this interpretation is correct becomes apparent, not only from the context, but also from the original German text which links the content of the sentence to that of the preceding one by the word "auch" ("also") which suggests that Berger intended to refer specifically to the patient whose case he is discussing here.

T63 The word "arrangement" was added in the English translation to clarify the meaning of the sentence. (In modern E.E.G. terminology one would perhaps here say "montage".)

T64 The original text in German says "andere Untersuchungen", *i.e.* "other investigations". It seems highly probable that what Berger meant was "other E.E.G. investigations" and that he did not have in mind other investigations of a different kind; hence "further" was used in the translation instead of "other".

T65 The letter *a* refers to the schematized record on the top of the right side of Figure 3. The phrase "schematized record" does not appear in the original text and was added for the sake of clarity.

T66 The original text, instead of reproducing the symbol *1″* used in the figure, says "1 sec". Although the symbol does indicate this time measure, it seems preferable to use the actual symbol appearing in the figure in order to avoid any confusion. The same applies to the next sentence.

T67 The letter *d* refers to the schematized record on the bottom of the right side of Figure 3. Again the phrase "schematized record" does not appear in the original text.

T68 In the original text *J.S.* appears, but Figure 3 to which the text refers shows *I.S.* which must be the correct symbol, since the two letters undoubtedly represent the abbreviation of "innere Schwelle" ("internal threshold").

T69 The original says "inhibition of the course ("Ablauf") of the E.E.G." The word "course" is frequently used by Berger in the sense of "pattern" (see T20), but in this case "pattern" would be an inadequate translation. "Activity" seems to render as closely as appears feasible the meaning which was intended.

T70 The original German text uses the term "periodische Veränderung" ("periodic change"). In the English translation "periodic" was not used but rather "intermittently recurring", since it was assumed that this rendered the intended meaning more accurately.

T71   The original text only says "course" ("Verlauf"), not "time course". It seems likely that the latter translation renders accurately what Berger intended to say, but the meaning of the original text is somewhat unclear.

T72   The meaning of the term "course" ("Ablauf") is not very clear in this instance. Berger may have meant what today we call the background activity of the E.E.G. Since he never uses this expression or one that comes close to it, it did not seem justified to use this modern term, especially since one cannot be certain about the precise meaning which Berger had in mind.

T73   It is probable that this attenuation refers to the processes that take place when attention is aroused, but the original German text is ambiguous in this respect.

T74   This sentence is a very free translation of the original one whose precise meaning had to be guessed. In order to convey the meaning presumably intended by Berger, additions such as "as compared with a startle" and "to a lesser degree of arousal" had to be made.

T75   The German terms used by Berger are "Empfindung, Gefühl und Streben". It is difficult to find the appropriate equivalents in the English language for these words commonly used in German psychiatric terminology. "Empfindung" does not present too much of a problem; the English term "sensation" probably renders the intended meaning quite accurately. With "Gefühl" and "Streben" the difficulties are however great. In the English translation of Karl Jaspers' *Allgemeine Psychopathologie* (K. JASPERS: *General Psychopathology*, translated from German into English by J. Hoenic and Marion W. Hamilton, University of Chicago Press) "Fühlen" is translated, depending upon the context in which it appears, by "feeling", "emotion" or "affect". Similarly, "Streben" is translated by "striving", "drive (but only when used in a sense synonymous with the German word "Trieb")", "goals", "setting of goals", "will power" or "psychic energy". In the present translation, the term "emotion" was chosen for "Gefühl", because it seems to fit best into the context, although it should be noted that Berger elsewhere generally uses the word "Affekt" for "emotion". From the context in which the word "Streben" appears, it was very tempting to use "drive" as the English translation. However, this did not seem legitimate, because in all likelihood any German psychiatrist of the 1930s would have used "Trieb" and not "Streben", had he wished to express the meaning which "drive" conveys in the English language. The term "goal seeking" therefore seemed to be the most acceptable compromise[1].

T76   The German text uses the term "an Ort und Stelle". It does not specifically mention point *a*, but this is what the original text seems to imply.

---

[1] I am indebted to Dr. Karola Müller for her help in the translation of these German psychiatric terms.

T77 The term "metencephalitis" used by Berger probably indicates an encephalitis involving the metencephalon (cerebellum and pons). In this context the term is however a misnomer, for the oculogyric crises referred to are mesencephalic in origin, and the basal ganglia, also mentioned by Berger in this context, are prosencephalic and mesencephalic structures. It is therefore possible that "metencephalitis" is a misprint and should read "mesencephalitis".

T78 The German text only speaks of "Ausfälle" (defects or deficits) without specifying that they are neurological. Since in German clinical parlance "Ausfälle" is almost exclusively used to describe *neurological* deficits, the word "neurological" was added in the translation.

T79 What Berger probably means is that there are no corresponding variations of the amplitudes of the two sides, or, expressed differently, that there is no correspondence between the two sides in the amplitude modulation of the bilaterally synchronous E.E.G. background activity. It is very unlikely that Berger had intended to say that the amplitudes of the deflections on the two sides are unequal, for he would have been unable to compare the amplitudes of the E.E.G. records obtained from the right and left sides in terms of voltage or current intensity, since the upper curve was obtained with a current measuring device (coil galvanometer) whereas the lower curve was recorded with a voltage measuring device (oscillograph).

T80 The phrase "in order to verify this, records were taken in the following manner" does not appear in the original text and is used to translate the word "daher" ("therefore"), which in the German text introduces a very long and involved sentence. To clarify the multiple connections with the preceding sentence and translate this very unwieldy German sentence into readable English, it became necessary to break it up and to deviate in part from a faithful, literal translation of the original text.

T81 The original cyrtometer (from the Greek word κυρτόσ, vaulted) was an instrument which had been devised by the Parisian physician, Eugène Joseph Woillez (1811–1882), for determining the size and shape of the thoracic circumference. The Swiss surgeon, Theodore Kocher (1841–1917), devised an instrument serving a similar purpose for obtaining measurements of the skull which could be used to determine approximately on the surface of the skull the location of the main fissures and convolutions of the brain.

T82 The question mark also appears in the original German text and is grammatically no more justified there than in English. As in other similar instances Berger may have used it for the sake of emphasis.

T83 From the context, it is clear that Berger wished to refer to time measurements which would be applicable to the *normal* conduction between the motor cortex and those muscles which in the present pathological case were involved in the cortically induced movements elicited by epileptic discharge. He does not make this explicitly clear however.

T84   It is of interest that Berger, in tune with neuropsychiatric thought current in German speaking countries at that time, made in theory at least, a sharp distinction between epileptic and epileptiform attacks, no matter how difficult such a distinction might prove in practice. Focal seizures, such as the one exhibited by the paretic patient whose case he discusses in such great detail in this report, were not considered by him to be true epileptic seizures. Epilepsy according to a concept current in German speaking countries at that time was a disease *sui generis*, however ill defined, hence the term "genuine epilepsy" which was much in favor at that time. It is quite surprising that in all the theorizing on epilepsy and "epileptiform seizures" in which Berger engages here, and in some of his later reports (especially in the 9th and 14th reports) he never even once quotes Hughlings Jackson's views. In this neglect of Jackson's contribution to the understanding of epilepsy he was not alone. German neurology and psychiatry in the 1930s had yet to discover the outstanding contribution of this great British neurologist to our understanding of epileptic seizure mechanisms.

T85   F3 probably stands for "inferior frontal gyrus".

T86   The German term for "accessory waves" used by Berger is "Nebenwellen", which could also be translated by the term "secondary waves". Berger rarely used the word "Nebenwellen" in his earlier reports. It is evident that he refers to the "β-w", when using this term.

T87   The original German sentence starts as follows: "Im Hinblick auf die Beobachtung ("In view of the observation") und die schönen Untersuchungen von *Fischer*... etc.", and not "Im Hinblick auf diese Beobachtung ("In view of this observation")...". However, it seems that the intended meaning is better rendered by the latter translation, though a possible alternative would read: "In view of Fischer's observation and based upon his beautiful investigations... etc."

T88   The original text when translated literally says "... the two galvanometers, coil galvanometer and oscillograph, were connected together". The meaning of this sentence is unclear, but the caption of Figure 13 suggests that Berger meant that both galvanometers recorded from the same two needle electrodes. In that sense, they were connected together. The translation chosen is based on the assumption that this is the correct interpretation of the original German text.

T89   It is curious that apparently Berger did not consider the possibility that the 3 per second discharges shown in Figure 13 could have been generalized. This is all the more surprising in view of his overriding interest in E.E.G. phenomena which involved the entire cerebral cortex. What probably suggested to him that the discharges were localized and that they originated from the motor cortex was their association with small twitching movements of the left hand. Since in the paretic patient described before he observed similar high voltage discharges in association with focal motor seizures, this conclusion may have appeared justifiable to him.

T90   0.4 gram is probably an error and should read 0.04 gram, as suggested by the more pronounced sedative effect produced by 0.3 gram described in the following sentence.

T91   Avertine (tribromoethyl alcohol) was an anesthetic much used in the late 1920s and 1930s. It was usually given by rectum.

T92   Pernocton (butyl-beta-bromoallylbarbituric acid) is a rapidly eliminated barbiturate which was much used in the 1930s in psychiatry as an injectable hypnotic and was also used as a short-acting general anesthetic.

T93   The original text only says 5.0 Pernocton (or resp. 9.0 Evipan on page 213), without further specification. Usually these numbers refer to grams as was customary in Germany at that time (see T7) but in this case the numbers refer to milliliters, not grams. (Pernocton was usually injected in a 10% aqueous solution.)

T94   Evipan (sodium cyclohexenyl-methyl-*N*-methylbarbital) was one of the early intravenous short-acting anesthetics of the barbiturate group. It was usually injected as a 10% solution.

T95   The German term used by Berger is "Pfropfschizophrenie", from the verb "pfropfen", "to graft", which is sometimes used in its original German form also by English speaking psychiatrists. The term designates schizophrenia which has developed in a patient with congenital mental deficiency.

T96   This footnote probably contains a printing error or omission: "Nach *Pernocton*" appearing as it does after "260", makes no sense. Since it was impossible to check the original title for accuracy, the bibliographical reference was left in the original, probably partially erroneous form.

T97   Today one would speak of "the rhythmicity of the amplitude modulation of the α-rhythm", a phenomenon which Berger sometimes refers to as "the intrinsic rhythm" ("Eigenrhythmus") of the brain.

T98   The German phrase is "Überstürzen des Ablaufs der α-w", or later, "überstürzter Ablauf der α-w", which literally translated means "excessive acceleration of the course of the α-w" or "precipitate course of the α-w" respectively. These phrases, however, are not satisfactory translations and it becomes necessary to paraphrase as accurately as possible what Berger intended to say. Fortunately the meaning he wished to convey becomes evident from the diagrammatic representation of his concept of group formation shown in Figure 5. He thought that the α-w follow upon each other in accelerated sequences, inasmuch as each wave begins before the preceding one has run its full course. Hence the grouping (one could also say "incomplete fusion") of the α-w.

T99 The German original text speaks of "sensible und sensorische Reize" which can only be translated into English by the single term "sensory stimuli". In German "sensible Reize" is often applied to those stimuli commonly called "somatosensory" in English, whereas "sensorische Reize" is reserved to stimuli involving the special senses (auditory, visual, gustatory and olfactory).

T100 Berger does not give the reference to the original paper by Dusser de Barenne and Marshall. He probably knew of it only through a review article by Wachholder, to which he refers later. The reference to the original publication is as follows: DUSSER DE BARENNE, J. G. and MARSHALL, C.: On a release phenomenon of the "motor" cerebral cortex. *Science*, **1931**, *73*: 213–214.

T101 The German text says: "... während die Versuchsperson vor sich hindämmert". There is no way in which the phrase "vor sich hindämmern" can be translated into English in a reasonably literal way. The phrase, "to let the mind go blank" which was chosen, owes more to our present day knowledge of E.E.G. and its relation to phenomena of arousal, attention, etc., than is perhaps *a priori* justifiable. One cannot help wondering how a translator in the 1930s would have handled this problem.

T102 Berger merely says "a shortening of the rhythmic course of the altered α-w" ("eine Verkürzung des rhythmischen Verlaufs dieser abgeänderten α-w"). The difficulties in translation arise from the problem mentioned in T97. Hence the freer translation chosen in the present case.

T103 This statement is to be understood in the sense of a metaphor, rather than a factual account of the effects of pain. Here Berger makes use of a well known German idiomatic expression ("es vergeht einen vor Schmerz Hören und Sehen") which is commonly used to describe vividly an intense pain.

T104 The German word which Berger uses for "amplitude" in the original text is "Höhe" which literally translated means "height". The current neurophysiological meaning of "amplitude" is probably a little too specific and fails to render exactly what Berger had in mind. Another alternative would have been to translate "Höhe" by "intensity", but the meaning of this term is somewhat too general. From Berger's writings it can be concluded that he believed that the amplitude of the electrical activity of the brain was closely correlated with the intensity of the excitatory process. His usage of the word "Höhe" probably was meant to convey both the purely descriptive aspect, which is implicit in the original meaning of the word "height" as well as its derived connotation ("intensity"). It was felt that the English word "amplitude" was an acceptable compromise.

T105   The word "mental" was added in the translation. From the context it is certain that this is what Berger had in mind.

T106   The German poet, Friedrich Rückert (1788–1866) whom Berger quotes here, was his maternal grandfather.

T107   The German term for "active disconnection" is "aktive Abschaltung", which could also be translated, perhaps more accurately, by "active switching off". It is difficult to know which of the two translations is closer to the meaning Berger wanted to convey. The former was chosen because it appeared to be the more satisfactory English term from a stylistic point of view.

T108   The term appearing in the German text is "Fleischmilchsäure", which cannot be translated literally into English. This term must have originated when early bio-chemical work had shown that lactic acid can be produced by muscles ("Fleisch" in this instance is used in the sense of muscle tissue).

T109   Stimulation of the hypothalamus is implied here, although Berger does not explicitly say so.

T110   Berger probably has only the cerebral cortex and not the entire cerebrum in mind. The latter of course includes the thalamus. However, he does say "Grosshirn" and not cortex. The term "cerebrum" has therefore been retained in the translation, albeit reluctantly.

T111   In this instance the term "to switch off" would probably come closer to what von Economo had in mind. Since "to disconnect" or "disconnected" had been used before for translating the term "abschalten", which Berger repeatedly uses in connection with this hypothesis, this translation was retained here for the sake of consistency. (See also T107).

T112   The original says "the new process", but it is probable that "new processes" renders the intended meaning more accurately.

T113   The original text says "bei einer motorischen Innervation", which literally translated means "during a motor innervation". What is probably meant is "a voluntary movement".

T114   *i.e.* the potential decrease.

T115   It is evident that the absence of a potential decrease, which would have been indicative of a process of inhibition, applies to the response of the E.E.G. to a sensory stimulus. Certainly this is what Berger implicitly tried to say, although this passage and its meaning would have been clearer had he said so explicitly. The potential decrease referred to here would therefore be difficult to demonstrate in a state characterized by an already existing inhibition associated with a low voltage fast record and caused by such persistent stimuli as pain, uncomfortable positioning, etc., which are mentioned in the text.

T116   The German original says "Die beiden Herren *Adrian* und *Matthews*... etc.", which literally translated means "The two gentleman, Adrian and Matthews..." In contemporary English this phrase conveys an attitude of patronizing condescension, which it does not in the somewhat old fashioned German used by Berger. It seemed therefore best to eliminate the words "the two gentleman" from the English translation.

T117   It should be noted that Berger uses the term E.E.G. in a restricted sense here, *i.e.* as a synonym of α-rhythm. Adrian and Matthews do not use the term E.E.G. at all either to describe this or any other cerebral rhythm. They use the term "Berger rhythm" to describe the α-rhythm. (See also T119).

T118   The German word used by Berger is "allüberall", which is more emphatic than the English term "everywhere".

T119   It is very difficult and probably impossible to translate this sentence into English without losing some of the subtleties conveyed by the German original. The latter reads thus: "Ich halte es daher auch für richtiger, bei dem von mir, als dem Entdecker dieser Potentialschwankungen beim Menschen, gegebenen Namen des E.E.G. zu bleiben, als auf die von *Adrian* und *Matthews* so ehrenvoll für mich gewählte Bezeichnung überzugehen!" From the introduction in Adrian's and Matthews' paper in *Brain*, the reasons for choosing the term "Berger rhythm" are clearly explained, for they say: "Since the effect is so characteristic we shall refer to it in future as the Berger rhythm. Berger calls it electroencephalogram, but the shorter title avoids the suggestion that the rhythm is produced by the entire cortex." Thus, although Adrian and Matthews were ready to give credit where credit was due, their choice of the term "Berger rhythm" was not only motivated by their desire to honor Berger's name, but also by their unwillingness to accept the term "electroencephalogram" proposed by Berger, with all its far reaching implications. Particularly they were not prepared to accept Berger's view of the fundamental importance of this phenomenon for brain function in general. Berger was quick to sense this and he therefore responded rather sharply to the threat which Adrian's and Matthews' view posed to his concept of the significance of the E.E.G. In his refusal to accept the term "Berger rhythm", modesty certainly played an important part, but he also had more compelling reasons for not accepting Adrian's and Matthews' terminology. Certainly, however, he was also anxious not to ruffle Adrian's and Matthews' feelings, to whom he owed a great debt of gratitude, for here, at last, were two highly respected physiologists who had confirmed his findings and had given him credit for his discovery. This was the kind of recognition for which he had craved and which had been stubbornly denied him. The formulation of the last sentence of his 10th report reflects these feelings of ambivalence. (See introductory chapter.)

T120   Literally: "my β-w". (See T27).

T121   The term Berger uses is "Schnelligkeit", *i.e.* "velocity"; he still does not use the more modern term "frequency", which was chosen in the translation for the sake of clarity and better style. The term "frequency analysis" was chosen for the same reason. (See T55).

T122   The German term is "Lähmungssymptom". "Lähmung", *i.e.* "paralysis", is probably to be understood as a profound depression, but not necessarily as an abolition of function. Berger seems to use the term "Lähmungssymptom" as an antonym of the term "Reizsymptom" ("sign of irritation").

T123   In the German text the expression used is "psychische Reizerscheinungen", which translated literally means "phenomena of mental irritation". It is obvious that Berger likes to use the same word "Reizerscheinungen" (or its antonym "Lähmungs-erscheinungen" (see T122) for describing both the physiological changes which appear in the E.E.G. and their psychological correlates. It seemed, however, impossible to follow his example in the translation in this specific instance, for the term "mental irritation" could be misleading in the present context.

T124   The word "general" does not appear in the German text. Since "Betriebsstö-rung" presents great difficulties in translation (see T42) and otherwise is always used by Berger in the form of "allgemeine Betriebsstörungen" (a meaning also implied here), it seemed legitimate to add the word "general" in the English text.

T125   The German term is "Engraphiearbeit".

T126   The term "gallop rhythm" had never been used before by Berger in the series of papers entitled "On the electroencephalogram of man", which form the substance of this volume. (He may have used this term in a verbal communication or in some other publication with which this translator is not familiar.)

T127   The original text refers to Figure 4, but this reference is undoubtedly a printing error. It is most likely that Berger intended to refer to Figure 14 of the 7th report.

T128   The word "motor" does not appear in the German original and was added in the translation in order to avoid confusion. Berger only speaks of "discharge" ("Ent-ladungen"). He uses this word in a different sense from that which is customary today. Obviously, as is evident from his reference to Figures 10, 11 and 12 of the 7th report, he has *motor* discharges in mind, or in other words, the actual clonic jerks which involve the skeletal muscles, and not the cerebral discharges.

T129   The original text merely says "without insult" ("ohne Insult"). It is not altogether clear what Berger meant by this. The translation that was chosen paraphrases what appears to be the most likely meaning of this phrase.

T130   The word "mental" was added in the translation. (See also T41)

T131   Berger indeed says "in the different cortical layers" ("in den verschiedenen Rindenschichten") and not "in different cortical layers", even though the latter version would seem to be more consistent with the logical sequence presented in this and the preceding sentence. It is impossible to know for certain which version corresponds to what Berger intended to say and therefore the original one was retained in the translation.

T132   It is assumed that this is the correct translation of the German sentence which runs thus: "Ferner ist es nicht wunderbar, dass das Neugeborene noch keine α-w darbietet". The use of the word "wunderbar" in the sense of "surprising" rather than in the customary sense of "wonderful", "marvelous" or "miraculous" is however very unusual.

T133   The German term translated by "stimulants" is "Genussmittel". It has no exact equivalent in the English language. This term is generally used for beverages, foods and other items that are consumed for the stimulating or pleasurable effects they produce. It would *e.g.* include tea, coffee, alcoholic beverages; it may also be used for tobacco.

T134   The frequency of the alternating current in European countries is 50 cycles per second.

T135   The German word is "Fehler" ("error", "mistake"). (See T10).

T136   The slight differences in wording between this and the final sentence of the 12th report are also present in the original text.

T137   The German phrase for "disturbance of cortical function" is "kortikale Betriebsstörung". For a discussion of the problems arising from the translation of this term, see T42.

T138   Berger does not refer here to one of the original 14 reports translated in this volume, but to the Society Proceedings which he mentions in the text.

T139   The original text refers to Figure 7, but this is undoubtedly a printing error.

T140 What Berger undoubtedly means by "muscle activity" is not so much the actual contraction of the muscles, but the activity in the motor system, especially in the cerebral cortex, which causes the muscles to contract.

T141 The German phrase used by Berger is "Umschaltung des corticalen Betriebs". The word "Umschaltung" conveys the meaning of turning a switch or of shifting gears. For the difficulties arising from the translation of the word "Betrieb", see T42.

T142 The German term used by Berger is "sich erarbeiten" which is almost untranslatable. Using modern terminology, one could paraphrase what Berger meant by saying "which the healthy growing child probably only acquires through learning".

T143 Berger says: "Ich habe mit Vorliebe einen Imbezillen benützt". It is likely that he meant "a certain imbecile" rather than just "an imbecile", but the German phrase is somewhat ambiguous in this regard.

T144 The German term is "vor sich hindämmern". The English verb "to doze" used in the translation is a little too strong, for it implies that a state of drowsiness exists, whereas the German term only implies a passivity of mind.

T145 The word "physiological" does not appear in the original. It was added for the sake of clarity.

T146 It is an irony of fate that at the very end of his last paper of the series "On the electroencephalogram of man", Berger returned to this question of telepathy. For it was the conviction that telepathic phenomena were real, based on a personal experience in his youth, which had been the starting point for his abiding interest in psychophysical problems out of which had grown his discovery and the development of electroencephalography. (For more details, see introductory chapter.)

Index